A QUARTER CENTURY OF NEPHROLOGY

Commemorating
American Society of Nephrology's
25th Anniversary

A QUARTER CENTURY OF NEPHROLOGY

Commemorating
American Society of Nephrology's
25th Anniversary

EDITED BY THE

ASN HISTORICAL COMMITTEE

Richard L. Tannen, *Chairman*
Leon G. Fine
Carl W. Gottschalk
George E. Schreiner

Publisher: Deanna F. Gemmill
Associate Publisher: Carole E. Pippin
Copy Editor: Virginia Gerhart
Designer: Norman Och
Production Coordinator: Mary Lorenzen

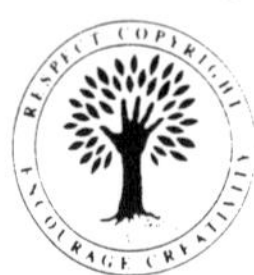

Printed in the United States of America

Library of Congress Cataloging-in-Publication Data

Tannen, R. L. (Richard L.), 1937–
A quarter century of nephrology—commemorating the American Society of Nephrology's 25th anniversary / Richard L. Tannen. p. cm.
Includes bibliographical references and index.
ISBN 0-683-08095-4
1. American Society of Nephrology—History. 2. Nephrology—United States—History. I. Title.
[DNLM: 1. American Society of Nephrology. 2. Nephrology—history—United States. 3. Societies, Medical—history—United States. WJ 1 T166q]
RC903.T26 1992
616.6′1′006073—dc20
DNLM/DLC
for Library of Congress 92-12310
CIP

PREFACE

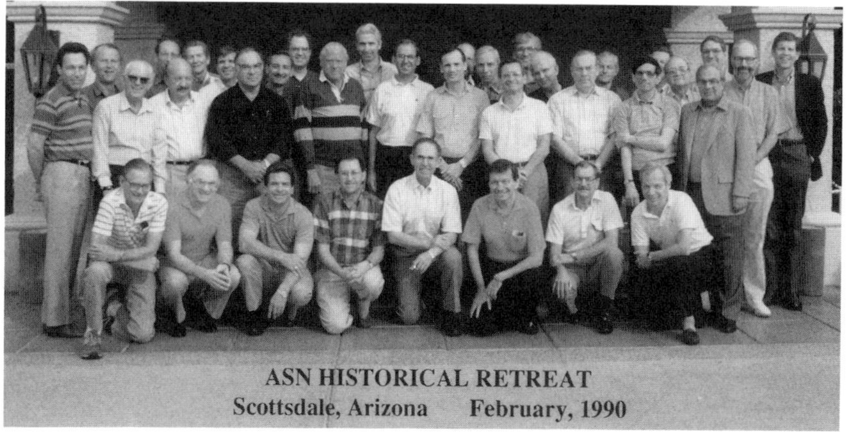

ASN HISTORICAL RETREAT
Scottsdale, Arizona February, 1990

The American Society of Nephrology

In 1986 Barry Brenner, the President of the American Society of Nephrology, charged an Ad Hoc Committee with planning the celebration of the Society's 25th Anniversary.

With the endorsement of the ASN council, this historical committee decided that a book reviewing the historical aspects of the scientific progress reported at the society's first quarter century of meetings would be one appropriate way to commemorate this event.

The chapters are organized to reflect the major abstract categories that characterized the majority of the first 23 meetings. An introductory chapter detailing the history of the Society and a closing chapter focusing on therapeutic advances are also included. The contributors to each chapter are distinguished members of the ASN, who have participated in the activities of the Society since its inception.

An initial planning meeting of all contributors was held in Scottsdale, Arizona, in February 1990 (Fig. 1.1) to coordinate the development of this text. It was agreed that the Abstract Book of the ASN would be the primary reference source for all contributions and that each chapter would begin by discussing the knowledge that was state of the art in 1967, the time of the first ASN meeting.

I would like to thank all the contributors and the members of the historical committee for their diligence in producing this volume.

Finally, I would like to thank Merck Human Health Division, for their generous contribution which helped make this volume feasible.

It is our hope that our members, and all others in the nephrology community, will find this historical overview to be enlightening.

Sincerely,

Richard L. Tannen, M.D.
President, ASN, 1992

CONTRIBUTORS

Thomas E. Andreoli, M.D.
Professor and Nolan Chair, Department of Internal Medicine
University of Arkansas College of Medicine
4301 West Markham, Slot 640
Little Rock, Arkansas

William M. Bennett, M.D.
Professor of Medicine and Pharmacology
Co-Head, Division of Nephrology, Hypertension and Clinical Pharmacology
PP262 Division of Nephrology and Hypertension
3314 SW Veterans Hospital Road
Portland, Oregon

Robert W. Berliner, M.D.
Professor Emeritus, Medicine
Yale University School of Medicine
333 Cedar Street
New Haven, Connecticut

Roland C. Blantz, M.D.
Professor and Head, Division of Nephrology and Hypertension
University of California at San Diego
School of Medicine and VA Medical Center
(911H)
San Diego, California

John W. Boylan, M.D.
Deceased

Maurice B. Burg, M.D.
Chief, Laboratory of Kidney and Electrolyte Metabolism
National Institutes of Health
Building 10, Room 6N307
Bethesda, Maryland

Charles B. Carpenter, M.D.
Professor of Medicine and Director
Laboratory of Immunogenetics and Transplantation
Brigham and Women's Hospital/ Harvard Medical School
75 Francis Street
Boston, Massachusetts

Ramzi S. Cotran, M.D.
Chairman, Department of Pathology
Brigham and Women's Hospital/ Harvard Medical School
75 Francis Street
Boston, Massachusetts

Gerald F. DiBona, M.D.
Professor and Vice-Chairman
Department of Internal Medicine
University of Iowa College of Medicine
Iowa City, Iowa

Michael J. Dunn, M.D.
Hanna Payne Professor of Medicine
Case Western Reserve University
Director, Division of Nephrology
Department of Medicine
University Hospitals of Cleveland
Nephrology RM 8124 Lakeside
2074 Abington Road
Cleveland, Ohio

Franklin H. Epstein, M.D.
William Applebaum Professor of Medicine
Harvard Medical School
Director of Renal Division
Beth Israel Hospital
Nephrology Division
330 Brookline Avenue
Boston, Massachusetts

Thomas F. Ferris, M.D.
Nesbitt Professor of Medicine and Chairman
University of Minnesota
Box 194, 14-106 PWB
516 Delaware Street
Minneapolis, Minnesota

Leon G. Fine, M.D.
Head, Department of Medicine
University College and Middlesex School of Medicine
The Rayne Institute, University Street
London, England, United Kingdom

Gerhard H. Giebisch, M.D.
Sterling Professor of Cellular and Molecular Physiology
Yale University School of Medicine
Department of Cellular Physiology
333 Cedar Street
New Haven, Connecticut

Richard J. Glassock, M.D.
Chairman, Department of Medicine
University of Kentucky College of Medicine
800 Rose Street
Lexington, Kentucky

Carl W. Gottschalk, M.D.
Career Investigator, American Heart Association
Kenan Professor of Medicine and Physiology
University of North Carolina at Chapel Hill
CD# 7155
3034 Old Clinic Building
Chapel Hill, North Carolina

Jared J. Grantham, M.D.
Professor of Medicine and Director
Division of Nephrology and Hypertension
Nephrology-Sudler 4015
Kansas University Medical Center
39th and Rainbow Boulevard
Kansas City, Kansas

Ronald D. Guttman, M.D.
Director, McGill Center for Immunobiology and Transplantation
Royal Victoria Hospital
687 Pine Avenue West
Montreal, Quebec, Canada

Lee W. Henderson, M.D.
Vice-President, Scientific Affairs
Director, Extramural Affairs
Baxter Healthcare Corporation
Route 120 and Wilson Road
Round Lake, Illinois

Lawrence G. Hunsicker, M.D.
Professor of Medicine
University of Iowa Hospitals and Clinics
Room E300F GH
Iowa City, Iowa

Saulo Klahr, M.D.
Simon Professor of Medicine
Co-chair, Dept. of Medicine
Washington University School of Medicine
Physician-in-Chief, The Jewish Hospital of St. Louis
Jewish Hospital at Washington University Medical Center
216 South Kingshighway
St. Louis, Missouri

James P. Knochel, M.D.
Chairman, Department of Internal Medicine
Presbyterian Hospital of Dallas
8200 Walnut Hill Lane
Dallas, Texas

Juha P. Kokko, M.D., Ph.D.
Chairman of Medicine
Asa G. Candler Professor of Medicine
Emory University School of Medicine
Suite F410, 1364 Clifton Road, NE
Atlanta, Georgia

Joel D. Kopple, M.D.
Chief, Division of Nephrology
Harbor-UCLA Medical Center
1000 West Carson Street
Torrance, California

Jacob Lemann, Jr., M.D.
Chief, Nephrology Division
Professor of Medicine
Froedtert Lutheran Memorial Hospital
Medical College of Wisconsin
9200 West Wisconsin Avenue
Milwaukee, Wisconsin

David Z. Levine, M.D.
Professor and Head, Division of Nephrology
Ottawa General Hospital and University of Ottawa
501 Smyth Road
Ottawa, Ontario, Canada

Norman G. Levinsky, M.D.
Wade Professor and Chair
Department of Medicine
Physician-in-Chief, The University Hospital
Boston University Medical Center
88 Newton Street
Boston, Massachusetts

Manuel Martinez-Maldonado, M.D.
Vice Chairman and Professor of Medicine
Emory University School of Medicine
Chief Medical Services
Atlanta VA Medical Center
1670 Clairmont Road
Decatur, Georgia

Shaul G. Massry, M.D.
Chief, Division of Nephrology
Professor of Medicine
University of Southern California
2025 Zonal Avenue
Los Angeles, California

Alfred L. Michael, M.D.
Regent's Professor of Pediatrics
Laboratory Medicine and Pathology
Chairman, Department of Pediatrics
University of Minnesota, Box 391, UMHC
Harvard Street at East River Road
Minneapolis, Minnesota

L. Gabriel Navar, Ph.D.
Professor and Chairman
Department of Physiology
Tulane Medical School
1430 Tulane Avenue
New Orleans, Louisiana

Karl D. Nolph, M.D.
Director, Division of Nephrology
Professor of Medicine
University of Missouri
MA 436 Health Science Center
Columbia, Missouri

Roscoe R. Robinson, M.D.
Vice Chancellor for Health Affairs
Professor of Medicine
Vanderbilt University Medical Center
D3300 Medical Center North
Nashville, Tennessee

James A. Schafer, Ph.D.
Professor of Physiology, Biophysics, and Medicine
University of Alabama at Birmingham
P.O. Box 10 SDB
Birmingham, Alabama

George E. Schreiner, M.D.
Distinguished Professor of Medicine
Georgetown University Medical Center
PHC F6003
3800 Reservoir Road, NW
Washington, DC

Belding H. Scribner, M.D.
Professor of Medicine
University of Washington
Division of Nephrology
Mail Stop Rm-11
BB1265 Health Sciences Building
Seattle, Washington

Eduardo Slatopolsky, M.D.
Professor of Medicine
Director, Chromalloy Kidney Center
Joseph Friedman Professor of Renal Diseases in Medicine
Barnes Hospital Plaza
Box 8129, One Barnes Hospital
St. Louis, Missouri

Jay H. Stein, M.D.
Professor and Chairman
Department of Medicine
University of Texas Health Science Center
7703 Floyd Curl Drive
San Antonio, Texas

Philip R. Steinmetz, M.D.
Professor of Medicine
Director, Division of Nephrology
University of Connecticut Health Center
263 Farmington Avenue
Farmington, Connecticut

Wadi N. Suki, M.D.
Professor of Medicine, Molecular Physiology, and Biophysics
Chief, Renal Section
Baylor College of Medicine
Renal Division, Suite 1275
6550 Fannin
Houston, Texas

Richard L. Tannen, M.D.
Chairman, Department of Internal Medicine
University of Southern California School of Medicine
2025 Zonal Avenue, Room 7900
Los Angeles, California

C. Craig Tisher, M.D.
Professor of Medicine and Pathology
Emminent Scholar, Central Florida Kidney Center
Chief, Division of Nephrology, Hypertension and Transplantation
University of Florida, Box J224, JHMHC
Gainesville, Florida

Robert L. Vernier, M.D.
Professor and Associate Head
Department of Pediatrics
Co-Director, Pediatric Nephrology
University of Minnesota, Box 491
Minneapolis, Minnesota

CONTENTS

1

The American Society of Nephrology and Its Beginnings

Carl W. Gottschalk, Robert W. Berliner, and George E. Schreiner

The American Society of Nephrology

The American Society of Nephrology was founded in 1966, and its first annual meeting was held October 18 and 19, 1967 in Los Angeles, California; President Neal S. Bricker presided. Annual meetings have been held each year since, except in 1972 when the International Society of Nephrology met in Mexico City.

The Society was founded in 1966 by 18 nephrologists assembled under the aegis of the Kidney Section of the New York Heart Association. The founding group was drawn from the Scientific Advisory Board of the National Kidney Foundation and the Renal Section of the Council on Circulation of the American Heart Association (Table 1.1, Fig. 1.1). The group wrote the Constitution and Bylaws, elected the first officers of what was to become the American Society of Nephrology, chose Los Angeles as the site of the first meeting, and then dissolved itself as the constitutional process took over.

The immediate stimulus for convening the group was to establish an American society to communicate with the International Society of Nephrology, which had decided to have its 1966 Congress in Washington, D.C. The first Congress of the International Society of Nephrology was held in 1960 in Evian, France, and the second, in Prague, Czechoslovakia, in 1963. The executive committee of the International Society of Nephrology extended an invitation to the Renal Section, Council on Circulation, American Heart Association, John P. Merrill, Chairman, to sponsor the 1966 Congress in Washington, D.C. Robert W. Berliner was President of the Third International Congress of Nephrology, and George E. Schreiner was Secretary-General. The Congress was well attended and enormously successful scientifically, socially, and financially.

The Constitution of the American Society of Nephrology states unambiguously the aim of the Society and the mechanism of its operation: "The purpose of this Society shall be to advance the knowledge of nephrology and

TABLE 1.1
The Founding Group

Henry L. Barnett	John P. Merrill
Robert W. Berliner	Solomon Papper
Stanley E. Bradley	Robert G. Petersdorf
Neal S. Bricker	George E. Schreiner
David P. Earle	Belding H. Scribner
James F. Glenn	Donald W. Seldin
Robert Alan Good	Daniel C. Tosteson
Charles R. Kleeman	Robert L. Vernier
Richard Malvin	Louis G. Welt

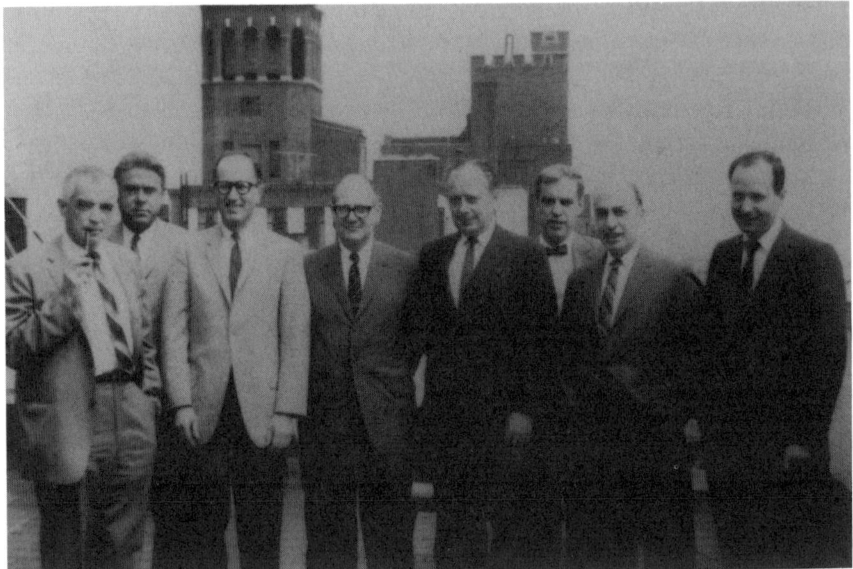

Figure 1.1. ASN Founding Group. Several members of the ASN Founding Group are pictured (*from left to right*): John Merrill, George Schreiner, Donald Seldin, Louis Welt, Neal Bricker, Robert Vernier, Robert Berliner, Richard Malvin.

to foster the dissemination of this knowledge (*1*) through national scientific meetings; (*2*) through cooperation with other national societies of nephrology; and (*3*) by other means approved by the members on recommendation by the Council." Membership was to be open and inclusive and not elitist. The annually elected officers of the society are President, President-Elect, and Secretary-Treasurer. They, along with the Past-President and four Councillors, elected for 4-year terms, are responsible for supervising the affairs of the Society, including electing members and arranging for the annual meeting (Table 1.2, Fig. 1.2).

TABLE 1.2
Past Presidents

1966–67	Neal S. Bricker
1967–68	Donald W. Seldin
1968–69	Robert W. Berliner
1969–70	Louis G. Welt
1970–71	George E. Schreiner
1971–72	Gerhard H. Giebisch
1972–73	Robert H. Heptinstall
1973–74	Jack Orloff
1974–75	William B. Schwartz
1975–76	Carl W. Gottschalk
1976–77	Floyd C. Rector, Jr.
1977–78	Laurence E. Earley
1978–79	Belding H. Scribner
1979–80	Robert L. Vernier
1980–81	Maurice B. Burg
1981–82	Roscoe R. Robinson
1982–83	Robert W. Schrier
1983–84	Richard J. Glassock
1984–85	Juha P. Kokko
1985–86	Saulo Klahr
1986–87	Barry M. Brenner
1987–88	Thomas F. Ferris
1988–89	Jay H. Stein
1989–90	Michael J. Dunn
1990–91	C. Craig Tisher
1991–92	Richard L. Tannen

The program format, initiated at the first annual meeting, is still employed: state-of-the-art addresses at plenary sessions, simultaneous symposia on a variety of topics selected to interest clinicians or basic scientists, and multiple free communications sessions. Originally, the President and advisors selected abstracts for presentation. In recent years, with much greater attendance and many more abstracts being submitted for oral and poster presentations, a program committee has assumed this responsibility.

The first meeting was very successful. Attendance, approximately 1250, was twice that originally projected. Planning for and financing the first meeting was made simpler by borrowing from a revolving loan fund established from unexpended funds generated by the 1966 International Congress of Nephrology. Also, there were 10 corporate sponsors of the first meeting, with the result that the meeting generated a surplus. These funds were later used in a similar fashion for the next International Congress of Nephrology held in the United States, the 1984 Congress in Los Angeles. The residual

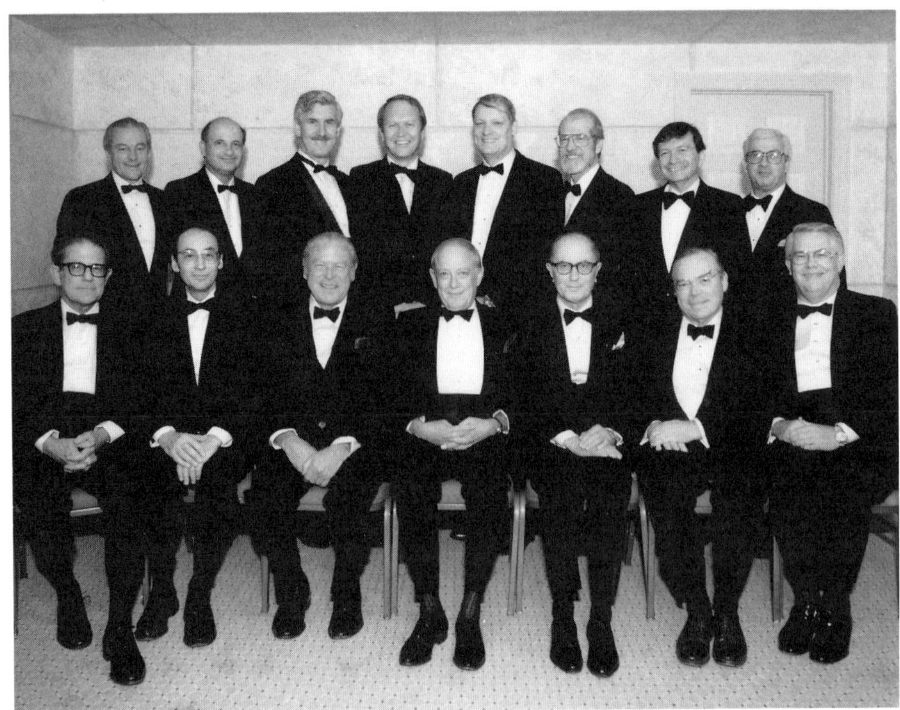

Figure 1.2. Presidents of the American Society of Nephrology. Photograph taken at the 20th annual meeting in 1987. *Front row, left to right*: Jack Orloff, Gerhard Giebisch, George E. Schreiner, Neal Bricker, Donald Seldin, Carl Gottschalk, Roscoe Robinson. *Standing*: Thomas Ferris, Jay Stein, Richard Glassock, Juha Kokko, Robert Schrier, Floyd Rector, Saulo Klahr, Barry Brenner. *Absent*: Robert Berliner, Lawrence Earley, Belding Scribner, Robert Vernier, William Schwartz, Robert Heptinstall, Maurice Burg, and Louis Welt, deceased.

was then turned over to the American Society of Nephrology, by which it is now administered.

It was apparent at the conclusion of the 1967 meeting that the American Society of Nephrology fulfilled a need. Even though it was established later than similar national societies in Europe, the Society provided an attractive forum for diverse groups, including clinicians, dialysis physicians, transplant surgeons, pathologists, urologists, and scientists interested in all aspects of the basic sciences relating to the kidney.

The roots of nephrology in the United States derive largely from a concern with the function of the kidney. Homer Smith led an entire school of renal physiology, involving clinicians in clearance studies on patients with a variety of renal disturbances. A. N. Richards led a group of renal physiologists who used micropuncture techniques to study glomerular and tubular functions, and E. K. Marshall led a group studying tubular transport and renal pharmacology. Robert Pitts led still another group in studies of acid-base balance and other aspects of tubular function. The rich tradition of clinical nephrology arose from cardiologists who extended their interests to patients with hypertension and then to patients with primary kidney diseases. Also, there was a strong tradition, originating with Henderson, Van Slyke, Gamble, Shannon, Albright, Peters, and others, of clinical and laboratory research on salt and water and acid-base balance and on metabolic disturbances, especially of calcium and phosphate. These investigators, clinical and basic, gravitated to the American Heart Association, the American Physiological Society, the American Society for Clinical Investigation, and the Nephrosis Foundation. The American Society of Nephrology provided a forum for productive interaction of these scientists and physicians with such diverse interests at a single meeting.

The major and only activity of the Society specified in the Constitution and Bylaws is an annual meeting "for presentation and discussion of papers by members and their guests at a time and place to be decided by the Council. . . . A business meeting of the Society will be held annually at the time of the scientific meetings." The Constitution is silent on publications and other possible professional activities, and until very recently, they were eschewed. The annual book of abstracts was the only publication until the Society established the *Journal of the American Society of Nephrology*, Jared J. Grantham, Editor. The inaugural issue was published in July 1990.

The Constitution is also silent on matters of public policy and professional activities. Again, quite recently, the Officers and Council broadened the scope of the Society and formed a number of new committees addressing public policy issues, including support of research, postgraduate education and certification, staffing needs, and other aspects of clinical practice. In 1987 the Society established its office in Washington, D.C., and retained a political consulting group to represent the Society in the fields of biomedical research and health care delivery.

For approximately 20 years, the annual meetings of the National Kidney Foundation and the American Society of Nephrology have been consecutive. This was a natural development, since many individuals were interested in the activities of both organizations. From its inception in 1964, the National Kidney Foundation has been primarily involved in fund-raising to support research on kidney diseases; many lay people have been in this effort. The Clinical Dialysis and Transplant Forum of the National Kidney Foundation was the bridge to its scientific counterpart, the American Society of Nephrology. The development and success of chronic dialysis techniques and the success of renal transplantation in the 1960s, followed by passage of the Social Security Amendment to Medicare in 1972, enormously increased the number of nephrologists, especially physicians and surgeons in the areas of dialysis and transplantation. These clinicians represent a significant portion of active members of both organizations. More recently, the Society has moved to further its relations with the Association of Renal Physicians.

The growth of the Society and attendance at the annual meetings have been extraordinary. There are now more than 4000 members. Attendance at the 1991 annual meeting in Baltimore exceeded 6000, including many from abroad attracted by the high quality of the program. The meetings have been lengthened from 2 to $3\frac{1}{2}$ days as the number of abstracts submitted has dramatically increased from 287 in 1967 to 2067 in 1990 (Fig. 1.3). Approximately two-thirds of submitted abstracts are presented orally or in poster sessions.

Several awards are presented annually. The Homer W. Smith Award, established in 1964 by the New York Heart Association to recognize outstanding achievements in renal physiology, was first presented at the annual meeting of the American Society of Nephrology in 1971 (Table 1.3). Since 1983 it has been cosponsored by the two organizations. Each recipient's address is now published in the *Journal of the American Society of Nephrology*.

The John P. Peters Award for Excellence in Clinical Research was established and first awarded in 1983 (Table 1.4). In 1985, the Young

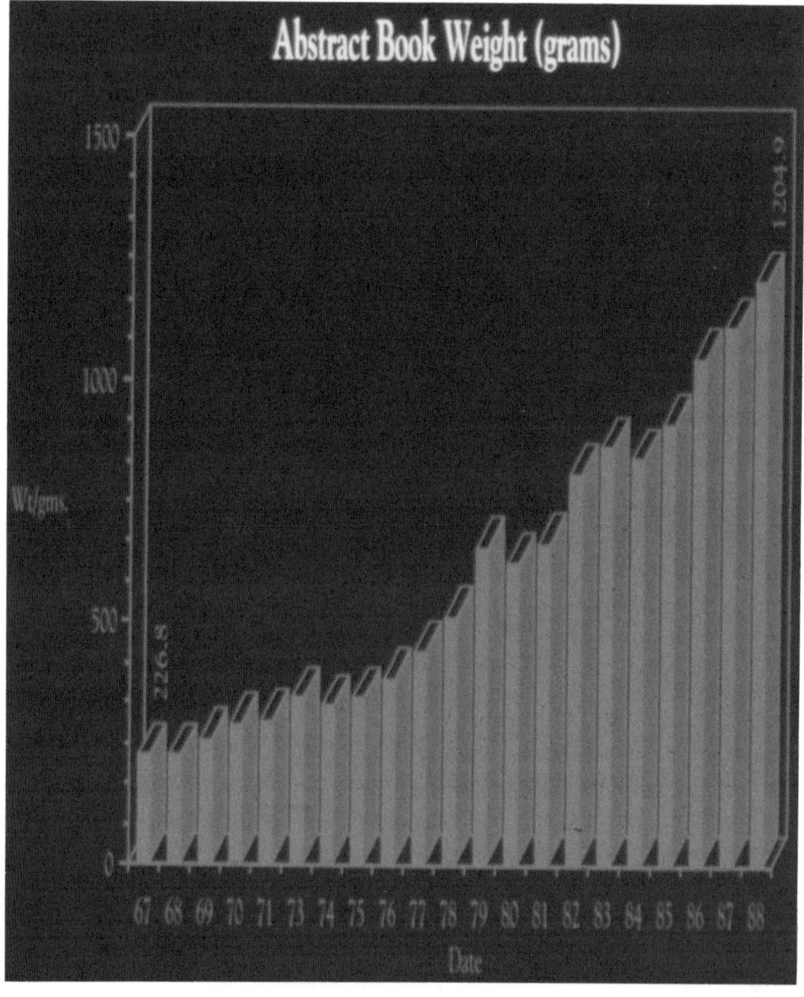

Figure 1.3. The growth of submitted abstracts as evidenced by the weight of the annual book of abstracts. (From presidential address of Jay H. Stein).

TABLE 1.3
Homer W. Smith Awardees[a]

Robert F. Pitts–1964	Erich E. Windhager–1978
Robert W. Berliner–1965	François Morel–1979
Hans H. Ussing–1966	Isidore S. Edelman–1980
Heinrich Wirz–1967	Alexander Leaf–1981
Jean R. Oliver–1968	Floyd C. Rector, Jr.–1982
James A. Shannon–1969	Eberhard Frömter–1983
Carl W. Gottschalk–1970	Barry M. Brenner–1984
Gerhard Giebisch–1971	Philip R. Steinmetz–1985
Hugh E. de Wardener–1972	Emile Boulpaep–1986
Jack Orloff–1973	Joseph S. Handler–1987
No award presented–1974	Marilyn G. Farquhar–1988
Karl J. Ullrich–1975	Rolf Kinne–1989
Frank J. Dixon–1976	Klaus Thurau–1990
Maurice B. Burg–1977	Heine H. Murer–1991

[a] Co-sponsored by the American Society of Nephrology and the New York Heart Association.

TABLE 1.4
John P. Peters Awardees

Donald W. Seldin–1983
John P. Merrill and Jean Hamburger–1984
Franklin H. Epstein–1985
Belding H. Scribner–1986
Conrad L. Pirani and Jacob Churg–1987
Renée Habib and Henry Barnett–1988
George E. Schreiner–1989
John H. Laragh and Louis Tobian–1990
Neal S. Bricker and Roscoe R. Robinson–1991

Investigator Award, cosponsored by the Council on the Kidney of the American Heart Association, was established (Table 1.5).

At the 1991 annual meeting, a new honor, the President's Award, was established to recognize outstanding service on behalf of the Society by a member of a standing committee exclusive of the Program Committee. The first recipient was Wadi N. Suki.

The 25 annual meetings (Table 1.6) of the Society have reflected and helped to shape the rapidly changing field of nephrology. It is interesting that with its astounding growth and diversity of content and with the addition of poster sessions, the basic format of the ASN meeting has continued the "unfolding" concept developed by Berliner and Schreiner for the 1966 International Congress in Washington, D.C.: state of the art in the major

TABLE 1.5

Young Investigator Awardees

Peter S. Aronson–1985
Walter F. Boron–1986
Eric G. Neilson–1987
Martin G. Cogan–1988
Rajiv Kumar–1989
Alan M. Krensky–1990
Stephen T. Reeders–1991

TABLE 1.6

American Society of Nephrology Annual Meetings

1.	October 18–19, 1967	Los Angeles, California
2.	November 25–26, 1968	Washington, D.C.
3.	December 1–2, 1969	Washington, D.C.
4.	November 23–24, 1970	Washington, D.C.
5.	November 22–23, 1971	Washington, D.C.
	No meeting in 1972	
6.	November 19–20, 1973	Washington, D.C.
7.	November 25–26, 1974	Washington, D.C.
8.	November 25–26, 1975	Washington, D.C.
9.	November 21–23, 1976	Washington, D.C.
10.	November 20–22, 1977	Washington, D.C.
11.	November 19–21, 1978	New Orleans, Louisiana
12.	November 18–20, 1979	Boston, Massachusetts
13.	November 23–25, 1980	Washington, D.C.
14.	November 22–24, 1981	Washington, D.C.
15.	December 12–14, 1982	Chicago, Illinois
16.	December 4–7, 1983	Washington, D.C.
17.	December 9–12, 1984	Washington, D.C.
18.	December 15–18, 1985	New Orleans, Louisiana
19.	December 7–10, 1986	Washington, D.C.
20.	December 13–16, 1987	Washington, D.C.
21.	December 11–14, 1988	San Antonio, Texas
22.	December 3–6, 1989	Washington, D.C.
23.	December 2–5, 1990	Washington, D.C.
24.	November 17–20, 1991	Baltimore, Maryland
25.	November 15–18, 1992	Baltimore, Maryland

subspecialties of nephrology, followed by controversies, panels, and seminars, followed by original communications, oral and poster. Most of the social features have also been maintained and have been an effective catalyst for lasting friendships and scientific collaborations. The remainder of this volume presents a review of the highlights of the meetings.

2

Mineral Metabolism

Jacob Lemann, Jr., Shaul G. Massry, and Eduardo Slatopolsky

Renal Osteodystrophy

Historical Background

It has been known for more than 50 years that patients with chronic renal failure have enlarged parathyroid glands often associated with unusually severe calcification of arteries and calcification of soft tissues. During the 1930s Fuller Albright and his associates postulated that the hyperplasia of the parathyroid glands was due to phosphate retention. Subsequently, studies by Liu and Chu in the early 1940s demonstrated impaired intestinal calcium (Ca) absorption in uremia that could not be corrected by physiological amounts of vitamin D that were sufficient to heal nutritional rickets. The overall concept of renal osteodystrophy was later classified by the work of Stanbury in the late 1950s. He pointed out that rickets and osteomalacia secondary to chronic renal failure was due to resistance to the action of vitamin D. He attributed the development of osteitis fibrosa to a skeletal manifestation of increased parathyroid activity. At the same time, Lichtwitz and his associates in France greatly contributed to the understanding of the alterations of mineral metabolism in patients with chronic renal failure.

With the development of the technique for radioimmunoassay, including the first radioimmunoassay for parathyroid hormone by Berson and Yallow, and with the extensive work of Reiss and Canterbury in patients with chronic renal failure in the late 1960s, physicians had, for the first time, the tools to quantitate the degree of secondary hyperparathyroidism in patients with renal insufficiency.

Work Presented at the American Society of Nephrology (ASN)

The Los Angeles group (Kleeman, Massry, Coburn, and associates) studied in great detail the clinical and biochemical manifestations of secondary hyperparathyroidism. They described alterations in mineral and bone metabolism in uremic patients during dialysis and after renal transplantation. They characterized the intestinal calcium malabsorption in renal failure and the beneficial effects of dietary calcium and vitamin D supplementation. They demonstrated that calcium malabsorption is an important pathogenetic mechanism in the development of secondary hyperparathyroidism in patients with renal insufficiency. In the late 1960s, the St. Louis group (Bricker, Slatopolsky, and associates) formulated a hypothesis that explained the mechanism of phosphate adaptation in chronic renal failure. These investigators proposed that as the glomerular filtration rate (GFR) diminished because of nephron destruction, renal phosphate excretion must decrease transiently and mild hyperphosphatemia ensue. The latter would, in turn, result in reduced serum ionized calcium levels. The decrease in ionized calcium rather than the elevation of phosphate per se would thus stimulate the parathyroid glands to increase the rate of hormone secretion. Thus, hyperparathyroidism would occur, in part, as a manifestation of an adaptive change in the control system, serving to promote the maintenance of external phosphate balance. It is important to emphasize, however, that when this hypothesis was proposed, it was not yet known that the kidney is responsible for the conversion of 25-hydroxycholecalciferol (25-OH-D_3; calcifediol) to 1,25-dihydroxycholecalciferol (1,25-$(OH)_2$-D_3; calcitriol), the hormonal metabolite of the vitamin D endocrine system. The original work of Frazier and Kodiceck first demonstrated the key role of the kidney in the metabolism of vitamin D. In addition to demonstrating alterations in vitamin D metabolism and phosphate retention, several investigators emphasized the role of metabolic acidosis. They showed that patients with renal metabolic acidosis characteristically have bone changes consistent with osteomalacia. Moreover, the correction of metabolic acidosis by the administration of sodium bicarbonate greatly improved the bone abnormalities. Thus, these studies emphasized the role of the skeleton in the maintenance of a normal acid-base status. It was clear that acidosis per se was responsible for the abnormal mineralization process and that this was independent of alterations in vitamin D metabolism.

At ASN meetings in the 1970s, numerous laboratories presented papers clarifying the different roles of vitamin D, calcium, and phosphorus in the pathogenesis of secondary hyperparathyroidism. The Los Angeles group demonstrated that calcitriol increased intestinal calcium absorption in renal insufficiency. With the consequent correction of hypocalcemia, these investigators showed a decrease in the levels of parathyroid hormone, radiological improvement of the skeletal manifestations of secondary hyperparathyroidism, and histological healing of osteitis fibrosa. Massry and Llach presented evidence for skeletal resistance to parathyroid hormone in renal insufficiency. They concluded that a deficiency of 1,25-$(OH)_2$-D_3 was partially responsible for the resistance. They also demonstrated that a low phosphate diet improved the response of the skeleton to the administration of exogenous parathyroid hormone. The low phosphate diet increased the production of 1,25-$(OH)_2$-D_3 in patients with early renal insufficiency. Consequently, the degree of secondary hyperparathyroidism improved. Several years later, Slatopolsky and associates further characterized the mechanisms responsible for the skeletal resistance to parathyroid hormone. These investigators studied the calcemic effect of parathyroid hormone (PTH) in dogs with chronic renal failure. The calcemic response to PTH in dogs with renal failure was abnormally low and not corrected by the administration of 1,25-$(OH)_2$-D_3. However, when uremic animals underwent parathyroidectomy 24 hours before PTH administration, the calcemic response increased to normal. This normal response occurred despite the continued uremic state and low levels of 1,25-$(OH)_2$-D_3. These results led to the conclusion that the deficiency of 1,25-$(OH)_2$-D_3 was not responsible for the resistance to the calcemic action of PTH. Rather, down-regulation or desensitization of PTH receptors by high circulating levels of endogenous PTH was responsible for the abnormal calcemic response. Thus, with secondary hyperparathyroidism, high levels of endogenous PTH bind to receptors in the skeleton, diminishing the response of the skeleton to the administration of parathyroid hormone.

The role of phosphate in the pathogenesis of chronic renal insufficiency was studied in great detail by the St. Louis group. In the late 1960s and early 1970s, they demonstrated that feeding a low phosphorus diet to dogs with experimental chronic renal insufficiency could prevent the development of secondary hyperparathyroidism. Subsequently, the same group demonstrated that a reduction of phosphate in proportion to the degree of renal insufficiency was also effective in controlling secondary hyperparathyroidism. Subsequent studies by Portale and associates demonstrated that the administration of a low phosphate diet to patients with renal insufficiency increased the production of 1,25-$(OH)_2$-D_3. Thus, the increase in calcitriol was, in part, responsible for the amelioration of secondary hyperparathyroidism in these patients. Further studies by Portale indicated that a low phosphate diet increased the production rate of calcitriol without changing the metabolic clearance rate. In the late 1980s, Slatopolsky and associates provided further evidence in uremic dogs that phosphate per se, independent of the levels of ionized calcium and 1,25-$(OH)_2$-D_3, had an important role in the development of secondary hyperparathyroidism. The precise mechanisms at the molecular level are still unknown.

In 1973, the American Society of Nephrology dedicated a workshop to vitamin D metabolism in uremia and its relation to calcium malabsorption and osteodystrophy. Coburn, Brickman, Sherrard, and associates presented extensive work on the treatment of renal osteodystrophy with 1,25-$(OH)_2$-D_3. They concluded that the effects of calcitriol were striking in patients with lesions attributable to hyperparathyroidism. After treatment with calcitriol, they found a remarkable decrease of 45% in resorptive surfaces. Marrow fibrosis fell from 11.5 to 3.0%. They observed, however, that 1,25-$(OH)_2$-D_3 failed to correct osteomalacia. They concluded that this failure may be due to inadequate doses or to end-organ resistance. In 1974, the St. Louis group presented a study titled "Long-Term Prevention of Secondary Hyperparathyroidism in Uremic Dogs." These studies were performed to evaluate the roles of phosphate retention versus calcium malabsorption in long-term observations on three groups of uremic dogs. Group I ingested 1200 mg of phosphorus per day. Group II was subjected to a reduction of phosphate intake in direct proportion to the decrease in GFR. Group III was maintained on a proportional reduction of phosphate plus 60 μg of 25-OH-D_3 three times per week. Uremic animals demonstrated low calcium absorption. This reverted to normal within 1 week of treatment with 25-OH-D_3. The animals maintained on a proportional reduction of phosphate in Group II had normal values for PTH after 1 year and only mild elevation at the end of the second year. Group III experienced no elevation of PTH levels after 20 months. These studies indicated that phosphate retention plays a role in the development of secondary hyperparathyroidism. However, on a long-term basis, vitamin D resistance appears to have a pathogenetic role. Correction of calcium malabsorption with 25-OH-D_3 in dogs maintained on a proportional reduction of phosphate completely prevented the development of secondary hyperparathyroidism of uremia. The St. Louis group demonstrated several years later that anephric patients can convert 25-OH-D_3 to 1,25-$(OH)_2$-D_3. It is now known that macrophages can convert 25-OH-D_3 to 1,25-$(OH)_2$-D_3. Thus, the effect of 25-OH-D_3 in chronic renal failure may be attributable, in part, to such further conversion into 1,25-$(OH)_2$-D_3.

In addition to playing an important role in calcium absorption and skeletal function, calcitriol has a direct effect on PTH secretion. The first conclusive experiments were performed in primary culture of bovine parathyroid cells. Although this field was studied by numerous endocrinologists, the St. Louis group's in vitro studies showed that 1,25-$(OH)_2$-D_3 has a direct suppressive effect on PTH release. Subsequently, other investigators have shown that calcitriol binds to receptors in the parathyroid cells and blocks gene transcription for pre-pro PTH mRNA. Thus, after numerous years of investigation, it has been unanimously accepted that calcitriol not only suppresses parathyroid hormone by increasing ionized calcium but also directly suppresses the synthesis of parathyroid hormone. Although it has been known for many years that patients with chronic renal failure have chief cell hyperplasia of all four parathyroid glands, which play a key role in the increased secretion of parathyroid hormone, other abnormalities have also been found in the parathyroid cells of uremic patients. It was shown that there is a shift in the setpoint for calcium-mediated suppression of PTH secretion. Thus, higher concentrations of ionized calcium are required to suppress secondary hyperparathyroidism. In part, this abnormal regulatory mechanism explains why nephrologists failed to correct secondary hyperparathyroidism by trying to correct only abnormalities in calcium and phosphate metabolism without providing calcitriol.

The laboratories of Malluche, Sherrard, Llach, Felsenfeld, and Goodman have greatly contributed to the understanding of the histological abnormalities in bone in patients with chronic renal insufficiency. These investigators clearly demonstrated a remarkable beneficial effect of calcitriol on those parameters characteristic of severe secondary hyperparathyroidism.

Subsequently, Alfrey, Llach, Coburn, Malluche, Sherrard, Felsenfeld, and other investigators have described a form of bone disease that did not respond to calcitriol treatment. They demonstrated the role of aluminum retention in the pathogenesis of osteomalacia. Characteristically, these patients presented with severe bone pain, pathological fractures, and normal or elevated serum calcium levels. The majority of these patients had relatively low serum PTH concentrations. Characteristically, there was increased deposition of aluminum at the mineralization front. Although the great majority of these patients have an increase in osteoid, some have a decreased amount of osteoid. This was termed aplastic or adynamic bone disease. Several groups presented results on the use of desferrioxamine (DFO) as a diagnostic tool. Although the "DFO test" provided important information, the studies by Malluche and others indicated that a bone biopsy was the only test that categorically could predict the degree of skeletal involvement. Moreover, the same group emphasized that it was not the amount of aluminum in bone but the presence of aluminum at the mineralization front (stainable aluminum) that best predicted the degree of bone involvement in patients with aluminum-induced osteomalacia. Many investigators showed that the majority of patients with pathological fractures and severe bone pain did not have secondary hyperparathyroidism but aluminum accumulation. On the other hand, tissue calcification and necrosis due to vascular calcification were associated, in general, with high calcium-phosphate products and high levels of parathyroid hormone.

In the late 1970s and early 1980s, numerous groups of investigators and clinicians demonstrated different approaches to the prevention and treatment of renal osteodystrophy. Although the control of phosphate was mandatory to prevent metastatic calcification and secondary hyperparathyroidism, physicians learned the side effects of aluminum administration. Thus, calcium carbonate ($CaCO_3$) became the main therapeutic tool in the treatment of hyperphosphatemia. It was shown that $CaCO_3$ is an effective phosphate binder when given with meals. Also, several groups noted hypercalcemia to be a consequence of the administration of large doses—6 to 8 g/day—of $CaCO_3$. Extensive work has shown that it is safe to decrease the amount of calcium in the dialysate from 3.5 to 2.5 mEq/L in those patients ingesting large amounts of $CaCO_3$. Recently, several groups presented evidence that calcium acetate is also an effective phosphate binder. The phosphate-binding characteristics of calcium acetate are greater than those of calcium carbonate, apparently because of the greater solubility of calcium acetate. Thus, theoretically, patients would require less elemental calcium when calcium acetate is administered instead of $CaCO_3$ to bind phosphate. Unfortunately, Delmez, Shafer, and others also have shown that despite the fact that the amount of elemental calcium could be reduced by half when given as calcium acetate than when administered as $CaCO_3$, the incidence of hypercalcemic episodes is similar. Thus calcium acetate, although a better phosphate binder, may be absorbed better than calcium carbonate. Further studies are necessary to clarify this issue. In addition, other investigators have shown that calcium citrate greatly increases aluminum absorption in normal volunteers as well as in animals with experimental chronic renal failure. These observations may explain the high levels of serum aluminum seen in children ingesting aluminum salts and Shohl's solution (citric acid 140 g/L plus sodium citrate 98 g/L, providing 1 mEq potential bicarbonate/mL). Thus, Alfrey, Molitoris, and associates recommended that calcium citrate should not be given if patients also ingest aluminum salts.

Several investigators, including Coburn, Llach, Sherrard, Malluche, and others, demonstrated a beneficial effect of desferrioxamine in patients with aluminum-induced osteomalacia. However, the initial enthusiasm to aggressively treat all patients with aluminum accumulation has decreased because of several reports indicating that 5 to 10% of patients receiving desferrioxamine develop fatal mucormycosis infections. Thus, unless patients have pathological fractures or severe bone pain secondary to aluminum accumulation, most investigators suggest elimination of aluminum in the dialysate and substitution of $CaCO_3$ for aluminum-containing phosphate binders to gradually ameliorate the side effects of aluminum without the need for desferrioxamine.

In the mid-1980s, an intravenous (IV) formulation of calcitriol became available. Several studies showed that IV calcitriol achieved suppression of parathyroid hormone in the great majority of patients. Moreover, it appeared that the degree of suppression of secondary hyperparathyroidism obtained with the IV calcitriol was greater than that observed with the oral calcitriol. In part, this may be due to the higher plasma levels of calcitriol obtained after the IV preparation. Several groups demonstrated that the number of receptors for 1,25-$(OH)_2$-D_3 in parathyroid tissue obtained from uremic patients or animals with experimental renal insufficiency is low. Because 1,25-$(OH)_2$-D_3 induces its own receptor number in the parathyroid gland, the high plasma concentrations of calcitriol achieved after intravenous administration may overcome the resistance of the parathyroid glands to calcitriol. Other investigators reported studies of "pulse therapy" with oral calcitriol. Thus, the dose was increased from 0.5 μg daily to 3.0 to 4.0 μg twice weekly. Using this therapy in patients maintained on continuous ambulatory peritoneal dialysis (CAPD), Martin observed an effective reduction of serum PTH levels. Delmez and collaborators and Dundlay and collaborators showed that the abnormal setpoint for calcium could be greatly improved with an intravenous administration of calcitriol.

The European literature and, more recently, numerous papers in our society have documented yet another form of bone disease in hemodialysis patients that is characterized by the accumulation of β_2-microglobulin. β_2-Microglobulin has been identified as a major component of amyloid deposits. Clinical manifestations include skeletal lesions, pathological fractures, and carpal tunnel syndrome. French investigators presented evidence that skin biopsies of patients maintained on hemodialysis, when examined by indirect immunofluorescence using an anti-β_2 monoclonal antibody, were more sensitive than staining with Congo red. The incidence of biopsy-proven β_2-microglobulin amyloid deposits in articular synovium increases with increasing time on dialysis. Zingraff, Drueke, and associates were unable to show in vitro generation of β_2-microglobulin from uremic blood during incubation with polysulfane membranes or with AN-69 polyacrylonitrile membranes. In addition, they showed that plasma β_2-microglobulin levels are lower in peritoneal dialysis patients, which is consistent with increased clearance of middle molecules by the peritoneal membrane. The investigators concluded that standard cuprophane membranes promote retention and possibly release of β_2-microglobulin in vivo, whereas AN-69 membranes lead to removal of β_2-microglobulins because of both transmembrane transfer and membrane binding.

In the late 1980s, several investigators, including Hercz, Andress, and Sherrard, presented evidence for the appearance of a low-turnover bone disease without aluminum in patients maintained on dialysis. The majority of these patients had relatively low values for PTH. The long-term consequence of low-turnover bone disease in asymptomatic patients on dialysis warrants further evaluation. At the 1990 meeting of the ASN, Slatopolsky and associates presented their innovative studies of a new, noncalcemic analog of 1,25-$(OH)_2$-D_3, 22-oxacalcitriol (OCT). This analog of calcitriol suppresses pre-pro PTH mRNA in uremic animals without inducing hypercalcemia. Further studies in patients with chronic renal failure are necessary to assess the role of OCT in the treatment of renal osteodystrophy.

Thus, in the past 25 years, ASN meetings have greatly contributed to the understanding of the pathophysiology and treatment of renal osteodystrophy. Currently, we have a better understanding of calcium malabsorption and phosphate retention. We are moving away from aluminum binders. We have decreased the amount of calcium in the dialysate and prescribed calcium carbonate and calcium acetate as phosphate binders. There is a better understanding of the regulation of PTH by calcitriol. The use of intravenous calcitriol or of oral "pulse" therapy appears to produce a greater suppressive effect on PTH than is obtained by small daily oral doses of calcitriol. Noncalcemic analogs of calcitriol are promising new tools in the treatment of renal osteodystrophy. The retention of β_2-microglobulins as a cause of bone disease as well as low-turnover bone disease will require further extensive study before physicians will have a way to treat these conditions.

Parathyroid Hormone

Historical Background

The existence of the parathyroid glands was first demonstrated in the rhinoceros by Owen in 1880. Vassale and Generali observed in 1900 that the removal of the parathyroid glands in cats and dogs caused tetany, and in

1908 MacCallum and Voegthlin found that the concentration of blood calcium fell in parathyroidectomized animals. Thus, the relationship between the parathyroid glands and calcium homeostasis was established. This relationship was further documented by the studies of Patt and Luckhardt, who demonstrated in 1942 that the blood levels of calcium control the secretion of PTH. The effect of PTH to augment renal tubular reabsorption of calcium was demonstrated in rats by Talmadge and Kraintz in 1959 and in humans by Kleeman and associates in 1961.

In 1911, Greenwald and Gross showed that the urinary excretion of phosphate is reduced and the blood levels of phosphate increased after parathyroidectomy. These observations pointed toward the important relationship between PTH and phosphate homeostasis. Munson and associates in 1955 demonstrated that pure PTH has a direct phosphaturic effect. Between 1948 and 1956, several investigators, including Barnicot and Chang, Gaillard, Talmadge, and Elliot, demonstrated that PTH exerts a direct effect on bone, causing bone resorption.

The first documentation of one of the biochemical mechanisms of action of PTH on kidney and bone was provided in 1967 by the classical studies of Chase and Aurbach, who demonstrated that the hormone stimulates adenylate cyclase and causes the generation of cyclic adenosine monophosphate (cAMP). Preparation of parathyroid extract in the early 1920s by Hanson and Collip, preparation of highly purified PTH by Aurbach and Rasmussen in 1959, and, subsequently, the synthesis of various forms of the hormone have permitted many physiological and biochemical studies clarifying the effects of PTH on organ function. In addition, the development of the radioimmunoassay of PTH in 1963 by Berson and Yalow provided a milestone in the studies of PTH secretion and metabolism and of the clinical disorders associated with PTH excess and deficiency.

In 1926, Mandel provided the first clinical description of hyperparathyroidism. He documented that the syndrome could be corrected by the removal of a parathyroid adenoma. Subsequent studies by Fuller Albright and associates and by Beginning greatly contributed to the detailed understanding of the clinical syndromes of PTH excess and deficiency.

Work Presented at the ASN

A series of studies presented at ASN meetings since 1967 have provided new information regarding parathyroid hormone and its actions. These data have dealt mainly with the effects of the hormone on the kidney; the mechanisms of secondary hyperparathyroidism in chronic renal failure, including derangements in parathyroid hormone secretion and metabolism in chronic kidney disease; and the effects of PTH on organs other than the kidney and bone. The effects of PTH on the renal handling of calcium and phosphate are discussed in the sections dealing with calcium and phosphate, respectively.

PTH also has been observed to alter sodium and bicarbonate reabsorption by the proximal tubule. Agus and associates demonstrated that PTH inhibits proximal sodium reabsorption. Suki and his group demonstrated that large doses of PTH decreased $TmPO_4$ in both intact and thyroparathyroidectomized (TPTX) dogs. Micropuncture experiments confirmed that PTH inhibits proximal bicarbonate reabsorption in dogs and in rats but that this effect of PTH was accompanied by either no change in urinary bicarbonate excretion or only a small increase. Other investigators have reported that the administration of PTH to TPTX dogs was associated with bicarbonaturia. Using microperfusion techniques, investigators found that this inhibitory effect of PTH on proximal bicarbonate reabsorption was also present in the proximal tubule of rabbits. PTH was also found to stimulate the renal 25-OH-D-1a-hydroxylase and thus the renal synthesis of 1,25-$(OH)_2$-D_3.

The mechanisms of action of PTH on the kidney are mediated by stimulation of an adenylate cyclase-cAMP system, alterations in cytosolic calcium, and/or an effect on phospholipid turnover. PTH-sensitive adenylate cyclase has been found in the glomeruli, the proximal convoluted tubule, the proximal pars recta or straight tubule, the cortical thick ascending limb of Henle's loop, and the distal convoluted tubule. PTH, through the stimulation of these adenylate cyclases, exerts at least in part its various actions on the kidney, including a reduction of ultrafiltration coefficient (Kf), inhibition of proximal tubular reabsorption of sodium, calcium, and phosphate, enhanced reabsorption of calcium by the cortical thick ascending limb of Henle's loop, (CTAL), and the stimulation of 1,25-$(OH)_2$-D_3 synthesis. The inhibition of proximal reabsorption of bicarbonate by PTH is apparently mediated by inhibition of the Na^+-H^+ antiporter in the brush border membrane of the proximal tubule. This inhibition of the Na^+-H^+ antiporter is probably also mediated by PTH-induced stimulation of renal cAMP.

The existence of secondary hyperparathyroidism in patients with chronic renal failure was known prior to the first scientific meeting of the ASN in 1967. Berson and Yalow had previously shown that blood levels of PTH are elevated in patients with chronic kidney failure and even in those with moderate renal insufficiency. Many studies have been presented at ASN meetings to dissect and elucidate the mechanisms of this phenomenon (see Renal Osteodystrophy).

The St. Louis group (Slatopolsky, Hruska, Martin, and associates) performed studies of the peripheral metabolism of PTH in normal animals and in those with chronic renal failure. Their data, as well as additional information provided by others, have indicated that about 60% of intact PTH is cleaved in the Kupffer cells of the liver into amino terminal (N-PTH) and carboxy terminal (C-PTH) fragments. The kidneys remove about 30% of the intact PTH as well as both N-PTH and C-PTH by glomerular filtration, tubular reabsorption, and, presumably, tubular catabolism. Contraluminal uptake of intact PTH and N-PTH, but not of C-PTH, also occurs, Bone, on the other hand, was found to remove only N-PTH. The half-life of

N-PTH in the circulation is very short (minutes), whereas that of C-PTH is much longer. Chronic renal failure interferes with the peripheral metabolism of PTH by both the liver and the kidney. Because the latter is the main site for the removal of C-PTH, the plasma concentration of C-PTH is markedly elevated in renal failure. Indeed, after kidney transplantation and restoration of normal kidney function, the blood levels of C-PTH fall rapidly. In 1974, Arieff and Massry presented the first observation that PTH may act on organs other than the kidney and bone. They demonstrated that secondary hyperparathyroidism in dogs with acute renal failure causes a significant increase in brain calcium content. This effect was prevented by parathyroidectomy and reproduced by the administration of PTH to TPTX dogs with acute renal failure. This increase in brain calcium appeared to be physiologically significant in that it was associated with abnormalities in the electroencephalogram.

These data and other clinical observations have led Massry to postulate that the elevated blood levels of PTH may be a factor in the pathogenesis of various manifestations of the uremic syndrome. He has considered PTH as a major uremic toxin. Massry and his group have presented a series of studies at the ASN demonstrating that brain and brain synaptosomes, heart, skeletal muscle, red blood cells, T and B cells, polymorphonuclear leukocytes, and pancreatic islets are targets for PTH action. Chronic exposure of these various cells to excess PTH has been observed to be associated with significant elevations in cytosolic calcium concentrations and with significant derangements in their functional integrity. These data have led to the suggestion that uremia may represent a state of generalized calcium toxicity. Parathyroidectomy, by preventing secondary hyperparathyroidism in renal failure, or treatment of animals with renal failure with verapamil that blocks PTH-induced increases in cytosolic calcium, corrects the cellular dysfunction in chronic renal failure.

The determination of the amino acid sequence of PTH has permitted the synthesis of various PTH fragments and PTH antagonists. In addition, the molecular biology of PTH synthesis has been clarified, and the PTH receptor has been cloned. These latter studies have been presented primarily at meetings of the Endocrine Society and of the American Society for Bone and Mineral Research.

Vitamin D

Historical Background

Knowledge of vitamin D evolved from studies of rickets in children, a disorder that became more common as populations shifted to smoky, dark cities during the industrial development that took place in the 18th and 19th centuries. Early pathological studies of the skeleton in rickets demonstrated impaired mineralization of newly formed bone (osteomalacia) as well as disordered epiphyseal cell organization and maturation. There were occasional reports of the healing of rickets by fish oils, predating both knowledge of vitamins as trace but essential dietary nutrients and subsequent knowledge of the availability of vitamin D in fish, milk, and eggs. Metabolic balance studies demonstrated lower than normal rates of net intestinal absorption of Ca and phosphate (PO_4) in children with rickets. At about the end of World War I, there were two major advances in the understanding of rickets. Mellanby developed a method to produce rickets in puppies and cured that experimental disease with cod liver oil, thus documenting the existence of a dietary antirachitic factor. At about the same time, it was observed that sun exposure or ultraviolet irradiation of the skin cured rickets in infants. Huldchinsky showed that irradiation of one arm could result in healing, thus providing the first clue that vitamin D is also a hormone produced in the skin. Subsequently, Steenbock and associates at the University of Wisconsin demonstrated that irradiation of the diet also resulted in the production of a factor that cured experimental rickets. In 1932, this lipid soluble factor was isolated and its chemical structure determined as vitamin D_2 (ergocalciferol), and in 1936 the structure of the naturally occurring vitamin D_3 (cholecalciferol) was determined.

With respect to the kidney, occasional patients with chronic kidney disease were observed to have either rickets as children or osteomalacia as adults. Liu and Chu in Beijing observed in the 1940s during metabolic balance studies among such patients that rates of net intestinal absorption of Ca were reduced in comparison to healthy adults. These abnormally low rates of intestinal Ca absorption in renal failure were not corrected by physiological doses of vitamin D_2 that were sufficient to heal nutritional rickets. These studies were among the first to detect vitamin D resistance in uremia, retrospectively indicating lack of further metabolism of vitamin D to a physiologically active form. Liu and Chu also demonstrated that intestinal Ca absorption could be increased by the administration of dihydrotachysterol (AT-10), a vitamin D analog whose structure contains a pseudo 1α-hydroxyl group, the 1α-hydroxyl group now known to be essential for the action of 1,25-$(OH)_2$-vitamin D_3 (calcitriol), the hormonal metabolite of the vitamin D endocrine system (see below). Further knowledge of vitamin D_3 lagged until the mid-1960s, when new knowledge of chemistry allowed the synthesis of radiolabeled cholesterol and radiolabeled vitamin D_3. Vitamin D_3 was shown to be produced in the skin by the enzymatic conversion of cholesterol to 7-dehydrolcholesterol and the subsequent conversion of dehydrocholesterol to vitamin D_3 under the influence of ultraviolet irradiation. In 1968, DeLuca and associates discovered the rapid metabolism of isotopic vitamin D_3 by the liver to 25-OH-D_3 (calcifediol; 25-OH-cholecalciferol), now known to be the major circulating and storage form of vitamin D_3. Progress in knowledge of the vitamin D endocrine system rapidly followed as a result of studies by biochemists, physiologists, endocrinologists, and nephrologists, with such advances being reported at subsequent meetings of the American Society of Nephrology, the Endocrine Society, and, since the mid-1970s, the meetings of the American Society for Bone and Mineral Research.

Work Presented at the ASN

With respect to the American Society of Nephrology, studies of Ca metabolism in relation to vitamin D in kidney disease were first presented at the third annual meeting in 1969. Koppel, Coburn, and Massry confirmed that Ca absorption, using ^{47}Ca, is low among patients with chronic renal failure and that pharmacologic doses of vitamin D_3 improved ^{47}Ca absorption.

In 1970, Kodicek and Fraser in Cambridge, England, and almost simultaneously DeLuca and associates at the University of Wisconsin and Norman and associates at the University of California, Riverside, made the key discovery of the synthesis of 1,25-$(OH)_2$-D_3 in the kidney and showed that this vitamin D metabolite could, within hours, increase to normal the impaired intestinal Ca absorption observed in vitamin D-deficient anephric animals, an action not achieved by the administration of vitamin D_3 or 25-OH-D_3.

Some of these data were first presented at the 1971 fifth annual meeting by Norman, Coburn, and associates. They showed that kidney homogenates from chick, rat, dog, and human could convert ^{3}H-25-OH-D_3 to ^{3}H-1,25-$(OH)_2$-D_3, an event localized to the mitochondria in the chick. They also demonstrated that the administration of 1,25-$(OH)_2$-D_3, but not vitamin D_3 or 25-OH-D_3, was capable of increasing intestinal Ca absorption in nephrectomized or ureter-ligated rats while all three vitamin D metabolites stimulated Ca absorption in normal control animals. Thus, the kidney was shown to play the major role in producing the biologically active form of vitamin D.

Because of these rapid advances, a symposium at the 1973 annual meeting was devoted to review of disordered Ca metabolism in uremia (Avioli), vitamin D metabolism (DeLuca), and the effect of the vitamin D metabolites on bone in organ culture, including the action of 1,25-$(OH)_2$-D_3 to augment bone resorption directly (Raisz).

During the 1970s, the metabolism of 25-OH-D_3 to 24,25-$(OH)_2$-D_3, currently believed to be a relatively inactive and degradative metabolite of 25-OH-D_3, was clarified. The transport in plasma of the lipid-soluble vitamin D metabolites by the vitamin D binding protein (DBP) was recognized. Studies by Haussler and associates and DeLuca and associates also demonstrated that 1,25-$(OH)_2$-D_3 became bound to a cytosolic and nuclear receptor in cells. Based on this knowledge, techniques were developed to quantitate 1,25-$(OH)_2$-D_3 by inhibition of binding to the cytosolic receptor, initially isolated from intestinal cells and subsequently isolated from the thymus. Subsequent studies since the 1970s have been devoted to anatomical localization of the site of production of 1,25-$(OH)_2$-D_3 together with studies of the regulation of synthesis and the sites and mechanism of action of the hormone.

Using conversion of ^{3}H-25-OH-D_3 to ^{3}H-1,25-$(OH)_2$-D_3, Brunette and associates localized the site of production of 1,25-$(OH)_2$-D_3 to the proximal tubule in microdissected segments of the vitamin D-deficient chick nephron, and Kurokowa and associates made similar observations in the rat.

Subsequent studies by Langman, Favus, and Coe demonstrated that isolated rat proximal tubular segments produced 1,25-$(OH)_2$-D_3 as quantitated by radioreceptor assay, and Korkor, Gray, and associates made comparable observations in primary cultures of mouse cortical cells that were characterized as proximal tubular cells. Studies by other investigators have localized the site of synthesis of 1,25-$(OH)_2$-D_3 to proximal tubular mitochondria and have shown that the 25-OH-D_3-1α-hydroxylase is a cytochrome P_{450} monooxygenase that requires as cofactors an iron sulfur protein and a nicotinamide adenine dinucleotide (NAD)–linked flavoprotein reductase. The 1α-hydroxylase has not yet been isolated, sequenced, and cloned.

A number of investigators have shown that among healthy adults, plasma concentrations of 1,25-$(OH)_2$-D_3 range from about 50 to 140 pmol/L (20 to 60 pg/mL). Chesney, DeLuca, and associates observed higher levels among children and rapidly growing adolescents. Plasma concentrations of 1,25-$(OH)_2$-D_3 are considered to principally reflect synthesis of the hormone rather than metabolic clearance. Many investigators observed plasma concentrations of 1,25-$(OH)_2$-D_3 to be generally undetectable in anephric patients on dialysis and very low in patients with advanced renal failure or on dialysis, thus emphasizing the kidney as the major site of 1,25-$(OH)_2$-D_3 production. In cross-sectional studies of patients with varying degrees of renal failure, serum 1,25-$(OH)_2$-D_3 concentrations were observed to fall as GFR declined, although plasma 1,25-$(OH)_2$-D_3 levels are not invariably low until GFR falls below the range of 30 to 50 mL/min.

Plasma 1,25-$(OH)_2$-D_3 levels have been found to be largely independent of precursor 25-OH-D concentrations but closely regulated by Ca, PO_4, PTH, and 1,25-$(OH)_2$-D_3 itself. Early studies by DeLuca and associates showed that dietary Ca deprivation increased renal synthesis of 1,25-$(OH)_2$-D_3. Hughes, Haussler, and associates subsequently demonstrated in rats that dietary Ca deprivation raised plasma 1,25-$(OH)_2$-D concentrations as a reflection of renal synthesis of the hormone, an effect that was abolished by parathyroidectomy, and that dietary PO_4 deprivation raised plasma 1,25-$(OH)_2$-D concentration independent of PTH. Bushinsky, Favus, Langman, and Coe subsequently demonstrated that plasma 1,25-$(OH)_2$-D levels in rats were inversely correlated to plasma ionized Ca concentrations in normal, PTX-, and PTX-PTH-infused rats among whom ionized Ca concentrations were chronically reduced by restriction of dietary Ca or metabolic alkalosis and increased by metabolic acidosis or Ca infusion. Additional studies by Langman and associates suggested that the rise in plasma ionized Ca associated with metabolic acidosis resulted in inhibition of 1,25-$(OH)_2$-D_3 synthesis by isolated rat proximal tubule segments as a consequence of mitochondrial Ca overload.

The control of 1,25-$(OH)_2$-D_3 by PTH has also been explored. Many, although not all, patients with primary hyperparathyroidism were shown to exhibit elevated plasma 1,25-$(OH)_2$-D concentrations despite hypercalcemia. Korkor, Gray, and associates demonstrated that bovine PTH added to the culture media augmented 1,25-$(OH)_2$-D_3 production from 25-OH-D_3 by primary cultures of mouse kidney cortical cells, an effect requiring 6 to 8 hours of PTH exposure and apparently mediated by PTH activation of adenylate cyclase because of the simultaneous accumulation of cAMP. Chen, Puschett, and associates made similar observations using primary cultures of rat proximal tubular cells. They also showed that a cAMP analog and prostaglandins (PGE_1, PGE_2) stimulated 1,25-$(OH)_2$-D_3 synthesis by a mechanism inhibited by cyclohexamide, implying that the increase in 1,25-$(OH)_2$-D_3 production requires new protein synthesis. Adams, Gray, and Lemann demonstrated that among healthy human adults, oral $CaCO_3$ supplements or dietary Ca deprivation reduced and increased plasma 1,25-$(OH)_2$-D concentrations, respectively, changes that were directly correlated to simultaneous changes in urinary cAMP excretion as a reflection of the effect of PTH on the kidney.

Other studies have been directed toward clarifying the regulation of 1,25-$(OH)_2$-D by PO_4. A series of elegant clinical studies during the 1980s by Portale, Morris, Halloran, and associates demonstrated that dietary PO_4 deprivation in children with moderate renal failure increased serum plasma 1,25-$(OH)_2$-D_3 concentrations, accompanied by a fall in serum PTH levels, while increased dietary PO_4 intake resulted in an opposite sequence. Extreme decrements or increments in dietary PO_4 intake as well as lesser variations within the range of normal among healthy adults had similar effects to increase and decrease plasma 1,25-$(OH)_2$-D levels, respectively. These increases or decreases in plasma 1,25-$(OH)_2$-D levels were shown to directly reflect changes in 1,25-$(OH)_2$-D_3 production as measured by the equilibrium infusion technique, and the changes were inversely correlated to the integrated mean plasma PO_4 concentrations prevailing throughout the day as measured hourly over 24 hours. In other correlative clinical studies, Gray, Lemann, and associates similarly demonstrated that the elevated 1,25-$(OH)_2$-D concentrations observed among some patients with idiopathic hypercalciuria were similarly inversely correlated to their slightly reduced serum PO_4 concentrations. Langman, Favus, and Coe demonstrated, using proximal tubular segments from rats fed normal diets, that 1,25-$(OH)_2$-D_3 production was inversely correlated to the PO_4 concentration prevailing in the incubation medium but that variation in Ca or PTH concentrations in the medium had little effect. These studies provide additional evidence for plasma PO_4 concentrations as a major and direct determinant of 1,25-$(OH)_2$-D_3 synthesis in the kidney. Gray and associates also showed that the effect of dietary PO_4 deprivation to augment renal synthesis of 1,25-$(OH)_2$-D_3 is abolished by hypophysectomy and is restored by growth hormone. Subsequent studies have indicated that the availability of somatomedin-C (IGF-1) is permissive for the effect of PO_4 deprivation to increase 1,25-$(OH)_2$-D_3 synthesis.

The administration of 1,25-$(OH)_2$-D_3 to animals was also shown to reduce renal 1,25-$(OH)_2$-D_3 synthesis, providing evidence for self-regulation of hormone production by induction of enzymes that further metabolize 1,25-$(OH)_2$-D_3, such as the 24-hydroxylase.

Additional studies were directed toward determining whether metabolic acidosis regulated 1,25-$(OH)_2$-D_3. Although metabolic acidosis had been shown to lower plasma 1,25-$(OH)_2$-D levels in vitamin D-depleted and -repleted animals, studies in vitamin D-replete normal humans by Kraut, Coburn, and associates and by Adams, Maierhofer, Lemann, and Gray showed that neither NH_4Cl acidosis nor increased dietary protein intake changed plasma 1,25-$(OH)_2$-D concentrations. Furthermore, Chesney, DeLuca, and associates showed that plasma 1,25-$(OH)_2$-D levels are not low among patients with renal tubular acidosis.

Hypercalciuria and, occasionally, hypercalcemia as a consequence of augmented intestinal Ca absorption, the classical expression of vitamin D action, had long been known to occur among patients with sarcoidosis, and in 1979 elevated plasma 1,25-$(OH)_2$-D levels in sarcoidosis were first observed as an explanation for disordered calcium metabolism. Moreover, it was observed that sun exposure to increase cutaneous vitamin D_3 production or the administration of 25-OH-D_3 raised plasma 1,25-$(OH)_2$-D_3 levels, an effect not detectable in healthy subjects. In 1981, Barbour, Slatopolsky, Coburn, and associates reported an anephric dialysis patient with hypercalcemia due to sarcoidosis who, unexpectedly, exhibited an elevated plasma 1,25-$(OH)_2$-D_3 level. This observation provided the first evidence in humans for extrarenal 1,25-$(OH)_2$-D production and rapidly led to the recognition that monocytes/macrophages may produce 1,25-$(OH)_2$-D_3. The St. Louis group, which subsequently demonstrated that the administration of 25-OH-D_3 to anephric patients was accompanied by a rise in plasma 1,25-$(OH)_2$-D_3 levels, more recently demonstrated that blood monocytes from dialysis patients exhibited an increased capacity to convert 25-OH-D_3 to 1,25-$(OH)_2$-D_3 in comparison to monocytes from normal subjects. These studies suggested that extrarenal 1,25-$(OH)_2$-D_3 synthesis is related to availability of precursor 25-OH-D_3. Speculatively, this increased capacity for extrarenal 1,25-$(OH)_2$-D_3 synthesis in uremia may account for earlier clinical observations showing that 25-OH-D_3 treatment of patients with chronic renal failure was capable of increasing intestinal Ca absorption and improving osteitis fibrosa (see Renal Osteodystrophy). Other studies have shown that cultured bone cells and keratinocytes are also capable of producing 1,25-$(OH)_2$-D_3, which may serve an autocrine or paracrine function.

Studies by many investigators during the late 1970s and 1980s that continue have provided evidence that the mechanism of action of 1,25-$(OH)_2$-D_3, a secosteroid, is initially effected by binding of 1,25-$(OH)_2$-D_3 to a specific cytosolic receptor protein. This receptor protein is now recognized as a member of the super family of steroid receptors that also bind glucocorticoids, estrogens, progesterone, and thyroxine. Following 1,25-$(OH)_2$-D_3 receptor binding, the receptor hormone complex is translocated to the nucleus, where it signals transcription and synthesis of new proteins, including at least the classical Ca binding proteins (CaBP) that have been found to be present in intestine, distal renal tubule, and brain. This process is termed the genomic effect of 1,25-$(OH)_2$-D_3. Expression of 1,25-$(OH)_2$-D_3 receptors appears to be directly regulated by the hormone. Apparent receptor numbers (Nmax) are high in parathyroid glands of patients with primary hyperparathyroidism and elevated plasma 1,25-$(OH)_2$-D and reduced in parathyroid glands of patients with chronic renal failure. The rapidity of onset of effects of 1,25-$(OH)_2$-D in several tissues, in time periods less than those required for new protein synthesis, provided evidence that 1,25-$(OH)_2$-D_3 might act on tissues in additional ways to change cell structure and function. Hruska, Kurnick, and associates provided evidence in a series of studies that exposure of cell membranes to 1,25-$(OH)_2$-D_3 rapidly alters their phospholipid structure and could account for the rise in intracellular Ca concentrations and in PO_4 uptake observed within a few minutes after exposure to 1,25-$(OH)_2$-D_3. This process has been termed the liponomic effect of 1,25-$(OH)_2$-D_3.

The effects of 1,25-$(OH)_2$-D_3 on a range of tissues in healthy individuals and in patients with kidney disease continue to be explored in vivo and in vitro. In the mid-1970s when 1,25-$(OH)_2$-D_3 first became available in sufficient quantities for clinical trials, Brickman, Coburn, and associates demonstrated the effect of the hormone in a dose-dependent manner to restore intestinal Ca absorption to normal among patients with chronic renal failure. Studies by Lee and associates and by Favus and associates have explored the effects of 1,25-$(OH)_2$-D_3 to alter Ca transport along the intestine. Following studies showing that 1,25-$(OH)_2$-D_3 stimulates resorption of bone in organ culture, the St. Louis group demonstrated specific uptake of 1,25-$(OH)_2$-D_3 by bone perfused in vitro. Metabolic balance studies by Maierhofer and associates among men eating low Ca diets also showed that the administration of 1,25-$(OH)_2$-D_3 caused net bone resorption, as evidenced by more negative Ca balances and increased urinary hydroxyproline excretion. Studies by other investigators have now demonstrated that osteoclasts possess receptors for 1,25-$(OH)_2$-D_3. Many clinical studies of the effects of 1,25-$(OH)_2$-D_3 in patients with chronic renal failure demonstrated reductions in serum immunoreactive PTH concentrations. Whether these decrements were mediated by an increase in serum ionized Ca concentrations, and thus the well-established effect of Ca to inhibit PTH secretion, or were a direct effect of 1,25-$(OH)_2$-D_3 on the parathyroid glands remained controversial until the mid-1980s. Following determination of the structure of PTH and isolation of its gene, Silver and associates in 1985 reported that 1,25-$(OH)_2$-D_3 directly inhibited pre-pro-PTH gene transcription. The effects of 1,25-$(OH)_2$-D_3 on the kidney have not yet been fully clarified. Bordeau and associates and Kumar and associates have provided evidence that vitamin D-dependent Ca-binding protein is present in the distal convoluted tubule and cortical collecting tubule, suggesting that 1,25-$(OH)_2$-D_3 may have an effect in these tubular segments where Ca^{++}-Mg^{++}-ATPase is also localized and where Ca transport is known to occur. Puschett and associates provided evidence that 1,25-$(OH)_2$-D_3 increased Ca delivery to the distal tubule in volume-expanded parathyroidectomized (PTX) dogs, but urinary Ca excretion increased only in the presence of antidiuretic hormone. Sutton, Dirks, and associates provided evidence by micropuncture studies in PTX dogs that 25-OH-D_3 reduced urinary Ca excretion by enhancing Ca reabsorption in the distal nephron. Although it is well known that 1,25-$(OH)_2$-D_3 administration to healthy adults and patients with chronic kidney disease not yet on dialysis increases urinary Ca excretion, the direct effects and mechanisms of action of 1,25-$(OH)_2$-D_3 on the kidney require further study.

Other studies have provided evidence for the presence of 1,25-$(OH)_2$-D_3 receptors in monocytes and macrophages as well as activated lymphocytes and have shown that the hormone enhanced cell maturation and differentiation. The potential clinical relevance of these effects continue to be studied.

Goldstein, Massry, and associates observed that plasma concentrations of 25-OH-D_3 were reduced among patients with the nephrotic syndrome, raising the possibility that vitamin D deficiency and consequent bone disease might develop. Studies by other investigators demonstrated that plasma 25-OH-D_3 concentrations were reduced among nephrotic patients because of a loss of vitamin D binding protein into the urine together with 25-OH-D_3. However, 1,25-$(OH)_2$-D_3 concentrations were found to be normal. Moreover, studies by the St. Louis group using bone biopsies showed no evidence of osteomalacia among patients with the nephrotic syndrome, despite reduced plasma 25-OH-D_3 concentrations. More recently, Freundlich, Hollis, Bourgoignie, and associates demonstrated that the kidneys from rats with experimental nephrosis retain the capacity to produce 1,25-$(OH)_2$-D_3 at normal rates.

The results of many studies documenting the effective therapeutic use of 1,25-$(OH)_2$-D_3 in the treatment and prevention of secondary hyperparathyroidism and osteitis fibrosa in chronic renal failure are considered under Renal Osteodystrophy. Also evaluated are the new analogues of 1,25-$(OH)_2$-D_3 that suppress PTH gene transcription but are less effective than 1,25-$(OH)_2$-D_3 in activating Ca transport.

Several additional invited lectures devoted to vitamin D have been presented: 1975–Vitamin D and the Kidney (DeLuca); 1986–Vitamin D Metabolism in Health and Disease (Bell); 1987–Effects of Calcitriol (1,25-$(OH)_2$-D_3) on the Synthesis and Secretion of Parathyroid Hormone (Sherwood); 1988–Use of 1,25-Dihydroxyvitamin D_3 in Early Chronic Renal Failure (Massry); and 1990–Vitamin D in Renal Failure (Slatopolsky).

Historical Background

Accurate chemical methods to measure Ca in biological samples were developed during the early decades of the 20th century. These techniques permitted measurement of Ca in blood (serum, plasma), urine, feces, and foods. Fuller Albright, the pioneer of modern endocrinology, together with his many associates, refined and applied the balance technique, especially to the quantitation of Ca and PO_4 metabolism in health and disease. Healthy subjects fed constant diets providing normal quantities of Ca (15 to 25 mmol Ca/day) were shown to be in approximately zero Ca balance, with urinary Ca excretion approximately equaling net intestinal Ca absorption (e.g., dietary Ca intake minus fecal Ca excretion). These and subsequent studies showed that normal daily rates of urinary Ca excretion among healthy adults average about 4 mmol/day, ranging up to 6.25 mmol/day in women, 7.5 mmol/day in men, and <0.1 mmol/kg/day regardless of sex or age. Balance studies demonstrated the following: the limited range of variation of daily urinary Ca excretion in response to extreme variations in dietary Ca intake, the effects of metabolic acidosis to increase urinary Ca excretion, and the increases in urinary Ca excretion generally accompanying diseases associated with hypercalcemia. Lichtwitz and his associates in France documented the decline in urinary Ca excretion occurring with early renal failure, now recognized as the consequence of the action of PTH to augment tubular reabsorption of filtered calcium. In addition, normal rates of urinary Ca excretion despite hypocalcemia were observed among patients with hypoparathyroidism, which provided an early clue that PTH acts to stimulate renal tubular Ca reabsorption. In the 1930s, Richards, Bott, Smith, and Shannon first developed techniques to accurately measure GFR using inulin. During the same era, McLean and Hastings developed a technique to measure blood-ionized Ca concentrations that subsequently led to understanding that of the total Ca concentration in plasma, averaging about 2.40 mmol/L in health about 60% is diffusible or ultrafilterable (1.44 mmol/L); 50% is ionized (1.2 mmol/L); 10% is ultrafilterable but complexed to citrate, phosphate, bicarbonate, and sulfate (0.24 mmol/L); and the remaining 40% is nondiffusible (0.96 mmol/L), being bound to serum proteins, primarily albumin. With the availability of methods to measure GFR and to prepare plasma ultrafiltrates for measurement of ultrafilterable Ca concentrations, rates of glomerular filtration of Ca could be estimated. Urinary Ca excretion could then be estimated in relation to filtration of Ca during clearance experiments and factors potentially affecting Ca clearance assessed. Among healthy adults, approximately 2.5% of filtered Ca was found to be excreted into the urine. Using these techniques, Walser first demonstrated that Ca clearance increased in proportion to Na clearance during NaCl infusion and that infusion of Na_2SO_4 caused an even greater rise in Ca clearance at any given rate of Na clearance, presumably because of Ca-SO_4 complex formation within tubular fluid. Using clearance studies combined with the "stop-flow" technique devised by Malvin and Wilde, Widrow and Levinsky demonstrated that parathyroid hormone stimulates renal tubular Ca reabsorption in the distal nephron. Dietary PO_4 deprivation was also known to increase urinary Ca excretion, whereas the administration of PO_4 diminished Ca excretion. Clearance studies also demonstrated that metabolic acidosis reduced renal tubular Ca reabsorption, an effect that was independent of PTH.

Subsequent studies have permitted evaluation of the sites and mechanisms for renal tubular Ca reabsorption along the nephron and their regulation.

Major technological advances have made such studies possible, including the renaissance of nephron micropuncture and microperfusion, the development of in vitro perfusion of microdissected specific nephron segments, bulk isolation of nephron segments, preparation of brush border and basolateral membrane vesicles and culture of cells from specific nephron segments together with analytical techniques to quantitate Ca in minute samples by electron microprobe, helium glow photometry or Ca-sensitive microelectrodes, and to estimate intracellular Ca concentrations using fluorescent complexing agents. Physiological studies of urinary Ca excretion and of Ca balance in humans as well as physiology studies of Ca transport in bone have also continued.

Work Presented at the ASN

Micropuncture studies, especially by Goldberg, Agus, and associates and by Dirks, Sutton, Quamme, Wong, and associates, have provided an overview of Ca filtration and segmental Ca reabsorption along the nephron. The Ca concentration in glomerular filtrate was found to be comparable to Ca concentrations measured in plasma ultrafiltrates prepared in vitro. Approximately 70% of filtered Ca was observed to be reabsorbed in the proximal tubule, about 15% in the ascending limb of Henle's loop, about 10% in the distal convolution and connecting tubule, and a final 2 to 3% in collecting ducts, leaving 2 to 3% in the final urine. Proximal reabsorption has been found to be largely passive based on parallel Ca, Na, and water reabsorption and the large Ca backflux in this "leaky" epithelium. In addition, the development of luminal Ca concentrations slightly above those of plasma ultrafilterable Ca and the development of a lumen-positive voltage along the proximal convolution establish an electrochemical gradient favoring passive Ca reabsorption. Bomsztyk and Wright have also provided evidence for active Ca transport in the proximal tubule. Ca reabsorption in the early proximal straight tubule (S_2) also appears to be passive, whereas that in S_3 is active. Studies by Suki and associates as well as by other investigators have shown that the thin descending and ascending limbs of Henle's loop are relatively impermeable to Ca. The considerable Ca reabsorption in the thick ascending limb of Henle's loop appears to reflect both passive and active transport. Using perfused medullary thick ascending loop of Henle (TALH), Suki, Rouse, Kokko, and associates concluded that Ca reabsorption in this segment is passive, being accounted for by the lumen-positive voltage. In perfused cortical TALH segments, Bourdeau and Burg and Shareghi and associates also concluded that Ca reabsorption was similarly passive, whereas Suki and associates, as well as others, have obtained evidence for additional active transport. Free-flow micropuncture and microperfusion studies by Costanzo and Windhager demonstrated active Ca reabsorption in the distal convolution and connecting tubule. Calcium was shown to be absorbed as ionic Ca. Because Ca remaining in the nephron at the end of the accessible distal convoluted tubule (DCT) is greater than that appearing in the final urine, Ca reabsorption must occur in the terminal nephron. Rochelle and associates recently demonstrated active luminal-to-basolateral Ca transport in primary cultures of rabbit cortical collecting duct cells, a process that was significantly stimulated by cAMP. Using retrograde microcatheterization, Bengele, Alexander, and Lechene observed Ca reabsorption in the medullary collecting duct.

Micropuncture and tubular perfusion have also been used to examine factors regulating segmental Ca transport along the nephron. Hypercalcemia has been shown to inhibit Ca reabsorption in the PCT, TALH, and DCT. Edwards, Sutton, and Dirks demonstrated that the effect of hypercalcemia to suppress Ca absorption in the DCT reflects suppression of PTH. Dietary PO_4 deprivation is accompanied by hypercalciuria, whereas PO_4 administration reduces Ca excretion. Quamme, Wong, Sutton, and Dirks have observed that the hypercalciuria of PO_4 deprivation is partially corrected by PTH, apparently by increasing Ca absorption in the TALH. Additionally, these investigators, as well as Lau and associates, have found that PO_4 administration to previously PO_4-deprived animals augments tubular Ca reabsorption beyond the DCT, presumably in the collecting ducts.

The critical role of PTH tubular Ca in augmenting reabsorption and thus maintaining normal serum Ca concentrations in health has been extensively studied. In 1971, Agus, Gardner, and Goldberg showed that PTH augments distal tubular Ca reabsorption. Subsequent studies from that laboratory as well as the laboratories of Dirks, of Costanzo, of Suki, and of Bourdeau have shown that PTH stimulates Ca reabsorption in the connecting tubule segment of the DCT as well as in the cortical TALH, an effect mediated by cAMP and consistent with the presence of PTH-sensitive adenylate cyclase in these tubular segments. Although PTH-activated adenylate cyclase is also present in the proximal convoluted and straight tubules, the effect of PTH on Ca reabsorption in these sites remains controversial.

The cellular mechanisms for PTH effects on Ca transport have been explored. In addition to activation of adenylate cyclase, the roles of intracellular Ca concentrations and the inositol phosphates as second messengers have been studied. Hruska observed that PTH rapidly increases proximal tubular cell Ca concentrations ($[Ca_i]$). Lau and Bourdeau also observed that PTH increases $[Ca_i]$ in connecting tubules, accompanying activation of Ca absorption. Hruska and associates observed that PTH activates Ca/Na exchange in renal cortical basolateral membrane vesicles (BLMV), and Sacktor and associates showed that PTH stimulates ^{45}Ca efflux from proximal tubular cells, also via Ca/Na exchange. Suki and associates showed that the absence of PTH results in inhibition of cortical cell BLMV high-affinity Ca-ATPase. More recently, Bourdeau and Eby have provided evidence that the activity of the basolateral cell membrane Ca/Na antiporter in connecting tubule cells is modulated by cAMP-dependent phosphorylation, presumably reflecting a sequence in the action of PTH to stimulate Ca reabsorption at this tubular site.

Vitamin D-dependent Ca-binding protein (CaBP) has been localized to the distal convoluted tubule and cortical collecting duct. The effects of 1,25-$(OH)_2$-D_3 to stimulate Ca reabsorption have remained controversial. In 1990, Bindels, Hartog, and van Os reported that exposure of primary cultures of rabbit connecting tubule cells to 1,25-$(OH)_2$-D_3 for 48 hours significantly increased transcellular Ca absorption. Kumar and associates have immunohistologically colocalized the Ca^{++}-Mg^{++}-ATPase present in red blood cell (RBC) to the DCT. Tsukamoto and Sactor have observed a Mg-independent Ca^{++}-ATPase in cortical BLMV that is stimulated by 1,25-$(OH)_2$-D_3. Recently, Sugimura, Abramowitz, and Suki reported partial purification of this Ca^{++}-ATPase and have shown that its functional properties differ from the RBC Ca^{++}-Mg^{++}-ATPase.

The augmentation of urinary Ca excretion caused by metabolic acidosis has been a subject of continuing study. Clearance and micropuncture experiments by several groups demonstrated that the administration of HCO_3^- to acidotic animals reduces urinary Ca excretion by increasing distal tubular Ca reabsorption. Sutton and associates and Kurtzman, Battle, and Arruda showed that the effect of acidosis to increase urinary Ca excretion was independent of PTH. Distal tubular microperfusion experiments by Miyakawa and Bomsztyk demonstrated that stimulation of distal tubular HCO_3^- absorption, but not the luminal HCO_3^- concentration, is accompanied by stimulation of distal Ca absorption. Sabatini and Kurtzman have used the turtle bladder as a model of the mammalian distal tubule and have demonstrated that serosal (basolateral) acidification inhibits mucosal to serosal Ca flux, and serosal alkalinization stimulates mucosal to serosal Ca flux. Earlier balance studies had demonstrated that the increase in urinary Ca excretion occurring during metabolic acidosis is derived from bone because significant augmentation of intestinal Ca absorption was not observed. Bushinsky and associates, using fetal rat bone in organ culture, demonstrated that acidosis produced by reducing the bicarbonate concentration of the medium (metabolic acidosis) stimulates Ca efflux from bone as well as loss of surface Na and K. Since earlier studies had shown that respiratory acidosis had little effect to increase urinary Ca excretion, the effects of respiratory acidosis on bone have also been evaluated. Bushinsky showed that acidification of the culture medium achieved by raising the pCO_2 (respiratory acidosis) does not alter surface Na and K in bone nor increase Ca efflux. Burnell, Madias, and associates also found that chronic respiratory acidosis in dogs increased the density and the percent of mineral/g bone, providing further direct evidence that chronic respiratory acidosis, unlike metabolic acidosis, does not stimulate bone resorption.

The effects of diuretics to modulate tubular Ca absorption have also been studied. Furosemide, bumetanide, and mercurial diuretics were known to increase urinary Ca excretion in humans. Quamme and associates demonstrated that furosemide inhibits Ca absorption in the TALH. The thiazide diuretics were known to reduce urinary Ca excretion. Costanzo and associates confirmed the effect of hydrochlorothiazide to augment net tubular reabsorption of filtered Ca in clearance studies and subsequently showed that luminal chlorothiazide enhanced Ca reabsorption in the early DCT. Brunette and colleagues observed that hydrochlorothiazide enhanced Ca uptake into distal tubular luminal vesicles, an effect that required Na and was inhibited by SO_4. Subsequently, Costanzo showed that amiloride enhanced Ca absorption in more distal DCT segments.

The administration of glucose has been found to be calciuric (as well as magnesuric). Clearance studies provided evidence that this effect is a consequence of inhibition of net tubular Ca reabsorption. Subsequent studies by DeFronzo and associates provided evidence that the effect of glucose to increase Ca excretion is probably mediated by insulin by inhibition of Ca reabsorption in the distal tubule. The detailed mechanisms have not yet been clarified. Diabetes is also known to be accompanied by increased urinary Ca excretion. Guruprakash, Rouse, and Suki observed impaired ^{45}Ca reabsorption in the loop of Henle and in the terminal nephron in diabetic rats based on increased recovery in urine of ^{45}Ca microinjected into serial sites along the nephron.

The administration of potassium chloride (KCl) or potassium bicarbinate ($KHCO_3$) to healthy adults by Lemann and associates was found to reduce daily and fasting urinary Ca excretion, whereas dietary K deprivation had an opposite effect. Recently, Brunette and associates showed that K enhanced Ca uptake into distal tubule luminal vesicles but not in proximal tubule luminal vesicles.

Ongoing studies of Ca transport across specific nephron segments and in specific cell types of these segments in tissue culture together with studies to characterize enzymes and ion channels should ultimately provide a detailed description of how tubular reabsorption of 98% of the Ca filtered across the glomeruli is accomplished.

At the 1971 meeting, Reiss, Kleeman, Kaye, and Coe presented a symposium devoted to Ca metabolism and the kidney. At the 1978 meeting, Lemann presented a review of urinary Ca excretion in humans and its regulation.

Urolithiasis

Historical Background

The ancient writings of Hippocrates and Hindu physicians first described urinary tract stones, especially bladder stones, and lithotomy for bladder stones was among the first surgical procedures to be devised. As knowledge of chemistry developed during the 19th century, the composition of urinary stones was determined. The amino acid cystine was first found in a bladder stone (from Greek: *kystis* = bladder), and cystinuria was among the first recognized genetic diseases described as inborn errors of metabolism by Garrod in the early years of the 20th century. The application of optical and x-ray defraction crystallography to the analysis of a large number of stones by Prien and Frondel during the 1930s demonstrated that in the modern era most urinary stones are composed of calcium oxalate mono- and dihydrates (whewellite and weddelite), alone or more often together with hydroxyapatite or carbonate apatite. Less frequently, stones are composed of uric acid, of cystine, or of magnesium ammonium phosphate hexahydrate (struvite), always together with apatite (hence the term "triple phosphates") that may form when the urinary tract is chronically infected by urease-producing bacteria. The limited solubility of these salts, of uric acid, and of cystine led to the understanding that increased daily rates of urinary excretion and thus of average prevailing concentrations could lead to increased rates of crystal nucleation and stone formation. It became known that diseases associated with hypercalcemia and thus hypercalciuria, exemplified by primary hyperparathyroidism, were sometimes manifested by nephrolithiasis. During the 1930s, Flocks recognized that hypercalciuria, without hypercalcemia, occurred frequently among patients with kidney stones. In the early 1950s, Albright, Henneman, and associates defined the syndrome of idiopathic hypercalciuria (IH), characterized by the occurrence of calcium stones in the absence of a history of excessive Ca or vitamin D intake, normocalcemia, hypercalciuria as a consequence of increased rates of net intestinal Ca absorption, and mild hypophosphatemia. Primary hyperoxaluria increased rates of cystine excretion in cystinuria and of uric acid excretion in some patients with gout, and increased urinary NH_4^+ concentrations and urine pH as a result of urea hydrolysis with urinary infection became known. The effect of urine pH on the solubility of stone constituents was also recognized: the persistently alkaline urine in distal renal tubular acidosis (RTA) favoring crystallization of brushite ($CaHPO_4 \cdot 2H_2O$) and apatite and persistently acid urine favoring uric acid crystallization. In addition, as a consequence of observations that a significant number of patients with Ca-containing kidney stones had no detectable abnormality in the composition of their urine, studies by Howard and associates provided evidence that the patients' urine lacked a normal inhibitor of crystal growth. Other studies, exemplified by Randall's anatomical observations, suggested that there could be alteration among stone formers in the surface structure of the renal papillae and pelvis that would favor crystal attachment and thus permit time for growth of initially tiny crystals into clinically symptomatic stones. Treatment of existing stones remained limited to endouroscopic removal from the distal ureters and bladder or surgical removal. Therapy to prevent Ca stones included increased fluid intake, dietary Ca restriction, and, as recognized by Yendt and associates, the sustained anticalciuric effects of the thiazide diuretics. Therapy to prevent uric acid stones, included increased fluids, alkali, and allopurinol; for struvite stones, antibacterial drugs and stone removal; for cystinuria, increased fluids, large doses of alkali, and D-penicillamine that was found to undergo a disulfide exchange reaction with cystine to form the more soluble cysteine-penicillamine mixed disulfide.

Work Presented at the ASN

Studies to clarify the pathophysiology of IH have continued. Whether hypercalciuria among Ca stone formers was a consequence of a primary increase in intestinal Ca absorption with excretion of the increased quantities of absorbed Ca into the urine or a renal Ca leak with compensatory augmentation of intestinal Ca absorption and whether resorption of skeletal Ca stores contributed to hypercalciuria remain controversial. In 1974, Pak reviewed significant new studies that provided a pathophysiological classification of the hypercalciurias into three major groups. Calcium stone formers in general were observed to exhibit increased intestinal Ca absorption. Most also had normal fasting serum Ca concentrations and normal rates of fasting urinary Ca excretion, thus defining absorptive hypercalciuria. A few patients exhibited fasting hypercalciuria despite normal or low normal serum Ca concentrations, thus defining renal hypercalciuria. Another small group exhibited fasting hypercalciuria and hypercalcemia defined as resorptive hypercalciuria and exemplified by patients with primary hyperparathyroidism because of the known effects of PTH to stimulate bone resorption. Shortly thereafter, when assays for plasma 1,25-$(OH)_2$-D_3 became available, Pak, Haussler, and associates observed that hypercalciuric stone formers may exhibit elevated plasma 1,25-$(OH)_2$-D concentrations without hypocalcemia or elevated serum PTH concentrations, known stimuli of 1,25-$(OH)_2$-D_3 production. Gray, Lemann, and associates also reported increased plasma 1,25-$(OH)_2$-D levels in Ca stone formers and observed an inverse correlation of plasma 1,25-$(OH)_2$-D levels with serum PO_4 concentrations. Broadus and associates also observed elevated 1,25-$(OH)_2$-D_3 levels in IH and demonstrated increased 1,25-$(OH)_2$-D_3 production using the equilibrium infusion of ^{3}H-1,25-$(OH)_2$-D_3. Although PO_4 is now known to be perhaps the most important determinant of 1,25-$(OH)_2$-D synthesis, the prevalence and mechanisms for mild hypophosphatemia in some patients with hypercalciuria remain controversial and to be clarified. Intestinal Ca absorption became known to be directly correlated to prevailing plasma 1,25-$(OH)_2$-D concentrations, but Pak and associates observed that ^{47}Ca absorption was increased out of proportion to prevailing (although normal and not suppressed) plasma 1,25-$(OH)_2$-D concentrations in patients with absorptive hypercalciuria, an observation confirmed in subsequent Ca balance studies by Lemann, Gray, and associates. Whether this increase in intestinal Ca absorption occurs via augmentation of vitamin D-independent intestinal Ca transport, the now known capacity of 1,25-$(OH)_2$-D_3 to up-regulate its own receptor or other factors augmenting expression and activity of the receptor, remains unknown. Although there has been general agreement that intestinal Ca absorption is increased among hypercalciuric Ca stone formers, controversy continues with regard to the presence of abnormal renal Ca transport. Some investigators have more commonly observed fasting hypercalciuria despite normal serum Ca concentrations. Sutton and colleagues and Lau and associates, using diuretics as pharmacological probes, provided evidence for reduced proximal tubular reabsorption in patients with hypercalciuria. Although high dietary intakes of NaCl and/or of protein (especially animal protein) may exaggerate hypercalciuria, patients with IH generally continue to exhibit increased urinary Ca excretion rates even when dietary NaCl and protein intakes are controlled at normal levels. A review of Ca balance studies in patients with IH as compared with healthy adults by Coe and Favus demonstrated that despite higher than normal rates of intestinal Ca absorption among patients with IH, these patients exhibit even greater rates of urinary Ca excretion, thus causing negative Ca balances. The possibility that IH reflects, therefore, a more generalized abnormality of Ca transport including bone was provided by studies by Sutton, Walker, and associates, demonstrating increased urinary excretion of hydroxyproline in IH, a direct reflection of increased bone resorption, and by histomorphometric studies by Malluche and associates. Bianchi and associates have provided evidence for such a mechanism by a demonstration of a genetically determined increase in the activity of Ca^{++}-Mg^{++}-ATPase in RBC from patients with IH. Several investigative groups have attempted to develop experimental models of IH by selective breeding of rats for hypercalciuria. The hypercalciuric rats bred by Lau and associates demonstrated increased intestinal Ca absorption and elevated serum 1,25-$(OH)_2$-D levels. Following induction of vitamin D deficiency, these animals continued to exhibit increased urinary Ca excretion, providing evidence for an underlying activation of Ca transport. Other hypercalciuric rats bred by Bushinsky, Favus, and Coe exhibited increased intestinal Ca absorption but reduced plasma 1,25-$(OH)_2$-D concentrations, also providing evidence for vitamin D-independent absorption.

The therapy of patients with IH has continued to be studied. Coe, Parks, and associates provided evidence for the benefit of thiazide diuretics to reduce urinary Ca excretion and prevent stone recurrence, an effect confirmed by several subsequent prospective control studies. Micropuncture studies in rats by Costanzo and Windhager showed that chlorothiazide, when present in tubular perfusate, directly enhanced distal tubular Ca reabsorption. Comparable micropuncture studies in dogs by Sutton, Quamme, Wong, and Dirks showed that the effects of chlorothiazide to augment distal tubular Ca reabsorption are independent of PTH. Maierhofer, Lemann, and Gray showed that hydrochlorothiazide given to healthy men not only reduces urinary Ca excretion despite experimentally elevated serum 1,25-$(OH)_2$-D concentrations but also causes Ca balance to become more positive and reduces urinary hydroxyproline excretion, leading to the interpretation that the thiazides also inhibit bone resorption. Balance studies in patients with IH by Coe, Favus, and associates similarly documented that thiazides cause Ca balances to become more positive without affecting plasma 1,25-$(OH)_2$-D concentrations. Other diuretics, including indapamide, metolazone, and amiloride, were also shown to reduce urinary Ca excretion.

Among children, an association of hypercalciuria with initially detected hematuria was observed. Stapleton and the Southwestern Pediatric Nephrology Study Group reported in 1987 that 36% of 215 children and adolescents with unexplained hematuria exhibited urinary Ca excretion rates $>$0.1 mmol/kg/day. In these and other patients followed for 1 to 4 years, 8 of 60 with hypercalciuria formed stones, while only 2 of 125 without hypercalciuria formed stones.

L. H. Smith and associates reported that the capacity of urine to inhibit apatite crystal growth could be attributed to urinary magnesium (Mg), pyrophosphate, and citrate. Studies by Oh and associates and by Pak and associates demonstrated that urinary citrate excretion is reduced in some Ca stone formers, citrate being capable of forming soluble Ca complexes and thereby inhibiting Ca salt crystallization. Coe and associates observed that urinary citrate excretions are higher among women than among men, which may contribute to the lower frequency of kidney stones in women (M:F incidence of Ca stones is approximately 3:1). Subsequent studies by Pak and associates have provided evidence that Na-citrate or K-citrate administration augments urinary citrate excretion, an effect mediated primarily by the alkalinizing effects of the metabolism of citrate to bicarbonate and that K-citrate reduces the recurrence of Ca stones. The additional benefit of K appears to be related to observations by Jaeger and associates indicating that in rats, K administration augments distal tubular PO_4 reabsorption. Subsequent observations by Portale and associates showed that KCl or $KHCO_3$ administration subtly raises plasma PO_4 levels in men that are accompanied by small reductions in plasma 1,25-$(OH)_2$-D concentrations. Lemann and associates recently confirmed these relationships during studies of K-loading and K-deprivation in healthy adults.

Because of continuing observations that many Ca stone formers exhibit no currently detectable abnormality in their urine composition that would favor Ca salt crystallization, there has been renewed investigative interest in the possibility that the urine of stone formers lacks a normal inhibitor of crystal growth or that the functional activity of such an inhibitor might be abnormally low. Coe and his group have presented the results of continuing studies addressing this topic. In the mid-1980s, they provided evidence that the urine of normal subjects contains a protein, named nephrocalcin, that inhibits Ca-oxalate crystal growth. The protein was shown to be glycosylated and to contain γ-carboxyglutamic acid (Gla), the two adjacent carboxyl groups conferring Ca-binding properties. Nephrocalcin isolated from the urine of stone formers was shown to have a reduced capacity to inhibit Ca-oxalate crystal growth and to be deficient in Gla. Subsequent studies demonstrated that the protein is also phosphorylated (serine-PO_4, threonine-PO_4, phosphorylated carbohydrate), which contributes to inhibition of crystal growth.

Nephrocalcin has also been found to inhibit secondary Ca-oxalate crystal nucleation. Antibodies to nephrocalcin have been prepared, and immunohistochemical studies currently suggest production in the proximal tubule and thick ascending loop of Henle. Physiological studies by Coe and associates demonstrated increased urinary excretion of nephrocalcin during pregnancy, which is thought to counterbalance the hypercalciuria of pregnancy. Nephrocalcin has not yet been isolated, sequenced, and cloned. This information is needed to assess normal function and potential abnormalities of structure and function in patients with urolithiasis. Coe and associates have also presented evidence that Tammm-Horsfall protein isolated from stone formers has abnormal physical properties and is defective with respect to its capacity to inhibit Ca-oxalate crystal aggregation. Most recently, studies by Hoyer and by Worcester have documented that osteopontin, a protein first detected in and cloned from bone, is produced in the kidney, is present in urine, and is a powerful inhibitor of Ca-oxalate crystal growth. These continuing studies have initiated a new era in the study of nephrolithiasis. At the 1989 ASN meeting, Coe used published micropuncture data regarding the composition of tubular fluid along the nephron to estimate the relative degree of saturation of tubular fluid with respect to potentially insoluble Ca salts. The results indicated that such supersaturation exists at several sites, thus providing further indirect evidence for the potential importance of urinary proteins to normally inhibit crystal growth and crystal aggregation.

Interest also has been renewed in the problem of crystal attachment to urothelial surfaces as a factor in the pathogenesis of stones. Riese, Mandel, Kleinman, Woessner, and associates have recently demonstrated saturable and inhibitable attachment of Ca-oxalate crystals to rat papillary collecting duct cells in primary culture. The mechanisms for crystal-cell surface interaction and the potential for there being abnormal papillary and pelvic surfaces among stone formers remain to be clarified.

Efforts to improve the still difficult care of patients with cystinuria have continued. Dietary NaCl restriction has been observed to modestly reduce cystine excretion rates. Pak and associates introduced α-mercaptopropionylglycine into clinical use in the United States. This compound is another sulfhydryl (SH)-containing drug that is capable of reducing cystine excretion by forming a more soluble mixed disulfide. During the initial studies, this drug was associated with fewer side effects compared to D-penicillamine. More recently, the angiotensin converting enzyme inhibitor captopril, which also contains an SH group, has also been found to reduce cystine excretion rates in cystinurics.

Although virtually all studies of newer surgical techniques for stones have appeared in the urological literature, they require brief mention because of their great clinical importance. Extracorporeal shock wave lithotripsy (ESWL) was introduced into clinical use during the 1980s and has rapidly become a highly effective primary form of treatment for existing kidney stones. Because the mechanism of the effects and the consequences of shock waves on tissues are not yet fully known, studies of the effects of ESWL on the kidney continue. Nephrostolithotomy has also been developed for difficult large stones.

Future studies will evidently be directed toward further understanding of the alterations in Ca transport in IH, the role of inhibitors of crystal growth and crystal aggregation, and mechanisms for crystal adhesion to urothelial surfaces. Ultimately, such new knowledge of the probable genetic bases for urolithiasis will allow identification of individuals who are at risk for stones and in need of primary prevention.

Phosphate

Historical Background

The processes that maintain and regulate the concentrations of plasma phosphorus are multiple and complex. There are large stores of phosphorus in bone, and the exchange of phosphorus between the skeleton and the extracellular fluid (ECF) plays a major role in determining the plasma concentration of phosphorus. About 90% of phosphorus is lost from the blood into the glomerular filtrate, with the majority of the filtered load being reabsorbed, primarily in the proximal tubule. Therefore, alterations in glomerular filtration or tubular reabsorption of phosphorus affect its plasma level. Reduced dietary intake of phosphorus and/or a defect in its intestinal absorption can be followed by hypophosphatemia and can ultimately lead to phosphate depletion. The handling of phosphorus by the kidney is affected by multiple hormonal and nonhormonal factors. Greenwald and Gross reported in 1911 that "parathyroid deficiency" is associated with a decrease in urinary phosphorus excretion. Munson demonstrated in 1955 that pure parathyroid hormone (PTH) has a direct phosphaturic effect. Hyatt and Thompson observed in 1957 that the intravenous infusion of calcium is accompanied by a reduction in urinary phosphorus excretion. This effect was attributed to the suppression of PTH secretion because of hypercalcemia. This phenomenon formed the basis of a test devised by Howard for primary hyperparathyroidism.

The mechanisms of action of PTH on tubular reabsorption of phosphorus were first explored by Chase and Aurbach in 1967 in studies demonstrating that PTH stimulates a renal adenylate cyclase-cyclic AMP system that mediates the phosphaturic effect of PTH. Other hormones have been found to affect renal handling of phosphorus as well. Calcitonin, thyroid hormone, and glucocorticoids have been observed to be phosphaturic, while growth hormone and its mediator somatomedin C (IGF-1) decrease urinary phosphorus excretion.

In 1928, Schmitt and White first reported micropuncture techniques for the evaluation of the renal handling of phosphorus. These investigators measured the phosphorus concentration in glomerular filtrate of Necturus. In 1933, Walker made similar measurements in frogs as well as in Necturus. Those studies demonstrated that the phosphorus content of glomerular filtrate is 94% of that in plasma in Necturus and 100% of that in plasma in the frog. In 1964, Carone and Strickler and associates used micropuncture techniques for the study of the renal handling of phosphorus in mammals. Subsequently, Frick and associates in 1967 used the micropuncture technique to show that extracellular volume expansion in rats is associated with inhibition of phosphorus reabsorption in the proximal tubule. The tubular reabsorption of phosphorus has a maximum (Tm); however, this Tm is not fixed but, rather, varies in different clinical and experimental conditions.

Clinical disorders associated with chronically elevated plasma PTH concentrations are associated with phosphaturia. Indeed, the fractional excretion of phosphorus is increased in patients with primary hyperparathyroidism and in those with chronic renal failure who almost always exhibit secondary hyperparathyroidism. Several indices of urinary phosphorus excretion have been proposed to evaluate derangements in the renal handling of phosphorus in disease. The best index, developed by Bijvoet, is the measurement of maximum tubular reabsorption of phosphate per unit/GFR (TmP/GFR).

In 1969, Lotz, Zisman, and Bartter drew attention to the clinical syndrome of phosphate depletion secondary to the long-term administration of phosphate-binding antacids that render phosphate nonabsorbable by the intestine. Patients with phosphate depletion displayed weakness, anorexia, malaise, bone pain, and negative calcium balances caused by marked increments in urinary calcium excretion. Subsequently, hypercalciuria was also observed during experimental phosphate depletion in rats, dogs, and sheep.

Work Presented at the ASN

At the second meeting of the ASN in 1968, Massry, Coburn, and Kleeman provided evidence, using clearance methodology, that extracellular volume expansion in dogs suppresses tubular reabsorption of phosphorus and decreases TmP/GFR. They observed that phosphaturia occurs during volume expansion despite marked reduction in filtered phosphorus and that a close and direct relationship exists between the renal clearance of phosphorus and the clearance of sodium. Their data showed that the decrease in TmP is due to volume expansion itself as well as to stimulation of parathyroid hormone secretion as a consequence of the fall in plasma calcium concentration during volume expansion. The magnitude of the phosphaturia in TPTX dogs was observed to be smaller than that observed in intact dogs. These observations were independently and simultaneously confirmed by Suki and associates and subsequently by others. The Philadelphia group led by Goldberg, Agus, and associates used micropuncture techniques to demonstrate that extracellular volume expansion selectively inhibits phosphorus reabsorption in the proximal tubule of the dog and reduces TmP in this segment of the nephron.

The mechanisms for the inhibition of phosphorus reabsorption by volume expansion are not fully understood but are most likely linked to those affecting the tubular reabsorption of sodium. These may include, but are not limited to, renal vasodilation, diminished filtration fraction with lower tubular hydrostatic pressure, and, possibly, the secretion of natriuretic hormones. Many excellent studies exploring the renal handling of phosphorus and the effect of PTH to inhibit phosphorus reabsorption have been presented at ASN meetings. Goldberg and associates and Knox, Dousa, and associates have contributed important studies. Emerging from these studies has been the concept that phosphate reabsorption includes the following events along the nephron: (*1*) phosphorus is reabsorbed in the proximal tubule, the pars recta, the loop of Henle, and the terminal nephron; (*2*) there is heterogeneity in phosphorus reabsorption in superficial nephrons as compared to deep nephrons; (*3*) extracellular volume expansion inhibits reabsorption of phosphorus in the proximal tubule only; (*4*) PTH inhibits both proximal and distal reabsorption of phosphate, and the hormone reduces TmP in these two segments of the nephron, both of which possess a PTH-sensitive adenylate cyclase-cAMP system; (*5*) alkalinization of the urine during the administration of bicarbonate or during the administration of acetazolamide is associated with phosphaturia.

Dietary phosphate restriction is rapidly followed by avid renal conservation and disappearance of phosphorus from the urine as a consequence of enhanced tubular reabsorption of phosphate. This phenomenon is due to intrinsic changes in the reabsorptive capacity for phosphorus in the proximal tubule and is more pronounced in this segment of superficial nephrons than in that of deep nephrons. This adaptation in phosphate reabsorption has been demonstrated to occur in the brush border membranes of the proximal tubule of both superficial and deep nephrons. Neither PTH nor volume expansion produces phosphaturia in animals previously fed a phosphate-restricted diet, and such animals continue to reabsorb more than 90% of filtered phosphorus during acute elevations in plasma phosphate concentrations and the filtered load of phosphorus.

The mechanisms underlying the adaptive changes in tubular phosphorus reabsorption during phosphate deprivation remain to be clarified. The adaptive augmentation of tubular phosphate reabsorption does not appear to be related to abnormalities in the adenylate cyclase-cAMP system, the protein kinase system, or the renal tubular content of ATP, ADP, AMP, or inorganic phosphorus. A role for alkaline phosphatase present in the brush border membrane in this adaptive process has been proposed, but the increase in phosphorus reabsorption precedes the rise in alkaline phosphatase activity. Dousa and associates have suggested that the suppression of renal gluconeogenesis during dietary phosphate restriction plays a role in the adaptive enhancement of phosphorus transport. During the process of gluconeogenesis,

NAD is generated in the tubular cell cytosol, resulting in a rise in the NAD/NADH ratio. Either NAD, a rising NAD/NADH ratio, or inhibition of the activity of NAD hydrolyzing enzyme reduces renal tubular transport of phosphate. Suppression of renal gluconeogenesis would thus be associated with a fall in NAD and the NAD/NADH ratio, resulting in enhanced renal phosphate reabsorption. Indirect evidence supporting a role for such a sequence of events has been presented, but a cause-and-effect relationship has not been established.

Several studies of the effects of phosphate depletion on renal function as well as on other organs have been presented. These data indicate that (*1*) phosphate depletion is associated with a fall in the cellular concentrations of inorganic phosphorus and adenine nucleotides; (*2*) there is a rise in basal levels of cytosolic calcium in pancreatic islets and brain synaptosomes; (*3*) phosphate depletion is associated with hypophosphaturia, hypercalciuria, hypermagnesuria, hypomagnesemia, reduced Tm bicarbonate and bicarbonaturia, reduced Tm glucose and glucosuria, and increased production of the 1,25-$(OH)_2$-D_3 due to stimulation of the renal 25-OH-D-1a-hydroxylase; (*4*) inhibition of insulin secretion by pancreatic islets and abnormalities in norepinephrine metabolism in brain synaptosomes, the latter abnormalities being due primarily to the reduced ATP content and elevated basal levels of cytosolic calcium in these cells.

Magnesium

In the early 1960s, little was known about the renal handling of magnesium (Mg). At the first meeting of the ASN in 1967, Massry and collaborators presented their work on the renal handling of Mg in normal dogs. They concluded that Mg excretion, like that of Na and Ca, is determined by filtration and reabsorption alone. Subsequently, further evidence was presented from studies in rats indicating that Mg is not secreted with K. It was also shown that in dogs, glomerular-tubular balance exists for Ca and Mg reabsorption in the proximal tubule during an acute rise in GFR. In the late 1970s and early 1980s, several micropuncture studies clearly defined the participation of different segments of the nephron in the regulation of Mg excretion. The laboratories of Dirks, Quamme, Agus, and collaborators presented several studies indicating that the amount of Mg reabsorbed in the proximal tubule was much less than that of Na and Ca. Quamme concluded that the superficial and juxtamedullary proximal straight tubules possess a low Mg permeability and absorb Mg proportionately less than Na and Ca, active Mg secretion probably does not occur, and Mg transport is dependent on luminal Mg concentration. On the other hand, the investigators showed that the thick ascending loop of Henle plays a critical role in the reabsorption of Mg. Agus and collaborators showed that voltage-dependent Mg transport in CTAL is stimulated by PTH and dibutyryl cAMP. Quamme demonstrated that experimental hypermagnesemia causes a marked decrease in Mg reabsorption in the CTAL, with a consequent increase in urinary Mg excretion.

Several investigators demonstrated an association between PO_4 depletion and the renal handling of Mg. Massry and collaborators concluded that PO_4 depletion is associated with hypermagnesuria and hypomagnesemia due to a decreased tubular reabsorption of Mg. Apparently, the skeleton provides most of the magnesium lost into the urine. Subsequently, Lau and collaborators, using micropuncture techniques, characterized the renal transport of magnesium during chronic dietary PO_4 deprivation in rats. They found that the hypermagnesuria was independent of PTH, of plasma Mg concentration, and of Na excretion. Hypermagnesuria during PO_4 deprivation was found to be mediated by impaired transport of Mg in the loop of Henle. There was no appreciable Mg transport beyond the superficial late distal tubule, regardless of dietary PO_4 content. Because PO_4 depletion is also accompanied by hypercalciuria and decreased skeletal content of phosphate, magnesium, and calcium, all of these perturbations may be due to increased levels of 1,25-$(OH)_2$-D_3, which accompany PO_4 depletion.

Studies by Freitag and collaborators demonstrated a state of skeletal resistance to PTH in Mg deficiency in isolated perfused bone. These investigators found a decreased extraction of PTH and diminished cAMP production by bone during Mg depletion. In addition, Slatopolsky and collaborators demonstrated that Mg depletion in rats impairs renal reabsorption of PO_4; this was only partially reversed by parathyroidectomy.

Several investigators, including Sutton, Wong, Dirks, and Quamme, presented studies of the effect of cisplatin and cyclosporin on the renal handling of Mg. They concluded that cisplatin and cyclosporin increased the urinary excretion of Mg, resulting in hypomagnesemia and negative magnesium balance.

More recently, several groups have shown that magnesium citrate and magnesium oxide can decrease the amount of oxalate in the urine, thus providing a beneficial effect in the treatment of recurrent calcium oxalate nephrolithiasis.

3

Clinical Nephrology

Richard J. Glassock, James P. Knochel, and Roscoe R. Robinson

Nephrology was just beginning to consolidate its position as a recently emergent clinical specialty at the time of the American Society of Nephrology's (ASN) first annual meeting in 1967. The general outline of the nature and scope of nephrological clinical practice had begun to take its current form during the 10- or 15-year period prior to the 1967 meeting, in large part stimulated by the advent of percutaneous kidney biopsy and the successful application of dialysis to the management of acute renal failure. Then, shortly before the Society's formative meeting, the most powerful procedural ingredients of modern nephrological therapeutics were defined dramatically by the introduction of chronic dialysis and the growing reality of successful transplantation. It was an exciting time!

These circumstances were reflected clearly amid the program of the 1967 meeting: a state-of-the-art lecture with the formidable and all-encompassing title "Clinical Nephrology" offered quiet testimony to the importance of the emerging specialty as a distinct clinical entity; renal biopsy was used by at least 4 of 10 oral presentations in a single free communication session on "Clinical Nephrology"; descriptive studies of the relationship between underlying renal pathology and various aspects of clinical presentation or cause were commonplace; and "Chronic Dialysis" and "Renal Transplantation" provided the subject matter for two of six symposia. In 1967, any timely discussion of clinical nephrology included a lengthy consideration of dialysis, transplantation, and the application of renal biopsy.

The Changing Domain of Clinical Nephrology

The categorization of submitted abstracts and the organization of the scientific program at the Society's annual meetings have never been easy tasks.

Many submitted abstracts could have been suitably placed in any one of several categories. In any analysis of the Society's meetings, this difficulty is no better illustrated than by the choice or assignment of abstracts or presentations to the category of "Clinical Nephrology." In one sense, most, if not all, abstracts or presentations are theoretically relevant to clinical nephrology. Further, it is equally apparent that many abstracts of high and immediate clinical relevance were included in other categories, such as "Dialysis," "Transplantation," and "Immunology/Pathology." Hence, over the years, the topical assignment of abstracts to sessions entitled "Clinical Nephrology" has tended to be inconsistent, somewhat exclusionary, and always arbitrary. With this in mind, it is therefore important for the reader to understand that the purpose of this chapter is to focus mainly on those aspects of the annual meetings that were organized under the headings "Clinical Nephrology." Such an approach must then acknowledge that many specific diseases or conditions and other important facets of clinical nephrology will be treated more fully elsewhere.

Given the above caveat, what changes are most apparent on review of past sessions and submitted abstracts that were categorized as "Clinical Nephrology"? First, perhaps in deference to the reality of the specialty's clinical base, it is noteworthy that each year's annual meeting has generally included one or more free communication sessions (either oral or poster presentations, or both) under the heading "Clinical Nephrology." More recently, and perhaps reflective of the increasing difficulty in abstract classification, the heading "Clinical Nephrology" has sometimes been reserved mainly for large poster sessions containing a heterogeneous mixture of clinically relevant abstracts that do not fit neatly into other more circumscribed categories. Irrespective of such organizational dilemmas, one of the most immediately noteworthy trends is the dramatic increase in the volume of submitted and presented work. In 1967, the *total* number of submitted abstracts was 287. From that number, 10 were chosen for oral presentation in a single free communication session on "Clinical Nephrology." By way of comparison, in 1990, almost 250 of approximately 1950 submitted abstracts were categorized as "Clinical Nephrology" by their authors, and 151 were selected for oral or poster presentation. But beyond the obvious growth in volume of submitted work, what other trends or changes are portrayed by a review of 25 years of content among submitted abstracts or presentations on "Clinical Nephrology"? What new clinical advances, conditions, therapies, or diagnostic approaches have been described?

Treatment of Renal Parenchymal Disease

Prior to the first meeting of the American Society of Nephrology in 1967, interest in the therapy of renal parenchymal disease was just beginning. Anecdotal reports indicating a possible beneficial effect of glucocorticoids and various immunosuppressive agents had appeared, but randomized, prospective trials were rare. Nevertheless, several uncontrolled studies had generated considerable optimism that antiinflammatory and immunosuppressive agents might be beneficial in certain types of parenchymal renal disease, particularly minimal change disease, membranous glomerulonephritis, and systemic lupus erythematosus (SLE). Nevertheless, only one presentation dealing with the therapy of renal disease was included in the first program. This study described the clinical course and effect of high-dose glucocorticoids on the course of the nephritis of systemic lupus erythematosus in children. Although retrospective and uncontrolled, this study suggested a trend toward prolonged survival among the patients receiving high doses of glucocorticoids compared with those receiving no or low doses of glucocorticoids. The effect of glucocorticoids on the course of lupus nephritis was to become a recurring theme in subsequent meetings.

In 1968, the early results of prolonged therapy of renal parenchymal disease with azathioprine were described. A variety of renal diseases were included in this study, and it was, of course, retrospective and uncontrolled. A complete and partial remission rate of approximately 56% was similar to previously published anecdotal reports and provided additional encouragement for investigators to pursue the possible beneficial effects of this antimetabolite immunosuppressive agent on renal disease. Further retrospective studies of patients with idiopathic nephrotic syndrome suggested that glucocorticoids might have beneficial effects, particularly among patients with mild histological alterations. However, these studies also pointed out the extremely important effect of complete or partial remission of proteinuria, whether therapeutically induced or occurring spontaneously, on the later development of progressive renal insufficiency. Renal failure was extremely uncommon among patients whose protein excretion decreased to less than 2 grams per day. The importance of the quantity of urine protein excreted per day on the ultimate prognosis was repeatedly confirmed in subsequent observations.

In 1969, the growing importance of immunosuppressive agents in the management of parenchymal renal disease was recognized by a special symposium chaired by Dr. Robert Good. Also in 1969, the effects of immunosuppressive agents on a more homogeneous subset of patients with renal parenchymal disease were first described. Although again the study was uncontrolled, this description focused on a subset of glomerulonephritis characterized by persisting decrease in the serum C3 complement component concentration. This phenomenon was later recognized to be strongly associated with membranoproliferative glomerulonephritis. Thus, the program of 1969 signaled the beginning of a segmentation of glomerulonephritis into smaller and more homogeneous subsets that could then be more rationally studied in terms of therapeutic responsiveness.

The 1970 program saw the emergence of cyclophosphamide as a potential therapeutic agent in idiopathic membranous glomerulonephritis. The remarkable improvement in biochemical features,—including increased serum albumin, decreased serum creatinine, and decreased proteinuria—that developed in all treated patients, was greeted with some skepticism. Nevertheless, this study was remarkably prescient, in that it predicted the later results of rigorously controlled randomized trials. In my opinion, this seminal observation received insufficient attention, and had it been quickly followed up by appropriate controlled trials, our approach to the management of membranous glomerulonephritis would have evolved in a drastically different way.

The 1971 meeting was an extremely important one in the field of therapeutics, since the first controlled study of cyclophosphamide in relapsing minimal lesion nephrotic syndrome of childhood was presented. This study clearly demonstrated that a 16-week course of cyclophosphamide plus prednisone in a group of frequently relapsing children with minimal change disease and nephrotic syndrome significantly reduced the likelihood of relapses when compared with a group of patients treated with prednisone alone for a similar duration. These findings were amply confirmed in subsequent studies, which helped to resolve issues concerning a minimum effective dose and optimal duration of treatment with cyclophosphamide. The 1970 program can be regarded as ushering in the modern era of controlled clinical trials of therapy of renal parenchymal disease. Nevertheless, uncontrolled studies of combined immunosuppressive agent–low-dose glucocorticoid therapy of lupus nephritis and the idiopathic nephrotic syndrome continued to appear. These studies continued to suggest a possible beneficial effect of azathioprine, particularly in permitting reduced intensity of glucocorticoid therapy in both lupus nephritis and idiopathic nephrotic syndrome, especially in subsets of patients with proliferative as opposed to basement membrane lesions.

In 1973, the putative beneficial effect of cyclophosphamide on membranous glomerulonephritis was challenged by a randomized prospective study in which 1 year of treatment with cyclophosphamide was compared with no treatment. The lack of any significant differences between these two groups considerably dampened any enthusiasm that might have been generated from earlier observations concerning this mode of therapy. However, the number of patients in the study was small, and cyclophosphamide was not combined with glucocorticoids. In addition, the deleterious effect of cyclophosphamide on gonadal function in males was described. Reduced spermatogenesis and increased plasma levels of follicle-stimulating hormone (FSH) were frequently encountered in male patients receiving cyclophosphamide. No gonadal dysfunction was observed in females treated with this agent. This study, and other similar studies, began to raise significant caution concerning the unrestricted use of cyclophosphamide in the treatment of renal parenchymal disease, particularly in youthful males.

In 1974 the long-term effects of azathioprine in diffuse and focal proliferative glomerulonephritis accompanying systemic lupus erythematosus were described. Although this was a retrospective study, azathioprine therapy was accompanied by few side effects, and patient survival of 84% at 5 years was superior to other retrospective studies in lupus nephritis conducted in the early part of the 1970s. Serial biopsies demonstrated a decrease in subendothelial deposits, unchanged or decreased proliferation, and a tendency for an increase in glomerulosclerosis. This study acted as a stimulus for the wide application of immunosuppressive drugs in the treatment of lupus nephritis.

In 1975, one of the first prospective randomized trials of treatment of lupus nephritis was reported. In this trial, patients with lupus nephritis who had demonstrated deterioration of renal function were randomly allocated into two therapeutic groups. One group received high-dose oral prednisone (30 to 45 mg per day for 6 months), and the other group received oral prednisone in the same dose as before entry to the study (10 to 40 mg per day for 6 months) and cyclophosphamide (50 to 150 mg per day for 6 months). After 6 months of treatment, patients in both arms of the study showed similar improvements in systemic features, creatinine clearance, proteinuria, total serum complement, and anti-DNA antibodies. However, beyond the first 6 months of observations, patients who had received cyclophosphamide demonstrated a significantly lower likelihood of subsequent renal progression. Therefore, the combined treatment approach was favored, largely because of the lower rates of later progression. In addition, the results of a prospective randomized trial of glucocorticoid therapy of adult idiopathic nephrotic syndrome were reported. When alternate-day prednisone was compared with a placebo, patients with minimal change histology who received prednisone demonstrated a significant reduction in proteinuria as compared with the placebo group. Furthermore, patients with membranous histology who received prednisone also had a significant reduction in proteinuria and better maintained glomerular filtration rate as compared with control groups. In all other histological lesions, no differences in proteinuria or renal function were apparent between the treated and placebo groups. These two prospective trials were to be challenged by later observations.

The 1976 meeting saw the introduction of a new form of therapy for glomerulonephritis. A regimen of extensive exchange of endogenous plasma for a plasma protein fraction, combined with cytotoxic drugs and glucocorticoids, was studied in patients with rapidly progressive glomerulonephritis. Patients with antiglomerular basement membrane antibody-mediated nephritis who were not oliguric at the time therapy was begun all showed remarkable improvement of renal function and lung hemorrhage. Circulating antiglomerular basement membrane antibody levels fell promptly, but the degree of reduction showed only a variable relationship to disease activity. The majority of patients with immune complex mediated glomerulonephritis also showed improvement of renal function associated with striking reduction in levels of circulating immune complexes, as measured by a C1q binding assay. These seminal studies sparked a great deal of interest in the possible application of plasma exchange therapy to a wide variety of renal diseases.

In a long-term uncontrolled study, normalization of the total hemolytic complement level by aggressive glucocorticoid and cytotoxic drug therapy of lupus nephritis was associated with a greatly improved prognosis. No similar effect could be observed in patients whose anti-DNA antibody levels normalized but who continued to display hypocomplementemia. Therefore, it was suggested that monitoring of complement levels as a guide to the intensity of therapy in lupus nephritis might yield a better result in terms of reduction in protein excretion and improvement or stabilization of glomerular pathology.

In 1977, a further follow-up of the prospective randomized trial of alternate-day glucocorticoid therapy in adult idiopathic nephrotic syndrome was reported. In minimal change disease, despite the fact that treatment with glucocorticoids was associated with an early reduction in proteinuria, the difference in protein excretion rates between the treatment and placebo groups gradually disappeared with time because of the effect of spontaneous remissions in the placebo group and relapses of proteinuria in the treated group. Similarly, in patients with membranous glomerulonephritis, although there was an early effect of glucocorticoid treatment on proteinuria, subsequent relapses in the treated group resulted in no difference in the number of patients remaining in remission between the treated and placebo groups. Nevertheless, treatment with prednisone was associated with a significantly lower rate of progression to renal failure. This difference could not be explained by any prerandomization characteristics of the two groups. The apparent effect of glucocorticoids on maintaining renal function in patients with membranous glomerulonephritis was to become the focal point of the controversy concerning the utility of glucocorticoid therapy in membranous glomerulonephritis.

In an uncontrolled, nonrandomized study of alternate-day glucocorticoid therapy in membranoproliferative glomerulonephritis (MPGN), better preservation of renal function and improved renal histology were found in the treated group. This long-term study remains as the only study suggesting a beneficial effect of glucocorticoids in membranoproliferative glomerulonephritis. This study was composed of 15 children with type I (subendothelial deposit) MPGN, 11 with type II (intramembranous dense deposits) MPGN, and 10 with type III (subepithelial and subendothelial deposit) MPGN. A case control study, in which a change in the rate of progression of renal disease was assessed by longitudinal studies of the log of the serum creatinine versus time, showed that long-term administration of prednisone and/or cytotoxic drugs to a variety of patients with proteinuria secondary to glomerular disease was beneficial. Approximately 60% of patients were found to have a reduction in the rate of progression of disease coincidental with the administration of the immunosuppressive regimen. Because this was not a controlled or prospective trial, it is not possible to determine whether these changes in renal function were a part of the natural history of the disease or were the result of therapy.

Finally, additional long-term follow-up results were reported concerning a prospective randomized trial of therapy in diffuse proliferative lupus nephritis using prednisone compared with combined prednisone and cyclophosphamide. With a follow-up averaging 4 years, patients in both treatment groups showed similar improvements in clinical features after 6 months of therapy; however, the incidence and rate of further renal progression continued to be significantly lower in those patients treated with combined cyclophosphamide and prednisone.

During the 1978 meeting, the first symposium devoted entirely to the topic of treatment of glomerular disease was held. This symposium described the beneficial effect of intensive plasma exchange in glomerulonephritis, the influence of alternate-day glucocorticoid therapy in idiopathic nephrotic syndrome in adults, and the results of randomized trials of treatment of both membranoproliferative and minimal change lesion nephrotic syndrome in children. This meeting also contained information regarding three new therapeutic approaches to glomerular disease. A controlled trial of platelet inhibitor drugs (dipyridamole) and aspirin in membranoproliferative glomerulonephritis was reported. This treatment improved platelet survival and tended to stabilize renal function in patients with this disorder. A variation on this protocol, which involved long-term therapy of membranoproliferative glomerulonephritis with combinations of warfarin and dipyridamole, was also reported. Using a cross-over design, this combination of agents tended to stabilize renal function; however, bleeding complications were relatively common. Finally, large doses of intravenous methylprednisolone substantially improved the outcome of antiglomerular basement membrane antibody-induced crescentic glomerulonephritis of rabbits.

In 1979, further results of controlled trials of cyclophosphamide, warfarin, and dipyridamole in membranoproliferative glomerulonephritis were reported. No significant differences in renal function were found between the two groups after 18 months of continuous therapy.

A retrospective analysis of treatment and outcome in crescentic glomerulonephritis indicated superior outcome when administration of prednisone plus a cytotoxic agent was compared with no therapy. In addition, the use of combined regimens of plasma exchange, glucocorticoids, and cytotoxic drugs provided superior outcome even though the extent of underlying renal disease was more severe than in the other groups analyzed. This data tended to support earlier observations that immunosuppressive drugs and plasma exchange were beneficial in patients with extensive crescentic glomerulonephritis. In an uncontrolled trial of large doses of prednisone administered on an alternate-day basis over a prolonged period of time in patients with membranous glomerulonephritis, substantial improvement in renal function and proteinuria was observed. Patients were selected for this therapy from a larger group of patients with membranous glomerulonephritis because of declining renal function. Creatinine clearance and/or serum creatinine improved in all patients. The precise significance of this observation is uncertain, since declining renal function could have been due to complicating interstitial nephritis, at least in some patients. Finally, a symposium on the treatment of systemic lupus erythematosus complicated by nephritis was held.

During the 1980 meeting, additional reports appeared concerning the putative beneficial effect of high doses of intravenous methylprednisolone in crescentic glomerulonephritis. These studies demonstrated that such therapy was of little value in the treatment of antiglomerular basement membrane antibody-mediated crescentic glomerulonephritis; however, significant improvement occurred in 70 to 80% of patients with nonantiglomerular basement membrane antibody-mediated forms of crescentic glomerulonephritis including immune complex mediated and the so-called "nonimmunologically mediated" or "pauci-immune" form of crescentic glomerulonephritis. Because of a lower likelihood of serious complications, therapy with pulse methylprednisolone was favored over therapy with intensive plasma exchange.

By 1981, interest in glomerulonephritis and its treatment had grown to the point where both a state-of-the-art lecture (by Professor Stewart Cameron) and a separate free communication session on the topic of glomerulonephritis and its therapy were offered. Preliminary results of therapy of lupus glomerulonephritis by defibrination using ancrod (Maylasian pit-viper venom) was reported. Because intracapillary thrombosis was associated with later glomerular scarring, it was believed that early interference with coagulation using ancrod might prevent later development of glomerulosclerosis. These preliminary trials suggested that defibrination therapy was safe and was associated with improving renal function. A beneficial effect of intravenous cyclophosphamide in lupus nephritis was also reported. Better morphological outcomes, as assessed by repeat renal biopsy, were found among patients with lupus nephritis who received cyclophosphamide plus low-dose prednisone in comparison with other regimens. The most favorable outcomes were associated with intravenous cyclophosphamide given once every 3 months. A controlled trial of plasma exchange therapy in lupus nephritis was reported. This small trial suggested better preservation of renal function, fewer hospitalizations, a reduction of disease activity, and a diminution in medications in the plasma exchange group. Unfortunately, as will be noted later, these early preliminary observations could not be confirmed. In corroboration of similar studies using intravenous cyclophosphamide, intravenous mechlorethamine was also found to be effective in the treatment of selected patients with very severe systemic lupus erythematosus. Such therapy was associated with significant improvement in signs of disease activity, magnitude of proteinuria, and overall renal function. Nevertheless, because of moderate but transient side effects, intravenous cyclophosphamide became the preferred modality of cytotoxic therapy, when administered intravenously, for patients with SLE. Finally, the effects of alternate-day glucocorticoid therapy in membranoproliferative glomerulonephritis were reported in a prospective randomized trial. The results suggested that such alternate-day glucocorticoid therapy given over a prolonged period of time might slow the rate of progression of type 1 MPGN, but this treatment was often associated with substantial side effects and was therefore not an entirely satisfactory approach to overall management.

During the 1982 meeting, results of the only randomized prospective trial of plasma exchange in antiglomerular basement membrane antibody-induced nephritis were reported. Patients who received plasma exchange combined with immunosuppression had a more rapid decline in circulating antiglomerular basement membrane antibody and had an improved outcome. Nevertheless, no patient who required dialysis therapy at the initiation of treatment recovered renal function. Also, the results of a randomized prospective trial of platelet inhibition therapy in membranous glomerulonephritis were reported. Data presented in 1978 were extended with conclusions similar to the previous report in that combinations of dipyridamole and aspirin for at least 1 year significantly prevented further deterioration of renal function with type 1 MPGN.

In 1983, the value of plasma exchange therapy in thrombotic thrombocytopenic purpura and hemolytic uremia syndrome was first reported. Although this was an uncontrolled study, rapid relapse following discontinuation of plasma exchange in several patients provided substantial evidence that plasma exchange therapy was, at least in part, responsible for the improvement in renal function and normalization of the platelet count in the patients. Reports describing the results of controlled trials of chronic plasma exchange therapy in the diffuse proliferative glomerulonephritis of SLE continue to appear. Although these trials included relatively small numbers of patients, there continued to be a trend favoring a more rapid improvement and better preservation of renal function in those patients receiving intermittent plasma exchange than in those who received only glucocorticoids and cytotoxic therapy. Immune complex levels, as measured by C1q binding, fell to a greater extent in patients receiving plasma exchange. Additionally, another report described the long-term benefits of alternate-day prednisone therapy in membranoproliferative glomerulonephritis. This report, which extended the information reported at the 1980 meeting, continued to demonstrate a favorable outcome for those patients receiving long-term alternate-day prednisone therapy. Life-table analysis indicated an 86% survival after 11 years, which was significantly greater than that described in other reports of untreated patients. The reasons underlying the favorable results reported in this trial and the lack of beneficial effect of alternate-day prednisone as reported in previous meetings in control prospective trials remain unclear.

During the 1984 meeting, the ongoing immunosuppressive trials of lupus nephritis conducted at the National Institutes of Health were described. Continued superiority of intravenous cyclophosphamide over all other regimens continued to be documented after a median follow-up of 75 months. In addition, any regimen that incorporated cyclophosphamide appeared to be superior to regimens of glucocorticoids alone or glucocorticoids combined with azathioprine. The intravenous (IV) cyclophosphamide regimen was associated with fewer side effects, particularly hemorrhagic cystitis.

The 1985 meeting was particularly noteworthy for the field of therapy of glomerular diseases. One of the first reports describing the effects of cyclosporine in nephrotic syndrome was presented at the plenary session. This report described the effects of an 8-week course of cyclosporine in doses sufficient to maintain levels of 100 to 200 nanograms per mL (as assessed by high-pressure liquid chromatography) for 8 weeks. All patients were in the pediatric age group and had previously demonstrated resistance to or dependency on glucocorticoids. Sixteen of the 20 patients had either focal sclerosis or IgM nephropathy. Six of nine patients with focal sclerosis, six of seven patients with IgM nephropathy, and two of four patients with minimal change or mesangial hypercellularity achieved a remission. Fifty percent of the patients continued to remain in remission; the remaining patients had a relapse following discontinuance of cyclosporine. Although the study was uncontrolled, this report clearly demonstrated the potential of cyclosporine as a new immunosuppressant agent in the therapy of idiopathic nephrotic syndrome. Similar encouraging but very preliminary reports on the effectiveness of cyclosporine in treatment-resistant idiopathic nephrotic syndrome were also presented.

The notion that cyclophosphamide therapy of membranous glomerulonephritis might be beneficial was resurrected in a controlled clinical trial. Patients with membranous glomerulonephritis and impaired renal function demonstrated improvements in proteinuria and in creatinine clearance following prolonged therapy (16 months) with cyclophosphamide (1.5 mg/kg/day), often in combination with low-dose prednisone. This study was one of the first to recognize the potential for aggressive cyclophosphamide therapy for patients with membranous glomerulonephritis and impaired renal function. Finally, additional reports confirming the efficacy of aggressive high-dose "pulse" methylprednisolone therapy of crescentic glomerulonephritis were presented. These studies, and others previously reported, firmly established a role for high-dose intravenous methylprednisolone therapy in patients with crescentic glomerulonephritis, particularly in subgroups failing to demonstrate significant glomerular deposition of immunoglobulins (so called "pauci-immune" necrotizing and crescentic glomerulonephritis).

During the 1986 meeting, the conventional view that intensive plasma exchange was beneficial in severe lupus nephritis was challenged by the report of a large controlled clinical trial In this trial, 45 patients with severe lupus nephritis were randomized to receive standard immunosuppressive therapy plus twice weekly intensive plasma exchange, and 41 patients were randomized to a standard regimen of immunosuppressive therapy without plasma exchange. After a mean follow-up period of 80 weeks, no significant differences were found between the groups in terms of death or renal failure rate. This study considerably dampened enthusiasm for this modality of therapy in patients with severe lupus nephritis, but anecdotal reports continued to appear regarding the potential efficacy of this form of therapy in highly selected patients with SLE uncontrollable by other more conventional approaches. In a retrospective analysis, the putative beneficial effects of fresh frozen plasma infusions on the outcome of hemolytic uremic syndrome were studied. The outcome of the disease in 12 children who received fresh frozen plasma infusion were compared with a group of 31 children who did not receive this therapy. The outcome, as assessed in terms of thrombocytopenia, anemia, and renal failure, was not different between the groups. On the other hand, a preliminary trial of high-dose immunoglobulin infusions in hemolytic uremic syndrome was very encouraging.

During the 1987 meeting, the clinical effectiveness of combinations of cyclophosphamide and prednisone on the course of membranous glomerulonephritis was further demonstrated. These observations provided further weight to the growing body of evidence that an aggressive approach using combinations of alkylating agents and glucocorticoids in patients with membranous glomerulonephritis and declining renal function was of value. In addition, studies were reported that corroborated the widely held view that intravenous pulse cyclophosphamide was of benefit in severe lupus nephritis. Nevertheless, despite clinical and serological improvement with such therapy, repeat biopsies often demonstrated evidence of continued progression of interstitial fibrosis and glomerulosclerosis. The results of a preliminary and uncontrolled trial of combined prednisone and azathioprine therapy of children with severe and progressive IgA nephropathy were reported. Although proteinuria improved and chronic alterations in renal biopsy stabilized, 29% of the treated patients progressed to renal insufficiency.

The results of a multicenter controlled trial of plasma infusion therapy for hemolytic uremic syndrome were also reported. After an average of 16 months, there were no significant differences in the outcome between the two groups of patients. Because renal biopsies demonstrated predominately glomerular involvement in the patients studied in this trial, it was not possible to conclude whether plasma infusion therapy (or plasma exchange therapy) might be beneficial in the group with more significant vascular involvement. It has been known for some time that this latter group generally carries a more ominous prognosis.

The 1988 meeting was a particularly rich year for studies of the treatment of parenchymal renal diseases. The results of a prospective randomized trial of alternate-day prednisone in membranous glomerulonephritis were reported. Eighty-one patients were randomized to receive 6 months of prednisone 45 mg/m^2 on alternative days, and 77 patients were randomized to no therapy. After an average follow-up of approximately 4 years, actuarial patient survival was the same in both groups (93%), and there were no differences in the development of progressive renal insufficiency. This study placed serious doubt on the significance of earlier studies purporting to demonstrate that alternate-day prednisone protected patients with membranous glomerulonephritis from progressive renal insufficiency. A prospective randomized trial of cyclosporine and low-dose prednisone therapy versus conventional prednisone therapy in patients with the recent onset of idiopathic nephrotic syndrome was reported. The prevalence of complete remissions was significantly higher in the group receiving cyclosporine. Patients with high levels of lymphocyte stimulation with phytohemagglutinin A and high production rates of interleukin 2 tended to have more sustained remissions. Unfortunately, the patients admitted to this study had a variety of underlying renal histologies, and it was not possible from this study to identify whether renal histology was an important parameter influencing the ultimate outcome of therapy with cyclosporine. Long-term therapy with cyclosporine may be associated with progressive tubulointerstitial alterations, particularly in focal and segmental glomerulosclerosis. Therefore, long-term assessment of response, including serial biopsies, was viewed as necessary before the proper place of cyclosporine in the management of idiopathic nephrotic syndrome could be established.

A study of long-term therapy of minimal-change lesion associated nephrotic syndrome with low to moderate doses of alternate-day prednisone suggested that this regimen may maintain patients in remission at an acceptable level of side effects. Therefore, prolonged courses of alternate-day prednisone may be preferable to treatment with cyclophosphamide in selected patients with steroid-sensitive or steroid-dependent minimal change disease. A long-term follow-up of an earlier report examining the clinical utility of normalization of total hemolytic complement in the course of lupus nephritis was reported. As had been observed in earlier studies with shorter term follow-up, therapy designed to maintain serum complement levels within the normal range was associated with significant improvement in the long-term outcome of lupus nephritis. This study suggested that monitoring of serum complement levels may have clinical benefit and may provide a useful guide for the intensity of therapy. Finally, in an uncontrolled trial, the beneficial effect of intravenous cyclophosphamide therapy and rapid tapering of glucocorticoid dosage in patients with crescentic glomerulonephritis was examined. A favorable short-term outcome was observed; however, later progression of disease, as assessed by repeat renal biopsy, led to some caution regarding the overall long-term effectiveness of this approach. No data were presented that would allow a comparison of the approach using intravenous cyclophosphamide with the more conventional approach of initiating therapy with intravenous methylprednisolone and maintenance therapy of oral prednisone and oral immunosuppressive agents.

During the 1989 meetings, a new approach to the management of IgA nephropathy was introduced. In a preliminary study, patients with IgA nephropathy at high risk for the progressive loss of renal function received large doses of omega 3 polyunsaturated fatty acids. With the onset of this therapy, proteinuria declined and renal function improved modestly. These results were sufficiently encouraging to justify a larger scaled prospective and randomized clinical trial. Additional uncontrolled studies of the efficacy of long-term cyclosporine therapy of glucocorticoid unresponsive nephrotic syndrome in children and young adults were presented. Long-term therapy with low-dose cyclosporine (approximately 3 to 4 mg/kg/day) was associated with prolonged remission and no evidence of deterioration of renal function. Repeat biopsies were not performed. Complications of therapy were minimal. These and similar studies continued to demonstrate a possible role for cyclosporine in the treatment of steroid-unresponsive idiopathic nephrotic syndrome; however, because of the continued concern regarding cumulative nephrotoxicity a long-term prospective trial will still be needed to confirm efficacy and safety among homogeneous subsets of patients with well-defined renal histology. As an indication of the continued interest in treatment strategies for glomerular nephritis, a symposium on therapeutic approaches to glomerulonephritis was held during the 1989 meeting. Topics included membranous nephropathy, renal vasculitis, and related forms of crescentic glomerulonephritis and the nephropathies of systemic lupus erythematosus.

During the 1990 meeting, several novel approaches to the therapy of glomerulonephritis and vasculitis were introduced. In a preliminary trial of high-dose intravenous immunoglobulin (0.4 mg/kg/day for 5 days), beneficial effects were suggested in patients with severe active vasculitis. This form of therapy may be a useful adjunct to other modalities of therapy, such as high-dose intravenous methylprednisolone, alkylating agents, and plasma exchange. Intravenous immunoglobulin G was also demonstrated to be quite effective in inducing remissions in patients with thrombotic thrombocytopenic purpura. Such therapy could be considered as an alternative approach to intensive plasma exchange or plasma infusion therapy. 6-Thioguanine resulted in prolonged remission in patients with steroid-dependent nephrotic syndrome who continued to relapse after steroids and cyclophosphamide therapy. The worldwide results of the use of cyclosporine in idiopathic nephrotic syndrome were reviewed. In steroid-resistant patients, complete remissions were obtained in 14% of patients and partial remissions in 25% of patients. Only 20% of patients with an initial remission continued to be in remission 6 months after discontinuance of therapy. Adverse events requiring discontinuance of cyclosporine occurred in approximately 8% of patients. Renal functional deterioration occurred only when renal function was abnormal initially. Overall efficacy of cyclosporine seemed to be improved when therapy was combined with low doses of oral glucocorticoids. In a long-term prospective collaborative study, the efficacy of cyclosporine depended both on previous response to glucocorticoids and on glomerular histology. In steroid-responsive or steroid-dependent minimal change disease, the complete and partial remission rate was 70%, whereas in steroid-resistant focal sclerosis, the complete and partial remission rate was only 22%. Repeat biopsies demonstrated that interstitial and vascular lesions developed rapidly in patients with focal sclerosis treated with cyclosporine. Therefore, the success rate was low and toxicity was high in focal sclerosis. These studies concluded that steroid-resistant nephrotic syndrome due to focal and sclerosing glomerulonephritis is a contraindication to treatment with cyclosporine A.

Previous studies demonstrated striking beneficial effects of cyclophosphamide and prednisone in the treatment of Wegener's granulomatosis. Studies were presented indicating that follow-up measurement of antineutrophil cytoplasmic antibody (ANCA) levels in Wegener's granulomatosis could be used as a guide to relapses that were likely to occur on discontinuance of cyclophosphamide therapy. Finally, several studies challenged the opinion that intensive plasma exchange was of value in patients with crescentic glomerulonephritis. However, relatively few patients in these studies were dialysis-dependent at the onset of plasma exchange therapy. Nevertheless, these studies would seem to indicate that intensive plasma exchange therapy is of little value in the therapy of crescentic glomerulonephritis (or vasculitis) if it is instituted prior to the onset of dialysis-dependent renal failure. Therapy with high doses of oral or intravenous glucocorticoids, combined with oral cyclophosphamide and perhaps supplemented by intravenous immunoglobulin, appears to be the treatment of choice for these patients.

This review has focused primarily on studies dealing with the specific therapy of several glomerulonephritides and vasculitides. Nevertheless, it is important to recognize that in recent years, considerable attention has been focused on the putative beneficial effect of other "nonspecific" therapeutic modalities on the outcome of a variety of renal parenchymal diseases. These therapies include antihypertensive drugs, including angiotensin-converting enzyme inhibitors, low-protein diets, lipid-lowering agents, and other inhibitors of inflammation or inflammatory mediators. It is anticipated that future meetings of the American Society of Nephrology will deal increasingly with these "nonspecific" therapeutic modalities, particularly because they seem to be applicable to a group of patients for whom no form of specific therapy has yet been well delineated. Examples might include IgA nephropathy, diabetic nephropathy, and focal sclerosis. In addition, the burgeoning evidence from fundamental studies of experimental models of disease would indicate the likely possibility that new immunomodulating agents, such as monoclonal antibodies, antiidiotypic antibodies, immunotoxins, eicosanoid receptor antagonists, and other specific inhibitors of inflammation mediators, may eventually reach clinical trials. Overall, the meetings of the American Society of Nephrology over the last 25 years have provided a microcosm of clinical studies into the therapeutics of renal parenchymal disease.

Clinical-Pathologic Correlations/Natural History/Prognosis

At the time of the first meeting of the American Society of Nephrology in 1967, the field of clinical-pathologic correlations in renal disease and studies of natural history were rather rudimentary. Although percutaneous renal biopsy had been introduced some 15 years previously, the immense heterogeneity of glomerulonephritis was still being recognized, and a paucity of studies had been published in which detailed clinical descriptions of disease had been related to underlying morphology. The classic text on renal pathology by Heptinstall had been published only 1 year before the first meeting, and Strauss and Welt's *Classic Diseases of the Kidney* had appeared only 4 years earlier. Nevertheless, ever wider application of renal biopsy to the study of renal disease, including use of the newer techniques of immunofluorescence and electron microscopy, added greatly to the dissection of renal disease into increasingly homogeneous entities. In parallel, rapid advances in serological techniques (such as assays for serum complement and autoantibodies) and more refined approaches to the assessment of renal function and glomerular permeability permitted more extensive correlations between morphologic findings and renal disease. As more patients were studied in detail, follow-ups extending over years or even decades became possible. Thus, the stage was set for careful analysis of the natural history of well-defined entities.

During the first meeting in 1967, a total of six studies were presented that dealt with clinical-pathologic correlations or natural history. The clinical and pathologic features of medullary cystic disease and familial juvenile nephronophthisis were compared and found to be virtually identical. In a renal biopsy study of patients with idiopathic hematuria and proteinuria, the lesion of focal proliferative glomerulonephritis was frequently encountered. Unfortunately, immunofluorescent studies were not included in this study, and it is very likely that many, if not all, of these patients would now be included under the rubric of IgA nephropathy or Berger's disease. The syndrome of rapidly progressive glomerulonephritis associated with extensive crescent formation was delineated. The value of renal biopsy in classifying various renal lesions in lupus nephritis as an aid to the determination of prognosis was reported.

In 1968, the renal morphologic findings associated with the hypersensitivity interstitial nephritis due to penicillin and methicillin were described. In addition, the glomerular and vascular alterations that accompanied the hemolytic uremic syndrome were delineated.

In 1969, further studies of rapidly progressive glomerulonephritis were presented, and the clinical spectrum of the subgroup-associated antiglomerular basement membrane antibodies and lung hemorrhage (Goodpasture's syndrome) was reported. Electron microscopy observations of the dense deposits seen in lupus nephritis were presented, and the significance of these deposits on prognosis was analyzed in detail. Long-term studies of sporadic poststreptococcal glomerulonephritis in children were presented. Initial renal biopsies in many of these children suggested that preexisting renal disease (perhaps IgA nephropathy) accounted for the majority of those patients who later developed progressive renal disease. Additional renal biopsy studies of childhood nephrotic syndrome emphasized the broad spectrum of renal lesions encountered, thus emphasizing the notion that not all childhood nephrotic syndrome was accompanied by minimal changes on light microscopy.

During the 1970 meeting, a report on the natural history of infantile polycystic kidney disease in children was presented. Neonates typically had severe respiratory distress, and deaths due to pulmonary insufficiency were common. Of survivors, renal insufficiency gradually ensued, and portal hypertension and hypersplenism were common. The value of serological monitoring in rapidly progressive glomerulonephritis was demonstrated by a clinical-pathologic study using assays for antiglomerular basement membrane antibody. Electron microscopy of renal biopsies in patients with persistent hypocomplementemia revealed a new variant of membranoproliferative glomerulonephritis in which dense intramembranous deposits were found. Renal biopsy studies of glomerulonephritis associated with bacterial endocarditis demonstrated a variety of glomerular lesions.

In 1971, studies of clinicopathologic correlations continued with description of unique glomerular basement membrane abnormalities in the nail patella syndrome, specific ultrastructural abnormalities accompanying glomerular disease due to sickle cell disease, and further descriptions of the variation in dense deposits seen in membranoproliferative glomerulonephritis. In addition, glomerulonephritis accompanying hepatic cirrhosis and the Guillain-Barré syndrome was described. A long-term follow-up study of 61 children with steroid-responsive nephrotic syndrome was reported. At the end of the follow-up (averaging about 14 years), 6% had died, 57% had sustained a remission of at least 2 years' duration, 33% continued to have relapsing nephrotic syndrome, and 5% had persisting proteinuria.

In 1973, studies relating complement activation to glomerulonephritis were reported as well as the evolution of an immune complex glomerulonephritis into an antiglomerular basement membrane form of glomerulonephritis. Careful studies of the glomerulopathy associated with neoplasia were presented. Also in 1973, the first American report of IgA nephropathy appeared. In a study of idiopathic hematuria of young adults, diffuse IgA deposition in the glomeruli was found frequently. Finally, in a renal biopsy study of patients with idiopathic nephrotic syndrome, the poor prognosis of patients with focal and segmental glomerulosclerosis was observed.

During the 1974 meeting, the importance of focal sclerosing glomerular lesions among patients with nephrotic syndrome was again reemphasized. Further electron microscopic analysis of renal biopsies in patients with lupus nephritis provided additional evidence that extensive subendothelial electron-dense deposits correlated with evidence of disease activity, and the disappearance of these deposits during treatment was associated with clinical improvement and a good prognosis. Finally, the first report of a highly sensitive radioimmunoassay for circulating antiglomerular basement antibodies was presented.

In 1975, additional long-term studies of the prognosis of sporadic acute poststreptococcal glomerulonephritis in children were reported. Serial renal biopsies demonstrated that histological healing occurred within the first 2 years after onset in 20% of patients, by 3 years in 30%, by 4 years in 43%, and by 5 years in 75%. Overall complete histological healing was eventually seen in 97% of patients, indicating the highly favorable long-term prognosis of this form of acute glomerulonephritis, at least among children. Electron microscopic analysis of patients with membranoproliferative glomerulonephritis and hypocomplementemia revealed a third variant in which subendothelial deposits were widespread, frequently disrupting the basement membrane. Duplications of basement membrane material in response to disruption of a capillary wall by deposits were widespread.

In 1976, a renal biopsy study of patients with systemic lupus erythematosus without evident clinical renal involvement clearly demonstrated that diffuse proliferative glomerulonephritis can develop even in the absence of abnormal clinical findings. Further long-term study of poststreptococcal acute glomerulonephritis in adults demonstrated a benign prognosis. Studies of plasma renin activity and plasma volume in patients with nephrotic syndrome delineated two forms of nephrotic edema. One was associated with high renin and normal or low plasma volume. These patients typically had minimal change lesions. The other form was associated with normal or high plasma volume and low renin. These patients typically had membranous glomerulonephritis or other structural renal changes. In 1977, an ultrastructural and functional correlative study of cysts from human polycystic disease was reported. The solute composition of the cyst fluids from patients with adult polycystic kidney disease and the ultrastructure of the cyst walls from these patients were studied. "Proximal" and "distal" cysts were described based on their functional and morphological characteristics. Immunofluorescent studies of complement deposits in membranoproliferative glomerulonephritis delineated a specific pattern of C3 deposition with mesangial "rings" and "railroad tracks." The entity of crescentic glomerulonephritis without immune deposits ("pauci-immune glomerulonephritis") was first described during the 1977 meeting. The presence of circulating immune complexes in many forms of glomerulonephritis was also described. Finally, an excellent clinical pathologic study of renal disease in adults over age 60 was reported. Among 82 patients 60 years of age or older, primary glomerular disease was diagnosed in 44 patients. Particularly common was crescentic glomerulonephritis, membranous glomerulonephritis, and minimal change nephrotic syndrome. Systemic diseases involving the kidney were found in 23 patients with vasculitis: amyloidosis and Wegener's granulomatosis were the most common. Arteriosclerosis and global glomerulosclerosis were the only findings in nine patients.

During the 1978 meeting, new studies emerged attempting to relate patterns of glomerular permeability to specific glomerular diseases. In addition, ongoing studies monitoring circulating immune complexes in various renal diseases, including lupus nephritis, were reported. In a noteworthy presentation, renal failure was observed in 14 patients with minimal change disease associated with nephrotic syndrome. The majority of these patients were elderly, and many manifested oliguria and severe edema. Improvement of renal function occurred in association with an induction of a diuresis, regardless of whether remission of proteinuria was achieved. The authors postulated that renal interstitial edema with resulting increased hydrostatic pressure in proximal tubules and in Bowman's space was responsible for a decrease in net filtration pressure, decreased GFR, and reversible renal failure.

The meeting of 1979 saw a distinct shift in focus away from clinical pathologic studies in human subjects and toward experimental models of renal disease. Much attention was focused on the mechanisms that underlie the formation of immune deposits in glomerular capillaries and the mechanisms underlying altered glomerular permeability.

During the 1980 meeting, an increased interest in studies of kidney disease of diabetes mellitus was evident. A symposium dealt with the relationships of glucose homeostasis to glomerulopathy in animals with diabetes mellitus and the natural history of diabetic nephropathy in human beings. In 1980, a careful analysis of the serological features that distinguished diffuse proliferative from membranous glomerulonephritis in systemic lupus erythematosus was reported. Higher levels of anti-DNA antibody were found in diffuse proliferative glomerulonephritis, and these antibodies were typically highly efficient at fixing complement in vitro. Further studies of the long-term prognosis of epidemic poststreptococcal glomerulonephritis continued to confirm the relative benign nature of this disorder.

During the 1981 meeting, the International Study of Kidney Disease in Children reported on their extensive study of the primary nephrotic syndrome in children. In a histopathological study of renal biopsy specimens from 389 children with minimal change nephrotic syndrome, 56% had entirely normal glomeruli by light microscopy, 25% had focal glomerular obsolescence, 4% had mild mesangial thickening, 8% had focal tubular changes, and 7% had mild mesangial hypercellularity. There were no significant differences among the groups in the clinical or laboratory characteristics at the time of diagnosis. Initial nonresponse to steroid therapy was found with greater frequency among those patients with minimal mesangial hypercellularity as well as in a separate group of patients with diffuse mesangial hypercellularity. Nevertheless, after 1 year of observation, there were no significant clinical differences between these two groups of patients. There was also a high proportion of initial nonresponse to steroids in patients with focal tubular changes.

Additional studies were reported on nephrotic syndrome with underlying focal and segmental glomerulosclerosis in children. Fourteen of 24 children were steroid resistant, and 10 children were initially sensitive. This latter group of patients had initial renal biopsies showing minimal change lesion, which later evolved into focal and segmental glomerulosclerosis. Finally, the initial reports of glomerulonephritis associated with extensive mesangial IgM deposits in the mesangium appeared. Subsequent analysis of this group of patients by others led to controversy as to whether a specific entity known as "IgM mesangial nephropathy" existed.

During the 1982 meeting, there was a continued strong emphasis on pathophysiology and experimental studies of renal disease. Nevertheless, several interesting studies concerning the prognosis of lupus nephritis were presented. One study analyzed the application of modified World Health Organization (WHO) histological criteria as a guide to prognosis. Thirty-seven patients were followed an average of 10 years following initial renal biopsy. Transformation from one category to another was uncommon. Overall survival was significantly improved from observations made in the mid-1970s. Long-term prognosis was distinctly related to WHO classification in that most patients with class II and class III lesions did well, whereas patients with class IV and V lesions frequently progressed to renal failure. In a separate study, 21 patients with class V lupus nephritis (membranous glomerulonephritis) were studied to determine prognostic factors. The distribution of electron-dense deposits and the degree of cellular proliferation were analyzed. The overall 5-year patient survival was 90%. Patients with severe proliferation were more serologically active than those in whom proliferation was absent. The prognosis was much poorer in those with extensive proliferation; however, occasional subendothelial deposits did not seem to alter the prognosis.

During the 1983 meeting, interest in the natural history of diabetic nephropathy emerged, stimulated in large part by new observations on the pathophysiology of diabetic glomerular disease in experimental models. One such study analyzed retrospectively the clinical course of 52 patients with type I diabetes mellitus. Significant correlations were found between median plasma glucose and the median duration of diabetes until the onset of persistent proteinuria. However, the time interval between the onset of persistent proteinuria and the first elevation of the serum creatinine was significantly shorter for diabetic patients whose blood pressure was elevated at the onset of persistent proteinuria. Thus, hypertension seemed to influence the rate of progression of diabetic nephropathy but was not a major factor in its induction. Several papers were presented describing early observations in a new nephropathy associated with the human immunodeficiency virus. In an interesting study, decision theory and analysis were applied to the question of whether renal biopsy is needed in the initial evaluation of adult patients with idiopathic nephrotic syndrome. No significant differences were found in the quality-adjusted survival between a strategy of empiric steroid therapy versus renal biopsy in patients with idiopathic nephrotic syndrome. This analysis included therapy with steroids only and did not take into consideration the possible beneficial effects of the use of alkylating agents, depending on the outcome of renal biopsy. Nevertheless, the analysis did point out the limited clinical utility of renal biopsy in patients with adult-onset idiopathic nephrotic syndrome. In a further study of diabetic nephropathy, percutaneous renal biopsies from 48 insulin-dependent diabetic patients with normal or mildly reduced glomerular filtration rates were studied by light and quantitative electron microscopy. There was no strong relationship between glomerular basement membrane or mesangial thickness in the duration of diabetes. Increased mesangial volume had a strong inverse correlation with the peripheral capillary surface area and glomerular luminal volume. These changes in turn were also inversely correlated with glomerular filtration rate. Clinically overt diabetic nephropathy always reflected far-advanced glomerular lesions. In the author's opinion, it was not possible to estimate the risk of subsequent serious diabetic renal disease without the performance of a renal biopsy. Finally, in an excellent study of crescentic glomerulonephritis in children, severe and progressive crescent formation was directly related to the extent of gaps in Bowman's capsule.

During the 1984 meeting, important new observations relating idiopathic hemolytic uremic syndrome to infection with virotoxin-producing *E. Coli* were presented. This linkage provided one of the first pieces of evidence for a specific pathogenetic mechanism for this type of renal disease. Also, during the 1984 meeting, several papers were presented that emphasized the role of tubulointerstitial changes in the prognosis of various glomerular lesions. These studies, and other published manuscripts, added considerable weight to the growing body of evidence that chronic interstitial changes were more predictive of long-term outcome than glomerular lesions in many forms of chronic glomerular disease. Studies on the value of renal biopsy analysis in the determination of long-term prognosis of lupus nephritis continued to appear. In a landmark study, the relationship of autoantibodies to granulocyte cytoplasm in active Wegener's granulomatosis was described. This study clearly identified that the antineutrophil cytoplasmic antibodies were a new and highly specific marker for active Wegener's granulomatosis. In a continuation of earlier studies, the relationship of urinary albumin excretion to glomerular structure was examined in insulin-dependent diabetes mellitus. In this study, urinary albumin excretion correlated poorly with the underlying diabetic glomerular pathology. Thus, the mechanism by which increased albumin excretion is associated with the later development of overt diabetic nephropathy remained unclear. On the other hand, the total capillary surface area, as studied by quantitative electron microscopy, was highly correlated with GFR both at the hyperfiltration range and when the GFR was declining. Because mesangial volume is inversely correlated with total capillary surface area, it is presumed that reduction in GFR is the consequence of an ever-expanding mesangial volume in diabetic nephropathy. Finally, in a careful study of renal biopsies from 60 patients with focal and segmental glomerulosclerosis, the early lesion of this glomerular disorder was identified. It was concluded that severe and segmental epithelial cell injury was the initial event in the pathogenesis of focal and segmental glomerulosclerosis.

In 1985, a large multicenter study of the long-term prognosis of children with hemolytic uremic syndrome was reported. Over 90% of 155 children with hemolytic uremic syndrome completely recovered. No significant indicators of outcome could be determined from a careful analysis of features present at the time of the initial illness. In a further extensive study of gross hematuria in adolescence, a high frequency of IgA nephropathy (50%) was demonstrated. These studies emphasized the importance of renal biopsy in the evaluation of patients presenting with gross hematuria in this age group. Finally, in a long-term study of 47 adults with biopsy-proven focal and segmental glomerulosclerosis, the importance of magnitude of proteinuria was again confirmed. Patients with focal sclerosis who have persistent nephrotic range proteinuria and who do not respond to steroids manifest progressive deterioration of renal function.

The 1986 meeting was characterized by a dramatic increase in presentations of studies that used cellular and molecular biological techniques. Experimental study of messenger RNA levels for laminin and collagen type IV chains in streptozocin-induced diabetes mellitus provided an example of such studies. This presentation demonstrated that steady-state levels of messenger RNA for these extracellular matrix proteins are increased in the kidney relatively early following the onset of diabetes. Further long-term studies of the prognosis of children with IgA nephropathy were reported.

Patients with segmental or diffuse proliferative glomerulonephritis in association with IgA nephropathy frequently progress to chronic renal failure. The continued analysis of outcome of lupus nephritis demonstrated that patients with membranous glomerulonephritis with severe superimposed proliferative glomerulonephritis had a prognosis that was much worse than patients with either segmental proliferative glomerulonephritis or diffuse proliferative glomerulonephritis.

During the 1987 meeting, there was a significant increase in the number of presentations dealing with adult polycystic kidney disease, reflecting a growing interest in the pathogenesis, clinical features, and natural history of this important hereditary disorder. In addition, studies of the value of the chronicity and activity index in the prognosis of lupus nephritis were reported. These studies failed to confirm any significant value of these indices in estimation of long-term prognosis. In a very interesting presentation, elevated urinary C-5 b—9 excretion was found commonly in early and severe membranous glomerulonephritis in human subjects. These findings were comparable to those previously reported in experimental membranous nephropathy and gave rise to the proposal that measurements of excretion of C5 b—9 could be used as an indication of the "activity" of this form of renal disease. Finally, in an extensive serological study, it was found that antineutrophil cytoplasmic antibodies react with myeloperoxidase in many patients with idiopathic necrotizing and crescentic glomerulonephritis. These autoantibodies were particularly likely to be found in patients with the so-called "pauci-immune" form of crescentic glomerulonephritis.

During the 1988 meeting, there was a continued expansion of studies employing molecular and cell biological technique. Not unexpectedly, there was an increasing focus on hereditary diseases such as polycystic kidney disease and Alport's syndrome. A study defining the nature of the defect in type IV collagen in Alport's syndrome was reported. In addition, the genetic locus defining this disorder was mapped to a Xq 21.3-q 22. Furthermore, studies of autoantibodies in glomerulonephritis and vasculitis continued to appear. The antigenic targets of these autoantibodies came under increasing scrutiny. Studies of vasculitis, IgA nephropathy, and diabetic nephropathy continued to appear.

The 1989 meeting was characterized by a further rapid expansion of studies of molecular biology and their application to experimental renal disease. Morphometric studies of renal biopsies in patients with minimal change disease and focal sclerosis confirmed previous findings in experimental renal disease that glomerular enlargement was associated with the development of focal and segmental glomerulosclerosis. These important findings provided a new dimension to the study of the long-term prognosis of minimal change disease. Additional studies of IgA nephropathy identified the presence of focal and segmental glomerulosclerosis as an important indicator of a poor prognosis. In addition, the ominous prognostic indications of focal and segmental sclerosis in renal biopsies from black and Hispanic patients with nephrotic syndrome were noted. Critical clinical variables influencing the prognosis of idiopathic membranous glomerulonephritis were identified. A predictive model for prognosis was developed using variables of persistent proteinuria (above a certain quantity for a specific duration), initial creatinine clearance, and the slope of the change of creatinine clearance over time. These kinds of prognostic studies allowed for the development of criteria to identify patients with idiopathic membranous glomerulonephritis at high risk for subsequent progression. Additional studies on the linkage of adult polycystic kidney disease to markers on chromosome 16 were presented. New evidence appeared suggesting that the prognosis for patients with adult polycystic kidney disease linked to markers on chromosome 16 was different than the form of disease not linked to markers on chromosome 16. Finally, in studies of the glomerular sieving profile on patients with minimal change disease and focal sclerosis, a similar abnormality in the size selective barrier was identified. The main difference between minimal change disease and focal sclerosis was the severity of the abnormality rather than the character of the abnormality.

During the 1990 meeting, several new and interesting observations were reported. The urinary excretion of platelet factor 4 was elevated in IgA nephropathy but not in thin basement membrane disease. Assays for the serum concentration of IgA-fibronectin aggregates were useful in the diagnosis of IgA nephropathy. Very high levels were strongly associated with IgA nephropathy, as patients with non-IgA-mediated diseases tended to have low levels. Further studies of antiglomerular basement membrane antibody disease indicated that the need for dialysis, the extent for crescentic involvement, and the degree of elevation of antiglomerular basement membrane antibody titer all contributed toward a very poor prognosis in this disorder. The phenotypic heterogeneity of Alport's syndrome was studied by examining the different mutations in the COL 4a5 collagen gene. Several different phenotypes were related to specific genetic abnormalities, including single-based mutations and intragenic deletions. Additional studies emphasizing the clinical heterogeneity of X-linked Alport's syndrome were also presented.

In summary, over the last several decades, the meetings of the American Society of Nephrology have included studies of great importance to the field of clinical pathologic correlations and long-term prognosis. Particularly noteworthy have been studies that have elucidated the importance of renal biopsy information in prognostication in systemic lupus erythematosis and also in uncovering the limitations of renal biopsy in prognostication. The evolution of serological diagnosis of several forms of chronic renal disease has been very impressive. Major strides in the understanding of the phenotypic and genetic heterogeneity of several hereditary diseases, the most noteworthy being polycystic kidney disease and Alport's syndrome, have been presented at these meetings. The careful studies of the prognosis of IgA nephropathy, minimal change disease, and focal and segmental glomerulosclerosis have been scrutinized carefully at the national meetings. Finally, it is impressive how these studies have evolved from simple clinical analysis to highly sophisticated genetic, serological, and molecular biological approaches.

Descriptions of at least two new forms of kidney disease have been included among the scientific programs of sessions entitled "Clinical Nephrology" during the Society's first 25 years. The first of these, heroin-associated nephropathy, was described initially during the 1971 meeting. These authors described heroin addicts who had presented with the nephrotic syndrome and findings of "focal membrano-proliferative glomerulonephritis and interstitial nephritis" in each of seven kidney biopsy specimens. A known cause of the nephrotic syndrome could not be identified, which led to the speculation that heroin addiction itself might provide a causatory "antigenic stimulus." In 1973, a description of the "natural history of heroin-associated nephropathy" was described in 14 black men with heroin addiction and the nephrotic syndrome. "Focal and segmental glomerular sclerosis" was the most common underlying lesion, and 7 of the 14 patients had progressed to end-stage uremia within 6 to 48 months after the first detection of proteinuria. Again, the cause of the nephrotic syndrome was not evident, and the suggestion was made that "an undefined response of the addict to heroin or its vehicle" might well be causative.

The association of kidney disease with heroin addiction was not considered further until the 1978 meeting. These authors described 23 black male addicts who presented with the "nephrotic syndrome and/or renal insufficiency" and uniform evidence of "sclerosing glomerulonephritis" in all kidney biopsy specimens. Their observations confirmed the existence of heroin-associated "sclerosing glomerulonephritis" in black men and established that its incidence, at least in the author's environment, was 30 times greater in black male addicts than in black male nonaddicts.

The next and last selected presentation on kidney disease in heroin addicts occurred in 1985. Renal amyloidosis and the nephrotic syndrome were described in 20 patients who had abused heroin subcutaneously. In contrast to 40 other heroin addicts with "focal glomerulosclerosis" who typically abused heroin intravenously, those with amyloidosis were thought to have developed their condition in response to chronic suppurative skin infection induced by repetitive subcutaneous administration.

The cause of "heroin-associated nephropathy" remains uncertain even today. By definition, it is a condition limited to addicts, and it seems to present most often as the nephrotic syndrome in association with steady progression to renal failure with small kidneys and hypertension. A variety of glomerular lesions have now been described, but focal or glomerulosclerosis has perhaps been noted most frequently. In some patients, at least suggestive evidence of an altered immune response has been observed, perhaps indicating that the condition reflects a response to a contaminant of heroin or a viral, bacterial, or other infectious agent to which heroin addicts are usually susceptible.

The second new condition or entity has received much more attention during recent ASN sessions on "Clinical Nephrology." It was but a short time after the first description of acquired immunodeficiency syndrome (AIDS) in 1981 that its relatively frequent association with several forms of kidney disease was recognized. In fact, only 2 years later (and prior to the first appearance of any published report), the first descriptions of kidney disease in patients with AIDS were presented at the 1983 meeting. In separate presentations during the same session, three different groups from New York and Miami described approximately 35 patients with AIDS and associated kidney disease. The first group from New York described 13 patients with AIDS, proteinuria and/or renal failure, and several types of underlying renal pathology. A high incidence of opportunistic infection, shock, and nephrotoxic exposures led to the suggestion that AIDS-associated kidney disease was multifactorial in origin. The same conclusion was reached by the Miami group, who described 12 Haitians or homosexuals with renal lesions (10 of whom exhibited either "mesangial proliferation" or "focal and segmental glomerular sclerosis") and the presence or absence of proteinuria and mild renal insufficiency. None was a "drug abuser." In contrast, a report from New York described 10 black men and women with AIDS, 5 of whom were heroin addicts and most of whom exhibited the nephrotic syndrome with underlying focal and segmental glomerular sclerosis on renal biopsy. Kidney disease "progressed rapidly to uremia" in several patients. The latter authors speculated that rapid progression to uremia was glomerulosclerosis, perhaps facilitated by "repeated antigenic stimuli from multiple infections."

The following year at the 1984 meeting, an additional 17 patients with "AIDS-associated nephropathy" were described. The authors concluded that this new entity was "characterized by focal and segmental glomerulosclerosis and a rapid decline to irreversible renal failure with a high mortality." It was later to become significant that all of their 17 patients were black men and that 9 of them were drug addicts. At that time, drug abuse represented the major known risk factor, although it was recognized that other factors must also be operative.

Such a conclusion was reemphasized at the 1985 meeting, when 50 men with AIDS were described in whom the "usual infectious and neoplastic complications" were "infrequently associated with glomerular disease." They suggested that factors other than infection, such as "drug abuse or delayed treatment," might be responsible for previously reported glomerular lesions.

The 1986 meeting witnessed a sharp increase in the number of AIDS-related abstracts selected for presentation at both oral and poster sessions. In their summary of a growing clinical experience, one group described patients with AIDS and kidney disease, all of whom were black. Most of them exhibited the nephrotic syndrome with rapid progression to normotensive renal failure. Many were intravenous drug abusers, and underlying focal and segmental glomerulosclerosis was noted in the majority of patients in whom kidney tissue was obtained by biopsy and/or autopsy. And, for the first time, the investigators described a group of "formerly nephrotic IV drug addicts" with end-stage renal disease who developed AIDS after 2 to 76 months of maintenance hemodialysis, thereby suggesting that the disease could antedate the onset of clinical AIDS. The importance of IV drug use as a risk or pathogenetic factor was confirmed by investigators from Miami, who also provided further "strong evidence for the existence of AIDS-related glomerulopathy independent" thereof.

Other 1986 presentations offered further confirmation to the fact that AIDS was associated with a more rapidly progressive form of focal and segmental glomerulosclerosis than that observed in other settings, including glomerulosclerosis associated with heroin abuse. Because "AIDS-associated nephrology" was increasingly noted to appear in advance of clinical AIDS, it was first suggested during the 1986 meeting that the new entity should be identified with the associated viral infection rather than with the occurrence of clinical AIDS. Hence, use of the term "HTLV III" or "HIV" (human immunodeficiency virus)-associated nephropathy" was recommended.

The characteristic ultrastructural features of HIV-associated nephropathy were first described in 1986. It was emphasized that the electron-microscopic observations of such alterations as tubuloreticular structures were typical of those often associated with an antecedent viral invasion. Finally, at the same meeting, the occurrence of hyponatremia in patients with AIDS and its association with hypoadrenalism and the syndrome accompanied by the inappropriate release of antidiuretic hormone (ADH) were described. Last, and most fortunately, the results of early epidemiological studies revealed that seropositivity for AIDS was infrequent or rare in such high-risk populations as dialysis and transplant patients.

The 1987 annual meeting was the banner year for presentations on AIDS and HIV-associated nephropathy (10 posters and two oral presentations). One of the most important presentations described for the first time a high incidence of AIDS on the West Coast. The data failed to confirm the "high incidence of malignant nephrosis and renal failure" that had been noted on the East Coast, and it was first suggested that the latter finding might rather reflect "a greater predilection" for the disease in blacks. For the first time, drug abuse was joined by race as an important and recognized risk factor for the development of HIV-associated nephropathy.

Other presentations in 1987 generally confirmed earlier descriptions of the clinical manifestations and various presentations of the new condition. Legitimate concerns with respect to the potential transmission of AIDS to patients or staff during dialysis were reflected in three presentations. Investigators from Brooklyn reported a 10% incidence of HIV seropositivity in their own dialysis population (69% of whom were drug abusers) and recommended that mandatory HIV testing be carried out routinely in hemodialysis units, especially in those dealing with inner-city populations. Observers from Miami described a similar incidence of HIV infection in their dialysis patients but found no evidence of high transmissibility. Last, a survey of 1412 hemodialysis centers established that approaches to the control of HIV infection were "heterogeneous," perhaps "reflecting a lack of satisfaction with Centers for Disease Control (CDC) recommendations."

Selected presentations on AIDS and HIV-associated nephropathy reached a numerical plateau in 1988. However, for the first time, the importance of the new condition was emphasized dramatically by the inclusion of six oral presentations in a single session entitled "AIDS and the Nephrologist." One presentation in this session described the occurrence of hypouricemia in AIDS and its claimed association with increased mortality. Another group described the frequent occurrence of a milder form of renal disease in children with HIV infection and suggested that it was expressed more prominently as a form of proliferative glomerulonephritis than as focal and segmental glomerulosclerosis. Another group reported the results of a CDC survey of HIV seropositivity among 1219 patients on hemodialysis at 27 centers in 10 states; only 10 patients were found to be Western blot positive (a seropositivity rate of 0.77%). All 10 patients "had recognized risk factors for HIV infection." A paper from New York City confirmed the unlikely occurrence of nosocomial transmission of HIV infection in a population of dialysis patients with a relatively high incidence of seropositivity. Finally, a model of "sclerosing glomerulopathy" was described in rhesus monkeys infected with a closely related AIDS virus that perhaps set the stage for the first and future experimental studies of the nature of HIV-associated nephropathy.

In contrast to the years 1986 to 1988, the 1989 meeting witnessed a dramatic fall in the number of presentations on HIV-associated nephropathy. No abstract was chosen for presentation, perhaps reflecting the fact that the central clinical manifestations and presentations of the new condition had already been outlined fully by earlier presentations and that they were therefore generally well known. However, HIV-associated nephropathy again rose to visible prominence during the 1990 meeting. A group from New York documented a high incidence of asymptomatic proteinuria in HIV-infected patients with minimal symptoms. Contrary to earlier reports, the investigator, were unable to confirm the frequent occurrence of hypouricemia in such patients. Another presentation described an interesting patient with "HIV-associated immune complex glomerulonephritis" and demonstrated the existence of the viral genome in renal biopsy tissue and eluate therefrom. They suggested that HIV-associated nephropathy may sometimes be of immune complex origin and that the cellular incorporation of viral products played an important pathogenetic role. Another study described the limitations that surround our current ability to detect HIV in paraffin sections of kidney tissue and suggested that in situ hybridization may offer greater potential specificity than does immunohistochemical methodology. But perhaps the most important paper, mainly because it offered promise of future benefit, reported on a study of associated kidney disease in mice transgenic for HIV genes. This was the first truly experimental study of possible pathogenetic mechanisms. In this animal model, the investigators documented the occurrence of a segmental increase of mesangial matrix, tubular atrophy, and interstitial fibrosis with increased glomerular deposition of laminin, collagen IV, and heparin sulfate proteoglycan. They concluded that the expression of HIV genes was responsible and that the resultant pathology closely resembled that of HIV-associated focal and segmental glomerulosclerosis.

Patients with AIDS may manifest many forms of acute or chronic kidney disease, many of which bear no direct relation to HIV infection per se. However, it is clear from even a casual review of the annals of the Society's recent meetings that HIV infection is also associated with a new and special form of kidney disease. It is hoped that the Society's future meetings will witness the final description of the pathogenesis of HIV-associated glomerulosclerosis and the definition of successful approaches to its control.

Metabolic, Fluid, and Electrolyte Disorders

Uric Acid and Hyperuricemia

When the Society was organized 25 years ago, a number of prominent nephrologists believed that hyperuricemia could cause chronic renal failure. Textbooks at that time described urate deposition, interstitial nephritis, nephrosclerosis, and even changes resembling chronic glomerulonephritis. Claims were made that these lesions occurred independent of hypertension. Because of the foregoing and the fact that several uricosuric and antiuricosuric drugs had appeared, a number of nephrologists became interested in renal handling of urate. It had become evident that thiazide diuretics could cause hyperuricemia and in susceptible patients could precipitate or aggravate gouty arthritis. In 1967, studies explaining the cause of thiazide-induced hyperuricemia and hypouricosuria were presented. They showed clearly that volume depletion incident to diuretic therapy reduced urate clearance and caused hyperuricemia. If thiazide diuretics were administered along with sufficient sodium chloride to offset volume depletion, urate clearance remained normal and hyperuricemia did not occur.

If plasma levels of urate are increased, the kidney responds by increasing both urate resorption and urate secretion. In 1968, an interesting study was presented to explore the effects of hyperfiltration of urate. In eight normal subjects studied before and 10 days after donating a kidney, plasma urate increased from 4.7 to 5.6 mg%. Urate-filtered load rose by 44%. Fractional resorption of urate remained almost complete. Administration of the antituberculous agent pyrazinamide, an antagonist of urate secretion, showed that tubular secretion of urate had increased 74%. Thus, reducing renal mass by one-half increased secretion but not absorption of uric acid so as to double the net rate of urate excretion per nephron.

Patients with Wilson's disease (hepatolenticular degeneration) are often hypouricemic, which is presumed to be the result of reduced tubular resorption. In 1971, 10 patients were studied before and after administration of pyrazinamide. The study showed that hypouricemia was the result of increased tubular secretion rather than decreased resorption. In 1973, micropuncture studies employing rat kidneys showed clearly that filtered urate was completely resorbed in the early proximal tubules and that net secretion occurred in the late proximal tubule. There was no evidence for uric acid transport in more distal segments. Volume expansion decreased proximal tubular resorption and also decreased secretion. Because of this reciprocal relationship, clearance of urate cannot be used as a proximal tubule marker.

In 1975, a report described studies of hypouricemia in patients with the syndrome of inappropriate secretion of antidiuretic hormone (SIADH). In these patients, plasma urate was less than 2.0 mg/dL. When hyponatremia was corrected by water restriction, the fractional clearance of urate and plasma urate became normal. Under conditions of hyponatremia and volume expansion induced by water loading, clearance of urate nearly doubled, thus explaining hypouricemia.

Rhabdomyolysis

Our understanding of the causes and clinical implications of rhabdomyolysis has increased enormously during the past 25 years. The mechanism by which heme pigments cause acute renal failure has progressed to a much lesser extent. This particular topic will be discussed in the section on acute renal failure.

In 1969, 62 patients with posttraumatic acute renal insufficiency from the Vietnam Conflict were presented. Of interest, the causes for acute renal failure were thought to be hemorrhagic shock, sepsis, and transfusion reactions. Sixty-nine percent of these patients died from causes that today would be described as the multiple organ failure syndrome. It was interesting that the terms "rhabdomyolysis," "muscle necrosis," or "pigment-associated acute renal failure" were not mentioned in that presentation. In 1971, 47 military recruits were described, 11 of whom developed acute renal failure. Each of them had evident rhabdomyolysis. The three who died showed both myocardial and skeletal muscle necrosis. In 1975, a new culprit had arisen. A report from Los Angeles described 21 patients with nontraumatic rhabdomyolysis as a result of heroin and/or ethanol. Twenty-six additional cases were presented in 1977 that emphasized the characteristically high values for plasma uric acid concentration seen in patients with extensive rhabdomyolysis and, in addition, showed a rough correlation between uric acid levels and the extent of creatine kinase elevation. That injured muscle cells accumulated calcium was already well known. This was reemphasized in a 1978 report demonstrating new noninvasive techniques to detect muscle calcification, which included electron radiography and elevated muscle uptake of 99m technetium diphosphonate (TCDP). It was also shown that metastatic calcium deposits could be mobilized and disappear following recovery.

Interest shifted to other causes of rhabdomyolysis. In 1989, a number of patients with modest degrees of rhabdomyolysis were reported, and in these instances, there appeared to be some relationship to hyperosmolality. However, many of the patients had other conditions that are known to be causes of rhabdomyolysis, such as hypokalemia and hypophosphatemia. In 1989, there was also a report of reversible hepatic dysfunction in 25% of 119 patients with rhabdomyolysis. Of these, 34 had acute renal failure. Each of the patients had drug-related rhabdomyolysis. The fact that the liver functional abnormalities were worse in patients with acute renal failure probably speaks for more widespread tissue injury that may have occurred as a result of cytokine formation.

Older literature described numerous instances of rhabdomyolysis in patients as well as in experimental animals with potassium deficiency. In 1990, one report described 100 patients with hypokalemia, of whom 28 showed laboratory evidence of rhabdomyolysis. In the same year, a magnetic resonance spectroscopic study was described on potassium-deficient rats in an attempt to characterize metabolic abnormalities of skeletal muscle that could be responsible for rhabdomyolysis. The rats were subjected to exhaustion by swimming. The only abnormality observed was a reduction of intracellular pH in the potassium-deficient group despite coexistence of metabolic alkalosis. The intracellular acidosis was worse in the potassium-deficient rats. Of interest, the ratios of phosphocreatine to inorganic phosphate and phosphocreatine to ATP were not different in these rats. Perhaps this reflects the repeated observation that of all species, K-deficiency hardly ever causes rhabdomyolysis in the rat but does with great regularity in humans and dogs.

Disorders of Serum Sodium Concentration

Hyponatremia is one of the most common electrolyte disorders in clinical medicine. Because it is potentially fatal, it has always been a topic of great interest among nephrologists. One of the most interesting facets was the old observation that for any given reduction of sodium concentration, acute hyponatremia is potentially more serious and symptomatic than the chronic form. In 1974, studies on rabbits described some of the important adaptations undergone in the brain. Two hours after hyponatremia was induced in rabbits, they displayed seizures leading to coma. The brain water content was increased by 16%, and the brain electrolyte content (the sum of sodium, chloride, and potassium expressed as total mEq/unit of tissue dry weight) was normal. After 4 days, adaptive changes included a reduction of total brain electrolytes by 16% and a reduction in brain water. These changes would permit the cells to reduce their size compared to that during acute hyponatremia. This was one of the first studies reported involving brain cell adaptation to hyponatremia. Studies of brain adaptation to hypertonicity were also reported. In rabbits made acutely hyperglycemic with 25% glucose, brain cell potassium content rose from 404 to 440 mEq/kg dry weight within hours. When intracellular tonicity is increased, water moves into cells, thus restoring their size to normal. These two studies, the first describing the cellular adaptations to hyponatremia and the second the cellular adaptations to hypernatremia, are important because they both show a control system that is capable of modulating intracellular electrolytes in a manner such that cellular volume is regulated. In addition to cellular uptake of potassium, other major components that serve to increase intracellular osmolality include amino acids and "idiogenic" osmoles. At least in the case of hyperglycemia, a portion of the idiogenic osmoles includes metabolites of glucose.

In 1975, four patients suffering from tuberculosis and malnutrition were presented who showed findings suggesting a reset osmostat. Their extracellular volume, endocrine function, and renal function were normal. Their serum sodium varied between 126 and 131 mEq/L. Following administration of a 20-cc/kg water load, water excretion exceeded 80% in a period of 4 hours and thus was completely normal. During administration of a water load, urinary osmolality fell below 100 mosmol/kg. When supplemented with 300 mEq of sodium chloride per day, the salt was excreted quantitatively and resulted in no change in serum sodium. Water deprivation elevated urinary osmolality and elevated but did not correct plasma sodium concentration. Measurements of arginine vasopressin in plasma showed that it responded normally to changes in plasma osmolality. Treatment of the underlying disease led to correction of the serum sodium concentration. These studies corroborated those presented years before arginine vasopressin measurements were obtainable and thus suggest that severe chronic illness, for unexplained reasons, may indeed reset the hypothalamic osmostat.

In 1976, the first evidence was presented showing that demeclocycline blocked the action of antidiuretic hormone in patients with SIADH. It had already been demonstrated that lithium had this action, but its use was often associated with unacceptable complications of cognitive function. In patients with classic examples of SIADH, demeclocycline, an agent that interferes with the cellular action of antidiuretic hormone, led to complete correction of all findings. The use of this agent was prompted by the notation in the early 1960s that some patients receiving demeclocycline for infection developed polyuria and polydipsia.

For a number of years, it had been clearly appreciated that acute symptomatic hyponatremia, especially that form developing in the wake of excessive water administration to postoperative patients, responded favorably to rapid, partial correction with hypertonic saline. A number of critical issues dealing with management of acute hyponatremia and the possibility that the treatment itself may cause central pontine myelinolysis are discussed in detail in the chapters dealing with treatment of renal disease. The other interesting issue that remains is whether acute hyponatremia (or preferably acute water intoxication), even when recognized and treated appropriately, may lead to irreversible or even fatal cerebral damage in women but not in men. This issue was presented at the 1984 ASN meeting. It described previously healthy ovulatory women who became water intoxicated as a result of excessive administration of free water, usually following elective surgical procedures. Even though many of these patients improved after emergent treatment with hypertonic saline, they went on to develop neurological disability. This issue was explored further in 1987. Ten men whose prostatic bed was perfused with glycine during transurethral prostatic resection showed a fall in their serum sodium from an average of 139 to 102 mEq/L over a period of 4.5 hours. Six of the 10 developed seizures. Each was treated in a timely manner with hypertonic saline to an average serum sodium of 125 mEq/L. They all recovered without residual effects. Brain computed tomography (CT) scans were normal. In contrast, in 34 women whose serum sodium fell from 139 to 115 mEq/L within 31 hours postoperatively, elevation of serum sodium at a rate below 0.6 mEq/hour was followed by permanent brain damage or death in all patients. CT scans showed cerebral edema in all. The same investigator described studies in rabbits showing that acute hyponatremia led to greater accumulation of water in the brains of female rabbits than in male rabbits. Mortality was 86% in females and 24% in males. The male rabbits showed a lower brain sodium and potassium content than in females. The same group presented experiments in 1987 on brain synaptosomal sodium transport in normal and hyponatremic rats. The basal rates of synaptosomal sodium transport in males and females were similar. However, when the rabbits were stimulated with veratridine, sodium transport in the males was twice that of females within seconds, and sodium accumulation rose 353% in females but only 61% in males. The authors postulated that this could be the result of either increased sodium permeability in female synaptosomes or decreased capacity of sodium-potassium ATPase mediated transport. In 1989, two papers were presented from other centers that failed to show a difference in either brain water or electrolyte content between hyponatremic male and female rats.

Three papers between 1986 and 1989 described modestly severe hyponatremia in patients with AIDS. Some patients had findings typical of SIADH, others had hyponatremia due to adrenal insufficiency, and a third had hyponatremia on the basis of gastrointestinal losses in the face of continued water intake.

Several presentations dealt with the role of medications as factors responsible for the development of hyponatremia. In 1978, one report described chronic schizophrenic patients who had typical findings of SIADH. They were also medicated with fluphenazine, haloperidol, and thioridazine. Each of these drugs can stimulate inappropriate release of antidiuretic hormone. Discontinuation of the drug led to rapid reversal of hyponatremia. In 1978, another interesting paper dealt with psychotic patients who demonstrated findings compatible with a reset osmostat. Twenty patients with psychogenic polydipsia became hyponatremic while receiving fluphenazine, haloperidol, and thioridazine. Their water consumption averaged 7 to 20 liters per day. Their urine osmolality varied between 47 and 95 mosmol/kg, and their plasma osmolality ranged from 238 to 248 mosmol/kg. Under conditions of water deprivation, they increased their urine osmolality. They depressed their urinary osmolality if allowed to drink water freely. Yet, their serum osmolality was set between 245 and 246 mosmol.

Studies of patients medicated with chlorthalidone or hydrochlorothiazide who became hyponatremic were presented in 1979. Studies on these patients showed that free water clearance was reduced nearly 10-fold by either drug and that excretion of a water load of 20 cc/kg body weight over a period of 4 hours fell from 65% to 15%. It had already been appreciated that thiazide diuretics impaired formation of free water in the cortical diluting segment of the nephron. Thus, any patient medicated with thiazide diuretics who consumes sufficient water runs the risk of becoming hyponatremic.

Disorders of Renal Tubular Acidification

The pathophysiology of urinary acidification has always been a subject of interest and fascination to renal physiologists. Accordingly, numerous presentations have dealt with various forms of renal tubular acidosis (RTA).

In 1968, an important paper from San Francisco illustrated the potential potassium-wasting effects of bicarbonate treatment in patients with Fanconi syndrome. Studies on four patients showed that by restoring plasma bicarbonate to a level exceeding its maximum resorptive capacity (T_mHCO_3), the bicarbonaturia caused potassium wasting into the urine. In 1971, a paper illustrated helpful findings to identify the Fanconi syndrome in adults in the presence of chronic renal failure. Patients whose GFR values were similar with either chronic renal failure due to common causes of established Fanconi syndrome were compared. The Fanconi patients showed higher fractional clearances of calcium, phosphate, and urate and a disproportionate reduction in the tubular maximum resorptive capacity of bicarbonate. Aminoaciduria and "tubular" proteinuria were also observed. Distal tubular acidification defects were identified in two of three patients.

Evidence had been presented in 1969 that some patients with apparently classical distal tubular RTA may also show proximal defects. During bicarbonate infusions, bicarbonate appeared in the urine at filtered loads below the normal T_mHCO_3. The defect was seen in its most exaggerated form during water loading. In 1973, the first evidence was presented that urine pH in normal subjects could be reduced by a single intravenous injection of ethacrynic acid. The same response occurred in patients with distal RTA, although the minimum pH reached in the urine was not as low. One would postulate that delivery of sodium to the distal nephron would facilitate sodium:hydrogen exchange and thus acidification. If H^+ secretion occurred in the presence of bicarbonate, the resulting carbonic acid would decompose to CO_2. Thus, the urine minus blood pCO_2 gradient (U-B pCO_2) would rise. The fact that the pCO_2 difference between urine and blood did not rise after bicarbonate loading in these patients was unexplained. In 1982, two papers were presented illustrating reduction of urine pH in normal subjects following infusion of furosemide. In 1981, studies on four patients who had either persistent or intermittent hyperchloremic metabolic acidosis were reported. Each of these patients was capable of lowering urine pH below 5.3 units during metabolic acidosis induced by ammonium chloride. During bicarbonate loading, these patients were unable to generate the normal U-B pCO_2, thus implying limitation of their relative capacity to secrete hydrogen ions but no limitation in their capacity to generate a steep hydrogen ion gradient.

In 1984, a paper was presented showing that amiloride prevents reduction of urine pH by furosemide. Amiloride prevents furosemide-stimulated potassium excretion. Therefore, the effect of furosemide depends on an intact cortical collecting duct. Furosemide can be used to assess cortical collecting duct function because hydrogen and potassium secretion are sodium dependent in the cortical but not the medullary collecting duct. Therefore, inhibition of hydrogen and potassium secretion by amiloride is a cortical collecting duct event. Furosemide does not decrease urinary pH in patients with classical distal RTA, thus suggesting a defect in the cortical collecting duct. In 1987, a presentation illustrated that bumetanide, which is similar to furosemide and ethacrynic acid, is also capable of lowering urine pH from 5.4 to 4.9 in normal persons. In contrast, infusions of amiloride increase urine pH from 5.3 to 6.7 in normal subjects. These findings indicate also that bumetanide and amiloride apparently exert their action in the cortical collecting duct.

The role of sodium delivery in facilitating hydrogen exchange in the distal nephron and the importance of sodium delivery in certain patients with cirrhosis of the liver were discussed in 1970. Inability to adequately acidify the urine in patients with cirrhosis and ascites has been implicated as a primary etiological factor in the generation of ammonium intoxication. Most patients with cirrhosis and ascites have a low urine sodium concentration. Lack of sodium delivery to the distal nephron, impaired hydrogen secretion as a result, and decreased acidification of the urine impair ammonia trapping as ammonium ions. Thus, the increased ammonia production that usually prevails in the kidney in patients with cirrhosis of the liver because of potassium deficiency provides the source of ammonia destined to cause ammonia intoxication. Of course, this implies that impaired liver function prevents conversion of ammonia in the arterial blood into urea. Observations presented at that time illustrated that increased sodium delivery by means of administration of mercurial diuretics, Na_2SO_4, or mannitol facilitated sodium hydrogen exchange and reduced urinary pH to levels that would permit increased ammonium excretion into the urine. Thus, in a sense, patients with cirrhosis of the liver and ascites have a form of distal RTA.

An interesting paper was presented in 1974 concerning identification of RTA in patients with nephrolithiasis and simultaneous urinary tract infection with urea-splitting bacteria. Administration of ammonium chloride to such patients to assess urinary acidification would be futile because of alkalinization of the urine by ammonia. In these patients, administration of bicarbonate and measurement of the U-B pCO_2 difference retain its validity. In these patients, administration of sodium bicarbonate at a dosage of 2 mEq/kg increased the urine minus blood pCO_2 gradient to a normal level within 5 hours, which infers normal hydrogen secretion. In these patients, it was subsequently shown that normal acidification could be restored by successful elimination of the urea-splitting bacteria by antibiotics.

Urinary citrate excretion is sharply reduced in patients with distal RTA, and this has been implicated as one factor favoring development of nephrolithiasis and nephrocalcinosis. In a presentation in 1975, it was postulated that even in patients with incomplete distal RTA, citrate excretion should be low. Low citrate excretion would eliminate the requirement to induce metabolic acidosis with ammonium chloride to identify this disease. Six suspected cases in children showed uniformly low values for citrate excretion, and in the same patients, renal tubular acidosis was confirmed by conventional testing employing administration of ammonium chloride.

When the ASN began, the term "type IV renal tubular acidosis" was not widely employed, and many such cases were called "chronic pyelonephritis" associated with hyperchloremic metabolic acidosis. It was believed that renal ammonia synthesis and excretion of hydrogen ions were limited because of decreased renal mass. Some prominent nephrologists referred to this disease as the Willoughby-Lathem syndrome. Eventually, it was recognized that hyperkalemia reduced renal ammonia synthesis. Thus, hyperkalemia itself was at least partly responsible for inability to excrete hydrogen ions. It was soon shown that correction of hyperkalemia facilitated increased ammonia production, enhanced excretion of hydrogen as ammonium, and corrected metabolic acidosis. Such findings were responsible for a number of interesting studies and identification of several plausible mechanisms to explain the common disorder known as type IV RTA. Continued refinements in methods to differentiate abnormalities of tubular hydrogen secretion versus hydrogen-gradient defects ascribed to a back leak of secreted hydrogen ions have greatly increased our understanding of these important disorders.

Type IV renal tubular acidosis is characterized by hyperkalemic, hyperchloremic metabolic acidosis that usually occurs in the setting of mild to modest renal insufficiency in the elderly patient. It is commonly associated with diabetes mellitus in its classic form and is often precipitated by conditions that cause hyperkalemia; by medications that interfere with the production of renin, angiotensin, or aldosterone; or by medications that interfere with the action of aldosterone on the renal tubule.

It was first shown in 1977 that type IV RTA is ameliorated by administration of furosemide. In patients with classic forms of this disorder, furosemide reduced serum potassium, elevated total serum CO_2, and increased both urine potassium excretion and net acid excretion. It was also shown that furosemide stimulated ammonia production, which appeared to be inversely correlated with the reduction of hyperkalemia. A study presented in 1979 showed that adults with typical type IV RTA did not increase potassium excretion into the urine following infusions of either sodium bicarbonate or sodium sulfate. In the same patients, administration of flurohydrocortisone partially corrected the abnormality in potassium secretion. Just the opposite findings were described in 1980 in a study of apparently typical type IV RTA in patients with sickle cell hemoglobinopathy. In these patients, flurohydrocortisone did not increase potassium secretion, but one patient responded to sodium sulfate.

Phosphorus deprivation and depletion in normal human subjects usually does not lead to disturbances of acid-base balance. Although urine phosphorus excretion becomes virtually zero, thus reducing ability to excrete hydrogen ions as hydrogen phosphate buffer, kidney cells also elevate their pH and reduce ammonia production so that hydrogen ion excretion as ammonium also becomes sharply limited. Nevertheless, mobilization of bone releases carbonate ions to buffer retained hydrogen ions and thus prevents metabolic acidosis. Some investigators have reported tubular defects, including impaired hydrogen secretion in phosphorus-deficient dogs. However, in 1977, a report showed that even severe phosphate depletion in dogs had no effect on tubular hydrogen secretion as assessed by U-B pCO_2 or by means of measuring the tubular maximum resorptive capacity for bicarbonate. Another study in 1978 showed that rats made phosphorus deficient display impairment of hydrogen secretion by the tubule that resembles incomplete RTA in human patients. Thus, phosphorus-deficient rats displayed impaired reduction in pH but without evidence for decreased hydrogen ion secretion. The reduction in tubular capacity to resorb bicarbonate in the face of metabolic acidosis was apparently responsible for the inability to reduce urine pH to normal values. Urinary ammonium excretion in phosphorus-deficient rats fell, a response similar to that in phosphorus-deficient humans and dogs. Also, as in humans and in dogs, phosphorus-depleted rats do not spontaneously become acidotic, suggesting that retained hydrogen ion is buffered by bone. This is confirmed by the observation that urine calcium excretion increases in the face of phosphorus deficiency.

A number of fascinating subtypes of type IV RTA have been described at our meetings. A 1978 presentation described a patient with hyperkalemic hyperchloremic metabolic acidosis who had hypertension and normal renal function. Plasma renin activity and aldosterone excretion were very low; however both responded appropriately to sodium restriction. When the patient consumed a normal sodium diet, urinary potassium excretion was subnormal, and it responded only minimally to mineralocorticoid. If sodium delivery were increased with either sodium sulfate or sodium bicarbonate, the patient became dramatically responsive to mineralocorticoid. This response was not observed during administration of sodium chloride. The authors proposed that intrinsic potassium secretion was normal and that the major defect was an inappropriately high distal resorption of chloride, which facilitated sodium resorption electrically and resulted in an expansion of arterial volume, a reduction of plasma renin activity, and a reduction of aldosterone excretion with a net result of hypertension. The nature of this patient's illness seems to correspond to patients with Gordon's syndrome.

In 1978, studies were presented on seven boys and six girls varying between 2 and 23 months of age who presented with nonazotemic, normoreninemic, type IV renal tubular acidosis. The hyperkalemia, metabolic acidosis, and stunted growth rates were relieved by sodium bicarbonate administration. The condition spontaneously disappeared by the age of 3 to 5 years.

In 1981, a 33-year-old patient was described with hyperkalemic metabolic acidosis and hypertension. His inulin clearance was 88 mL/minute. The patient was able to acidify his urine normally. Potassium excretion during infusion of sodium sulfate or acetazolamide was below normal. Volume depletion resulted in an increase of plasma aldosterone but no change in the subnormal value for renin activity. Serum potassium concentration did not fall during an infusion of glucose or insulin. Apparently, insulin failed to induce muscle potassium uptake. The findings suggested a generalized defect in potassium transport.

An interesting paper was also presented in 1981 concerning renal hypoprostaglandinism reversed by furosemide in a patient with hypertension, hyperkalemia, and renal tubular acidosis. The patient's blood pressure was 240/140 mm Hg. Serum potassium was 8.6 mEq/L, chloride 112, and bicarbonate 14 mEq/L, respectively. Plasma volume was increased. Plasma renin activity and aldosterone excretion were both decreased. During infusion of hypertonic saline, fractional distal chloride resorption was 93.7%, as estimated by $CH_2O/CCL + CH_2O$. Urine prostaglandin E2 excretion was very low. Furosemide decreased fractional distal chloride resorption to 81% and reversed all abnormalities. This patient also appears to resemble other cases of Gordon's syndrome. Finally, another variant of this interesting syndrome was presented in a paper from France in 1984. A 22-year-old man presented with type IV RTA with hypertension, volume expansion, depressed renin activity, and *elevated* aldosterone levels in plasma (32 to 100 ng/dL). GFR was 136 mL/minute. Urine acidification was normal. Urinary ammonium excretion was below normal. Tubular maximum capacity to resorb bicarbonate was reduced. When plasma bicarbonate was elevated to a normal value, the excreted fraction in the urine was 20%. The U-B pCO_2 was normal. Acidosis disappeared following correction of hyperkalemia by administration of either a potassium-binding resin or diuretics.

Diagnostic Techniques and Methodological Advances

In 1967, the most important diagnostic tools employed in evaluating patients with renal disease included the plain film of the abdomen, intravenous pyelography, rather primitive isotopic scanning procedures of the kidneys, and renal biopsy. Ultrasonography was in its infancy.

In the 25 years that have elapsed since the beginning of the ASN, technological advances to identify the anatomy, structure, and function of the kidneys and urinary tract have progressed in a spectacular fashion. It had already been recognized that iodinated contrast media was potentially nephrotoxic in patients with multiple myeloma. Chemical relatives of these dyes were also known to be toxic when used to visualize the biliary tree under conditions of biliary obstruction whereupon the dye had no route for excretion other than the kidney. Because of the development of other techniques to visualize kidneys, the popularity of employing intravenous pyelography has fallen sharply. In fact, a number of experienced nephrologists and urologists have raised questions why we continue to employ this technique at all. In fact, at present, iodinated contrast media nephrotoxicity occurs more from extrarenal angiographic procedures than from pyelography.

Of all of the modern diagnostic tools, ultrasonography is probably the most important and practical because it is totally noninvasive; it induces no harm; it is comparatively cheap; the instrument is easily transportable; and the results are available immediately. Abnormalities of structure and function that cannot be discerned with accuracy with ultrasonography are clearly demonstrable either by computed tomography (CT scan) or even more so by magnetic resonance imaging (MRI) technology. The latter is not only important for identifying structural abnormalities of the kidney, but by exploiting its spectroscopic properties, MRI permits examination of intermediary metabolism in renal tissue. One of the most promising technologies on the horizon is the development of probes that will permit microultrasonography and Doppler flow methodology within blood vessels. It is hoped this latter procedure will greatly improve our ability to characterize renal vascular lesions as well as structural abnormalities in arterial venous shunts employed for chronic hemodialysis.

Unfortunately, very few presentations concerning novel instrumentation and diagnostic methodology have been presented at the ASN meetings. However, in 1989, a paper demonstrated enhanced images of MRI by the use of gadolinium-DTPA (diethylenetriaminepentaacetic acid). The resolution obtained by this methodology may make it possible to differentiate cortical versus medullary renal injury and, it is hoped, facilitate specific differentiation of acute tubular necrosis involving the proximal nephron as opposed to interstitial nephritis. Another presentation in 1989 dealt with H-1 nuclear magnetic resonance (NMR) spectroscopy of urine that could potentially permit a very rapid identification of substances such as methanol or ethanol and facilitate immediate treatment for acute poisoning.

Newer and simplified techniques to measure GFR have appeared on the ASN program throughout our history. In 1971, simultaneous estimates of GFR with ^{125}I-iothalamate and creatinine were compared to that of inulin. The clearance ratio of iothalamate to inulin averaged 1.09. In 1986, a study compared GFR estimated by ^{99}Tc-DTPA, ^{169}Yb-DTPA, and ^{125}I-iothalamate to inulin clearance. Once again, it was shown that each of these substances overestimates the clearance of inulin by about 8%; on the other hand, each of these isotopes is rather easy to measure, and therein lies the advantage over inulin. In 1990, an interesting paper confirmed older findings that the clearance of inulin is higher in healthy persons during the daytime than at night. However, of interest, the clearance of creatinine in about 75% of normal persons does not display diurnal variation. In the 25% without diurnal variation, the clearance is higher at night than it is in the daytime. Of further interest, it was also shown that cimetidine, which inhibits creatinine secretion by the proximal nephron, equalized the inulin creatinine: clearance ratio around the clock. Finally, in 1990 it was shown that the isotope ^{99m}Tc-mag 3 (mercaptoacetyltriglycine), which has similar kinetics to ^{131}I-hippurate, may be a satisfactory substance for renal imaging.

Even the most mundane testing procedure employed by nephrologists, examination of the urinary sediment, has undergone some interesting twists during the past 25 years. For example, the importance of eosinophils in the urine is widely recognized as an aide in the identification of interstitial nephritis. Unfortunately, eosinophils sometimes lose their staining properties. However, chances of recognizing them are improved by using Hansel's stain, as presented in 1985. In 1987, it was reported that the mean corpuscular volume of red cells ranges from 44 to 62 femtoliters (fL) in the urine of patients with glomerular hematuria. In contrast, patients with proven non-glomerular bleeding have urinary red cell mean corpuscular volume values that are within normal limits, namely 81 to 93 fL. No reason was offered for this interesting observation. In 1989, the term "acanthocyturia" was applied to the appearance of red cells seen in the urine in patients with glomerular bleeding. These cells with vesicle-shaped protrusions were seen in 82 of 105 patients with biopsy-proven glomerulonephritis and hematuria. A phase microscope must be employed to observe these changes.

Advances in Understanding of Common Renal Diseases

Nephrology has witnessed many advances during the first 25 years of the Society's life. Foremost among these have been major contributions to our understanding of two common forms of parenchymal kidney disease, namely, diabetic nephropathy and autosomal dominant polycystic kidney disease (ADPKD). It is further noteworthy that these advances have been relatively recent, a fact that is no better illustrated than by perusal of the programs of oral or poster sessions on "Clinical Nephrology" at the Society's annual meetings. For example, during the first 15 years of the Society's existence (1967 to 1982), sessions on "Clinical Nephrology" accommodated less than 10 presentations on diabetic nephropathy and less than 5 presentations on *any* form of polycystic kidney disease. The scientific programs of the next eight meetings (1983–1990) stand in sharp and dramatic contrast to those of earlier meetings. Counting only those presentations at oral or poster sessions on "Clinical Nephrology" (plus abstracts categorized as "Clinical Nephrology" but actually assigned for presentation at sessions with different headings), these most recent meetings included at least 65 to 70 presentations on both diabetic nephropathy and polycystic kidney disease. Such figures become even more impressive when one realizes that they do not include many presentations that were otherwise classified, for example, as "Renal Pathophysiology." In fact, the recent cascade of new information on these two forms of common kidney disease has been explosive since 1985.

The many recent contributions to an enhanced understanding of diabetic nephropathy are treated more fully elsewhere. In general terms, these advances have centered on much-improved understanding of important pathogenic mechanisms (with special emphasis on those of hemodynamic origin); predictors of future kidney disease (e.g., microalbuminuria); determinants or control of the rate of progression of established nephropathy; differences (or similarities) between the nature of underlying kidney disease in type I versus type II diabetes mellitus; and the development of improved approaches to the management of end-stage renal disease via dialysis or transplantation. Abstracts that were categorized and/or selected for presentation as "Clinical Nephrology" most often dealt with predictors or determinants of future nephropathy; determinants of its rate of progression and/or attempts at modification thereof; and comparative studies of the nephropathy of non-insulin-dependent versus that of insulin-dependent diabetes mellitus.

The explosive growth in our understanding of many facets of diabetic nephropathy was accompanied by a parallel and equally dramatic surge of new insights into the pathogenesis of polycystic kidney disease (PKD). The first hint that PKD was about to provide the setting for a new focus of intense research activity was perhaps afforded by a presentation in 1985. It was demonstrated that the gene for ADPKD is located on the short arm of chromosome 16 in 95% of European subjects. This important observation was confirmed in 1986. Recognition of the genetic basis for most instances of ADPKD was paralleled by a rising number of papers on its various clinical manifestations or expressions. Also in 1986, a presentation described familial clustering of associated intracranial aneurysms, a 30% incidence of associated mitral valve prolapse, and a direct relationship between altered renal structure and urinary concentrating ability. The renewal of interest in possible determinants of cellular proliferation and mechanisms of cyst development was reflected by a description of elevated levels of the C-*myc* protooncogene in an experimental model of PKD in mice.

In 1987, preliminary observations were presented on the applicability of the DNA probe described earlier to the evaluation of families with ADPKD in North America. No evidence of genetic heterogeneity was found. The same meeting included a description of the greater predilection of women for the development of associated hepatic cysts and documentation that the renal handling of urate was within normal limits in patients with ADPKD and normal renal function. A simple screening protocol was presented for the detection of ADPKD that proved to be effective in 61 of 62 patients. And, for the first time, a report described successful establishment of continuous tissue culture system from human polycystic kidney cells, thereby offering promise of a new setting for future investigation of pathogenic mechanisms.

Presentations during the 1988 annual meeting were perhaps most reflective of a renewed focus on mechanisms of cyst development. Alterations of membrane Na, K-ATPase in ADPKD epithelia were characterized, and it was suggested that epidermal growth factor is an abnormally potent mitogen for ADPKD epithelia in vitro. Others reported that the C-*myc* oncogene is a factor in the induction of renal cysts in transgenic mice. Another group of investigators provided evidence of cytokine-like substances and inhibitors in human renal cyst fluid. In another presentation, it was suggested that cyst-derived cells do not exhibit accelerated growth or other features of cellular transformation, thereby implying that an abnormal increase in the rate of cell growth may not be the cause of cyst development. A continuing cascade of clinical observations established that 50% of patients with ADPKD develop cysts before age 20 and that arterial pressure begins to rise during the second decade of life in advance of decreased renal function. It was observed by another group that the long-term outcome of kidney transplantation was no different in patients with ADPKD than in others and that a recurrence of renal cysts was not observed in the grafted kidney. Studies were also presented on the identification of antibacterial agents most useful in the treatment of infected cysts.

The scientific program of the 1989 meeting included 20 presentations on some facet of ADPKD. Heading the list were a number of presentations on various genetic relationships in such patients. On their way to cloning the gene for ADPKD, one group described their studies on the isolation of probable coding sequences from the region of chromosome 16-linked forms of ADPKD. Kinetic cRNA hybridization studies of human ADPKD concluded that a comparison of normal versus ADPKD kidneys exhibited at least 50 differentially expressed genes. In a study of genetic heterogeneity, another presentation stated that a second genetic locus may well exist but that it occurred infrequently (in no more than 2 of the 69 kindred). Another report described a new genetic marker of ADPKD (Lom 2B) on chromosome 16p close to the locus of PKD-1 that might prove to be a useful flanking marker. A family was described that did not exhibit linkage to PKD-1 at the expected distances, perhaps reflecting an alternative form of ADPKD. Observations such as these on the genetic origin of ADPKD were again accompanied by a large number of presentations on various clinical manifestations of the disorder. A study of the presymptomatic phase of ADPKD using both genetic markers and ultrasound concluded that patients with a 50/50 chance of developing the disease were unlikely to do so if ultrasound examination was negative at 30 years of age or older. It had been established that ADPKD does, in fact, begin during fetal life.

Factors relating to renal functional deterioration in ADPKD included age at diagnosis, hypertension, left ventricular mass, gender, and renal volume. It was concluded that high blood pressure is an early manifestation of the PKD-1 form of ADPKD but that the alternative genetic location on chromosome 16 (PKD-2) may be associated with a later onset of cyst development and a slower rate of clinical progression. Another presentation reported that cyst decompression surgery could effect immediate symptomatic improvement but that long-term benefit on renal function was not observed.

The 1990 annual meeting was a signature year for ADPKD in the sense that all presentations were grouped in one of two sessions entitled, "Polycystic Kidney Disease." The flow of new observations was now judged to be sufficient to justify the dedication of entire sessions to this interesting condition. Observers from one laboratory described a form of ADPKD in the rat that produced renal changes with some phenotypic similarities to human ADPKD. A large number of other presentations dealt with possible pathogenic pathways of cyst development. Suspecting that cyst formation is a function of active cellular proliferation, another group of workers examined the effect of epidermal growth factor (EGF) on membrane phospholipid in ADPKD cells and concluded that its effect resembled that observed in proliferating fetal cells. Others described "an increase in EGF receptor numbers and a translocation of the high affinity EGF receptors to the apical membranes" in cells from the early phase of ADPKD. Such changes could explain the observed increased sensitivity of ADPKD cells to epidermal growth factor. Another group described results establishing that cyst fluids from patients with ADPKD contained "potent cell growth and fluid secretory agonist(s)" capable of contributing importantly to the progressive renal enlargement of ADPKD.

In genetic and clinical studies, a kindred was described in whom ADPKD and Marfan syndrome were coexistent and in whom the genetic location of both mutations appeared to be linked on chromosome 16. In a further effort to narrow the genetic region in which the ADPKD gene might fall, others continued to identify new flanking markers with the hope of limiting the number of genes that will need to be studied in the continuing search for PDK-1. Using inulin clearance as an index of GFR, one group examined the utility of various indices of creatinine clearance as measures of filtration rate in ADPKD. All indices were unreliable markers of GFR when the serum creatinine concentration was higher than 1.5 mg/dL. Life-table analyses were performed on 174 affected members from 17 kindreds with ADPKD. It was concluded that factors associated with survival included genotype (PDK-1 versus PDK-2) and maternal versus paternal transmission. A high degree of intrafamilial variation in survival was also found. Finally, it was reported that blood pressures were higher in asymptomatic children with ADPKD from "families with more rapid progression to renal failure."

In closing, it must be emphasized that a number of additional and equally interesting observations on ADPKD have been presented at recent ASN meetings. But those cited above should at least offer some reflection on the current level of interest and excitement that surrounds the study of this condition. Among other advances, it is almost certain that the PDK-1 gene will soon be identified and cloned.

4

Dialysis

Lee W. Henderson, Karl D. Nolph, and Belding H. Scribner

A Quarter Century

In 1966–1967 when this society was founded, virtually the only avenue for scientific communication open to the dialysis community was the annual meeting of the American Society of Artificial Internal Organs (ASAIO). First, because the artificial kidney was an artificial organ, this society provided the natural venue for scientific papers on this subject. Second, through the genius of George Schreiner, the editor of ASAIO *Transactions*, the communication among investigators was both rapid and maximally informative. Not only did *The Transactions* appear within weeks after the annual meeting, but it also contained the pertinent discussion that followed each presentation.

It is, therefore, not surprising that the American Society of Nephrology (ASN) ran a poor second as a venue for communication in this field at a time of great scientific activity. For example a crisis of major proportions due to loss of sites for vascular access was avoided by the introduction of the Brescia-Cimino arteriovenous (A-V) fistula in 1966. The hemodialysis process was greatly simplified by the introduction that same year of on-line proportioning of dialysis fluid and the creation of a fully automated artificial kidney system for home use.

Despite these and other developments, the program for the first meeting of the ASN in 1967 contained only one free communication session, which covered both dialysis and transplantation, and only one paper worthy of mention.

Despite these shortcomings, the quality and size of the dialysis free communication sessions increased steadily. At present, the ASN and the National Kidney Foundation (NKF) Forum have become major venues for communication in dialysis research, providing both a fall and a spring meeting. There are several explanations as to why this change has occurred. One explanation is that some university promotions committees refused to recognize the *Transactions* of the ASAIO as a refereed publication, despite the fact that only papers selected by the program committee in a highly competitive arena were included in the publication, which also contained peer review in its best sense, namely discussion by the membership after each presentation. This policy of some promotion committees forced a number of investigators to seek another venue for presentation of their work. The ASN was the obvious answer, and the dialysis sessions evolved as outlined above and presented herewith.

These contributions are discussed in subsections that consider access to the circulation; dialysate composition and contamination; hemodialysis membrane development; topics that eventually bombed; peritoneal dialysis; chronic viral diseases in dialysis populations; anemia; iron overload, and erythropoietin; studies of dialysis populations; biocompatibility; and adequacy of dialysis.

Access to the Circulation

1968

Berne et al. from the University of Southern California gave an excellent analysis of the cause, diagnosis, and treatment of the multiple vascular lesions associated with Quinton-Scribner A-V shunts.

1971

Woodson and Shapiro from Toledo gave a paper on the important subject of the Brescia-Cimino A-V fistula. In this presentation, they described a new staple technique for reproducible surgical construction of A-V fistulas.

1975

Nash and Judy from Indianapolis described the adverse effect that high flow through A-V fistulas can have on patients with poor cardiac function.

1981

Fried from San Antonio described the very serious problems with loss of dialysis efficiency due to recirculation of blood when single-needle access is used. Spinowitz et al. stressed the importance of preventive dilation of the venous anastomosis of A-V fistulas in the prevention of clotting. They emphasized the advantage of using transluminal dilation for this purpose. Several additional papers stressing these points appeared in subsequent years.

1982

Bregman et al. from Pittsburgh found the Hickman double-lumen subclavian catheter a useful type of circulatory access, and Spinowitz et al. warned that thrombosis of the subclavian vein was a serious complication.

1985

Gersh et al. pointed out that recirculation of blood within the A-V fistula, especially Gortex® grafts, was a major cause of loss of dialysis efficiency.

1986

Guzzetta et al. described problems with excessive lower leg growth in children with femoral A-V fistulas in place. Cardiac complications also were described.

Dialysate Composition and Contamination

1969

Gordon et al. from Los Angeles introduced an ingenious device that regenerated dialysis fluid by recirculating it through a sorbent cartridge. This development led to the manufacture of a dialysis system that was very useful in remote areas where the tap water supply was unsatisfactory.

1974

Mahurker et al. from the Cook County Hospital in Chicago described a mysterious dementia and postulated deranged cerebrospinal fluid (CSF) hemodynamics as the cause. Novello et al. from Ann Arbor detected very high serum acetate levels in some patients when high-performance dialyzers were used.

1975

Alfrey et al. from Denver identified aluminum contamination in tap water as the cause of dialysis dementia in both Denver and Chicago.

1976

Graefe et al. from Seattle described several serious adverse effects of acetate intoxication during high-efficiency hemodialysis. In a carefully controlled double-blind study, they demonstrated elimination of or marked reduction in these problems on substitution of bicarbonate for acetate. In subsequent years there were many papers and symposia on the subject of acetate versus bicarbonate dialysate. Kjellstrand even argued that there was no difference. But Graefe's conclusions held up, and the issue was finally resolved from good with the introduction of high-flux–short-time hemodialysis, in which acetate could not be tolerated by any patient.

1985

Oettinger et al. from Emory University in Atlanta gave a very important paper, which has been largely ignored by the dialysis community. They demonstrated that a dialysate bicarbonate concentration of 40 mEq/L is well tolerated and usually completely corrects the chronic acidosis that persists in most chronic dialysis patients.

1989

Dalal et al. from Loyola in Chicago concluded that L-lactate was as well tolerated as bicarbonate during high-flux dialysis. If this conclusion is supported by other investigators, it could represent an important improvement in dialysis technology. It would mean return to a single concentrate system and the elimination of all the problems with sterility inherent in the use of bicarbonate.

Hemodialysis Membrane Development

1967–1971

Cellulosic membranes completely dominated the scene in this time frame, and the were configured either in tubular format as exemplified by the twin coil dialyzer or in sheet plate format as exemplified by the Kiil dialyzer. Priming volumes of 300 to 800 cc were the norm, and significant membrane compliance made extracorporeal sequestration of blood in response to ultrafiltration pressures a very real clinical concern. Available membrane area ranged between 0.5 and 2 m^2, with common clinical employment of approximately 1 m^2. The cellulosic membrane that was considered the standard of quality was Cuprophan PT150, produced by a single company in West Germany. Two landmark papers were reported at the ASN in 1971 (Gotch et al. from San Francisco and Roth et al. of Milwaukee), both employing capillary hollow-fiber dialyzers that were the product of Dow Chemical Corporation. The collaboration between industry and the academic world was well exemplified in this development process. It should be noted that hollow-fiber dialyzers had been under development and reported elsewhere prior to the 1971 report at the ASN meeting. These hollow-fiber devices had a prime volume of 80 to 100 mL for 1 m^2 in area and were made of cellulose acetate. The compliance of the blood path to increased pressure was virtually absent when compared with the coil or sheet plate dialyzers in common use. Compared with Cuprophan PT150, the cellulose triacetate fibers were more open both hydraulically and to solute transport, a point that was not lost on either Gotch or Roth, who identified that inulin (5200 daltons)-sized molecules traversed their membrane three to six times more swiftly than across Cuprophan PT150. Hollow-fiber format now virtually dominates the membrane market for hemodialyzers, and this technical innovation has been applied to virtually every membrane formulation available, such as Cuprophan polyacrylonitrile, polysulfone, polyamide, polycarbonate, and polymethylmethacrylate.

In this program year, hemodialysis employed the principle of diffusion for solute removal, and the limited amount of ultrafiltration performed served only to correct patient fluid balance.

1977

Three papers were reported in this program year (Johnson et al. from Rochester, Baldamus et al. from Frankfurt, and Sanfelippo et al. from San Diego) on a technique based on the convective transport of solute. Hemofiltration had been reported previously elsewhere, and these preliminary clinical observations resulted from the funding by the National Institutes of Health (NIH) Artificial Kidney Chronic Uremia Program of the development of this novel solute clearance method. Crucial to the ability to perform hemofiltration was the availability of membranes with a hydraulic permeability of ten or more times that currently available with Cuprophan PT150. Membranes with this high hydraulic permeability required special fluid-cycling equipment in order to control fluid balance in a way that had not heretofore been required with lower hydraulic permeability membranes. The rationale underlying this work was the fact that the natural glomerulus easily passes molecules in the range between 500 and several thousand daltons (middle molecules), whereas standard diffusive dialysis cannot remove significant amounts of these middle molecules, some of which might be toxic.

1986–1989

Information on membrane development during this time did not appear as direct reports to the ASN program. The design and use of more open membranes for hemodialysis, hemofiltration, continuous arterial venous hemofiltration, and other such techniques that depend on novel membrane design again have largely appeared elsewhere.

Controversy as to what constitutes adequate dialysis and its representation in the ASN program will be discussed in the last section, and the impact that membranes and choice of procedure have on adequacy will be touched on there.

Topics That Eventually Bombed

1967

It is of interest that of the five papers on dialysis that were presented at that first meeting at the Los Angeles Biltmore Hotel, two were on techniques that either had bombed already or soon did so. These topics were (*1*) lipid dialysis, a very messy procedure in which oil is substituted for dialysis fluid to try and enhance the removal of lipid-soluble overdose toxins such as glutethimide, and (*2*) dialysis through an isolated loop of intestine.

1969

A paper entitled "Lipid Dialysis for Glutethimide, Secobarbital and Phenobarbital" was presented. Only two more papers were presented in 1971.

1978

Nissenson and colleagues from Los Angeles, in a carefully controlled and costly double-blind study, finally discounted the claim that psoriasis is helped by hemodialysis. The first paper that purported to have devised a stable single concentrate of dialysate containing bicarbonate was presented. Subsequently, nothing ever materialized. Similar papers have appeared periodically, but nothing has materialized.

1979

The first of several papers describing carbon-coated transcutaneous access devices was presented. These devices, although they had enormous appeal, actually combined the worst features of the shunt and the fistula. Although there were several more presentations in subsequent years, these devices never gained acceptance and now have been abandoned.

1980

Can you imagine what it would have been like to have had 1 million or more schizophrenics on hemodialysis? Well it might have happened. Here is the story. During the 1970s, Cade from Gainesville, Florida, and Wagemaker from Louisville, Kentucky, had presented convincing evidence at the ASAIO that hemodialysis had a remarkably beneficial effect on schizophrenia. These claims were strongly supported by Kolff, who had visited Louisville to see for himself, and by a biochemist from Berkeley, who claimed to have isolated an endorphin that dialysis was removing from Wagemaker's patients. The NIH provided several hundred thousand dollars in grant support for controlled double-blind studies to try and settle this enormously important question. One of us (BHS) was on the study section that visited Wagemaker. We were duly impressed by the sequential videos and the patients presented. Wagemaker's application for grant support was approved. Our group in Seattle and Balow and his colleagues at the NIH also were given similar grants. Balow presented his negative results at our 1980 meeting, and I would guess that few in the audience realized how very important the paper was. A negative study from one of the author's (BHS) institutions was never published. When the psychiatrists eventually realized that the results were negative, despite early apparent success, they lost interest and never wrote up this exhausting investigation. (It is difficult to hemodialyze schizophrenics in a double-blind setting, see Figure 4.1.)

Peritoneal Dialysis

1967

In 1967, peritoneal dialysis was used primarily in patients with acute renal failure. Hypertonic solutions containing 7% dextrose were used to induce ultrafiltration. Nolph and Henderson presented the only peritoneal dialysis paper on the program at the first ASN meeting. They reported increased solute clearances, not only during the use of these very hypertonic exchanges (presumably primarily due to convection) but also with a series of 1.5% dextrose exchanges following exposure to the hypertonic solutions as compared to prehypertonic control values, also with 1.5% dextrose solutions. They postulated an effect of hypertonicity on membrane transport characteristics. In this paper, the concept of peritoneal dialysance (now usually termed the mass-transfer area coefficient) was introduced as a modification of

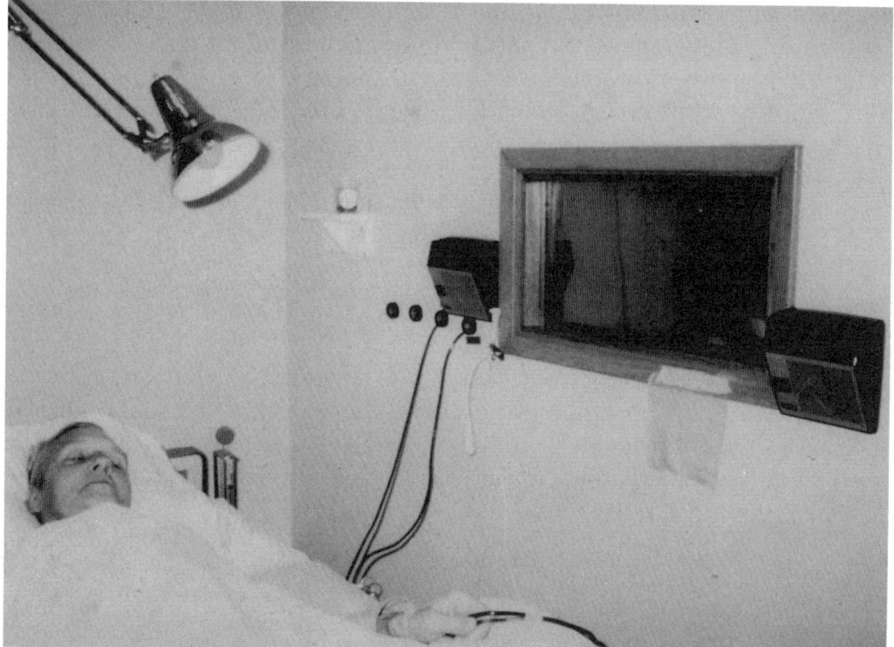

Figure 4.1. A patient being hemodialyzed in a double-blind setting. Note the blood lines passing through the holes in the wall. The window provides a one-way view into the patient area from the dialysis area on the other side of the wall. The two-way speakers facilitate communication between the two areas.

clearances that depended more on membrane area and/or permeability than on dialysis solution flow rate. These very hypertonic exchanges were later removed from clinical use because of problems of hyperglycemia with consecutive hypertonic exchanges and excessive ultrafiltration.

1968

Tenckhoff and Schechter presented the only peritoneal dialysis paper at the 1968 meeting, reporting on their experiences with peritoneal self-dialysis in the home. This presentation introduced the Tenckhoff catheter. Experiences with 10 patients who dialyzed themselves at home two or three times weekly with a closed automatic dialysis system were described. This was the era of chronic intermittent peritoneal dialysis, and this paper described its early days.

1973

At the 1973 meeting, experiences treating 75 patients in Seattle with chronic intermittent peritoneal dialysis for periods of 3 to 60 months were described. Patient well-being and rehabilitation were considered comparable to hemodialysis results. The patients used Tenckhoff catheters and automated peritoneal dialysis equipment; 80% did home peritoneal dialysis. An optimistic future for chronic peritoneal dialysis was predicted.

Shapiro and a group from UCLA studied the absorption of intraperitoneally administered insulin to dogs undergoing peritoneal dialysis. They warned of delayed absorption causing hypoglycemia when peritoneal dialysis is discontinued.

1976

In 1976, the group from Toronto documented an epidemic of aseptic peritonitis in patients undergoing chronic intermittent peritoneal dialysis. Solutions were shown to be contaminated with endotoxin. This was an important landmark because it highlighted the fact that peritonitis could not always be assumed to be infectious in origin.

1977

At the 1977 meeting, Popovich, Moncrief, and Nolph described clinical experiences with continuous ambulatory peritoneal dialysis (CAPD). Moncrief and Popovich began using CAPD therapy in patients in 1975 and submitted to first results with this new therapy to the American Society for Artificial Internal Organs in 1976. Their abstract was not selected for the program. Collaborative studies began with Nolph in early 1977 and were reported to the American Society of Nephrology that same year. This presentation took place at the first free communications session at the ASN ever devoted solely to peritoneal dialysis. Among the many papers in this session, the UCLA group documented the losses of serum proteins during maintenance peritoneal dialysis. Dr. Oreopoulos chaired this peritoneal dialysis session at the 1977 meeting and the next spring reported his new technique of CAPD using solutions in bags to the American Society for Artificial Internal Organs.

1978

In 1978 at a joint session of the Clinical Dialysis and Transplant Forum and the ASN, Oreopoulos and his colleagues in Toronto described their first year's experience with CAPD using their new technique with solutions in plastic bags. The technique was much less cumbersome and was associated with a lower peritonitis rate than had been observed using bottled solutions in the United States. Solutions in bags were approved for use in the United States approximately 1 year later, in late 1979.

During one of the free communication sessions at the 1978 ASN meeting, Blumenkrantz and the UCLA group described peritoneal clearances in 26 patients treated with chronic intermittent peritoneal dialysis for 1 to 38 months using indwelling chronic catheters and automated peritoneal dialysis machines. They found no differences in the peritoneal clearances of adult diabetic patients compared to nondiabetic patients of comparable age. They also noted no deterioration in the peritoneal transport characteristics over time in the total patient population.

1979

In 1979, Blumenkrantz and the UCLA group described glucose absorption during CAPD. Long-term effects of glucose absorption on appetite, total nutritional status, and hyperlipidemia are still under study today. At the 1979 meeting, The UCLA group also reported on metabolic balance studies in patients undergoing CAPD. They noted that protein losses in dialysate may alter nitrogen metabolism and reduce urea generation.

1980

At the 1980 meeting in a joint session with the Clinical Dialysis and Transplantation Forum, Diaz-Buxo described experiences with a hybrid of CAPD called continuous cyclic peritoneal dialysis (CCPD). Diaz-Buxo in North Carolina and Wadi Suki in Texas were the early pioneers in exploring the use of CCPD. The daytime freedom from manual exchanges was popular with some patients, especially with parents conducting peritoneal dialysis in children.

Also in 1980, there was an additional report on nitrogen balance studies in CAPD patients from Brzostowicz and the group at San Francisco. Kopple and the UCLA group also reported on studies of amino acid losses during CAPD. Delmez and his colleagues in St. Louis reported on the effects of CAPD on parathyroid hormone (PTH) and mineral metabolism. They noted that significant amounts of PTH were removed in drainage, that normal serum 25-$(OH)D_3$ levels were maintained despite large protein losses, and that substantial amounts of phosphorus were removed but not to the extent that precluded use of phosphorus binders. They recommended use of dialysis solutions containing higher calcium (to promote a more positive calcium balance) and lower magnesium concentrations (to promote better removal).

1981

In 1981, Williams and his colleagues from Toronto reported a discrepancy between changes in total body nitrogen and total body potassium in a

CAPD population. Many patients appeared to lose total body nitrogen in spite of what appeared to be adequate caloric and protein intakes; this was not associated with a decrease in total body potassium.

In the same year, Twardowski and colleagues from Missouri reported that sustained ultrafiltration could be produced during long-dwell exchanges in rats with dialysis solutions containing polyacrylate as the osmotic agent. Eventually, this particular polymer was shown to be toxic to the peritoneal membrane, but this presentation stimulated much of the polymer research that followed.

Teitelbaum and colleagues in St. Louis described the effects of CAPD on bone histomorphology. They found that, as with hemodialysis, worsening or improvement of osteitis fibrosa cystica was related to serum levels of parathyroid hormone. Osteomalacia did not progress during CAPD and, in some cases, improved.

Madden and the group from Wisconsin reported favorable results with intraperitoneal insulin for diabetics on CAPD. Falk and colleagues from Chapel Hill, North Carolina, showed that the addition of deferoxamine to dialysis solution was a simple and effective method for iron removal. Diaz-Buxo described stable peritoneal clearances in 10 patients on chronic peritoneal dialysis from 26 to 71 months.

Salusky and the group from UCLA described the nutritional status of

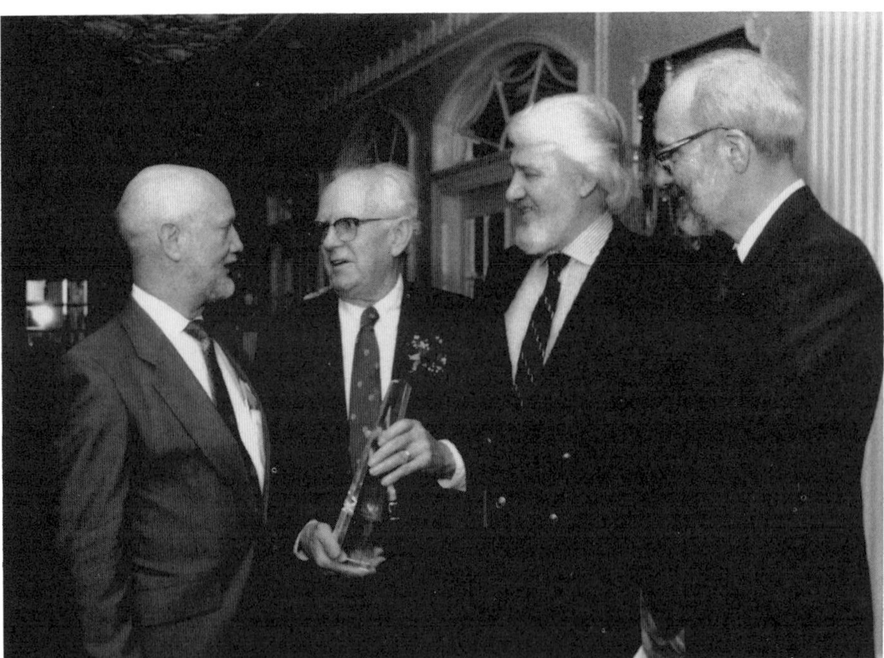

Figure 4.2. Recipients of the American Kidney Fund Torchbearer Award pictured at the 1991 award dinner in Nashville, Tennessee. From left: Jack W. Moncreif, Belding Scribner, Robert Popovich, Karl Nolph.

pediatric patients undergoing CAPD. Many of the children were growth retarded and malnourished, and the need for long-term studies to determine whether an increase in energy intake will improve growth in children undergoing CAPD was emphasized. The importance of adequate energy and protein intakes in children has received increasing emphasis since this presentation was included in a special seminar on this topic at the 10th Annual Peritoneal Dialysis Conference in Dallas in 1990.

At a joint session of the Clinical Dialysis and Transplant Forum, Raja and colleagues from Philadelphia described the enhanced glucose absorption and loss of ultrafiltration during acute peritonitis episodes.

1982

Verger and colleagues in Columbia, Missouri, showed that with peritonitis in a rat model of peritoneal dialysis, rapid glucose absorption was associated with mesothelial denudation and interstitial changes. A technique for damaging the mesothelium by dry heat exposure without inducing inflammatory interstitial changes also was associated with rapid glucose absorption. The importance of the mesothelial barrier was suggested.

At a joint session of the Clinical Dialysis and Transplant Forum, 4 years of CAPD experience in Toronto were summarized. Experiences with peritoneal dialysis in children were reported from Denver.

Keane and colleagues in Minneapolis reported on some of the early studies with the phagocytic function of human peritoneal macrophages. This paper helped to stimulate interest in interperitoneal host defenses.

A special session on CAPD moderated by Kopple focused on comparisons of CAPD and hemodialysis, nutritional requirements in CAPD, and disturbances in lipid metabolism in CAPD.

1983

At a slide forum on peritoneal dialysis, the first 5-year experience with CAPD at four institutions in Toronto was presented. Over the period from 1977 to 1983, 508 patients completed CAPD training. The cumulative patient survival was 94%, 82%, 72%, and 65% at 1, 2, 3, and 4 years, respectively. Peritonitis accounted for 42.6% of CAPD failures. Cardiovascular disease accounted for 42.7% of deaths. The overall peritonitis rate was one episode per 11.1 treatment months.

A report from the University of Wisconsin compared 37 diabetics started on hemodialysis and 34 diabetics started on CAPD between January 1978 and July 1983. Three-year patient survivals were 40% and 81% in the hemodialysis and CAPD groups, respectively. Hemodialysis patients had fewer initial hospital days but more follow-up hospital days.

Wells and colleagues from Omaha noted the tendency for the risk of atherosclerosis (as assessed by lipid profile) to increase with time on CAPD.

Wu and colleagues from Toronto noted two types of ultrafiltration failure in CAPD patients. These included (*1*) rapid absorption of glucose causing rapid dissipation of the osmotic gradient and (*2*) decreased glucose solute and water movement because of loss of peritoneal surface area and/or permeability.

1984

An entire slide forum was focused on peritoneal dialysis with an emphasis on loss of ultrafiltration. Great concern had developed over reports of ultrafiltration failure and the development of encapsulating peritoneal sclerosis in patients in France using solutions containing acetate as the buffer. In this session, Kwong and colleagues from Toronto found more rapid rates of glucose absorption in acute studies in rabbits with acetate solutions than with lactate solutions. Nielsen and the group from Columbia, Missouri, reported the results of studies in rats using acetate or lactate solutions for simulated CAPD over 3-month periods. At the end of the studies, four of seven rats in the group dialyzed with acetate were found to have sclerosing encapsulating peritonitis. No rat in the lactate group showed any gross pathology. Rats in the acetate group showed marked disruption of the normal mesothelial architecture by light microscopy. Acetate solutions were also found to be associated with protracted infections. Following these reports, other clinical studies continued to show the association of acetate-buffered solutions with ultrafiltration failure. A precise cause-and-effect relationship has never been established.

In studies of D-lactate and L-lactate balance in intermittent peritoneal dialysis, Richardson and Roscoe in Toronto showed that both isomers contribute equally to alkali gain.

Schilling and colleagues from Toronto reported on the nutritional status of patients on long-term CAPD. The authors suggested that total body nitrogen measurements are a better index of nutritional status than total body potassium. They also concluded that on a daily protein intake of 0.9 g/kg body weight (BW) for women and 1.0 g/kg BW for men, most patients will lose body nitrogen and equilibrate at a lower level. A higher protein intake was recommended. The question as to how much protein intake CAPD patients need is still under debate.

The group from UCLA found that aluminum removal was markedly augmented in CAPD patients by intravenous (IV) or intraperitoneal (IP) DFO administration. The effect of desferoxamine (DFO) persisted for several days after one dose. At comparable levels of serum aluminum, they achieved greater removal rates with CAPD than with hemodialysis.

At a joint session on peritoneal dialysis with the NKF, catch-up and normal growth were reported in infants receiving chronic peritoneal dialysis in combination with nasal gastric tube feedings. This report from Brewer and colleagues from Salt Lake City was an early report in what has evolved into a very active area. At the 10th Annual Peritoneal Dialysis Conference in Dallas, a special seminar was devoted to this subject.

Also, at this same joint session, Dasgupta and his coauthors from Alberta described biofilm-protected adherent bacterial microcolonies in Tenckhoff catheters. An equal prevalence of bacterial microcolonies were found attached to the surfaces of catheters whether or not the patient had had peritonitis. Since this 1985 report, this topic has received a great deal of attention. The clinical significance of the biofilm, particularly as it relates to the development of peritonitis, remains elusive.

Gallimore and associates from Montreal provided evidence in a mouse model that following the introduction of *Staphylococcus epidermidis*, the catheter biofilm is a probable site of protracted bacterial growth.

Mackow and colleagues from Georgetown reported the induction of sclerosing encapsulating peritonitis in rats with intraperitoneal chlorhexadine. These studies complimented clinical reports from Scotland associating an outbreak of sclerosing encapsulating peritonitis with a connector device that used chlorhexadine.

Twardowski and associates from Missouri summarized experiences with 83 Tenckhoff catheters, suggesting that exit-site infections are reduced and more responsive to treatment when subcutaneous tunnels are directed downward at the skin exit site. Catheter migrations seem less likely if the tunnel is directed downward at the abdominal cavity catheter entrance site. Rather than bend the Tenckhoff catheters to create an arcuate subcutaneous tunnel with ends pointing in the caudal direction, the authors suggested the need for a "swan neck" catheter permanently bent between cuffs to eliminate resilient forces and to avoid cuff extrusion while also minimizing exit site infections and migration. Since 1985, clinical experiences with permanently bent "swan neck" catheters support their clinical superiority.

Leypoldt and associates from San Diego proposed a dual-barrier model of peritoneal transport. They suggested that different barriers control convective and diffusive solute transport from blood to dialysate. Many analyses have emerged since this report supporting the concept of different barriers or different types of pores in the peritoneal membrane system.

Hirszel and his group from Bethesda, Maryland, noted that the clearances of high-molecular-weight dextrans from the peritoneal cavity were higher than the corresponding clearances from blood into the peritoneal cavity. They proposed that influx might proceed through more porous channels. Today we suspect that they were seeing absorption taking place through the very permeable lymphatic system mainly located on the subsurface of the diaphragm.

Nolph summarized the experiences with the Untied States NIH CAPD Registry from 1981 through 1985. This presentation reflected the interest of the ASN in monitoring the growth and development of this therapy.

1986

Mactier and colleagues from Columbia, Missouri, reported lymphatic absorption rates in 10 patients on CAPD during 4-hour exchanges with 2.5% dextrose dialysis solutions. The absorption was estimated by instilling albumin in the dialysis solutions and monitoring the albumin clearance from the peritoneal cavity. Lymphatic absorption averaged 89.6 mL/hour; the authors estimated that this rate could potentially reduce daily net ultrafiltration rate by 83%. Using similar techniques, the same group reported on the kinetics of peritoneal ultrafiltration in rats and found that lymphatic absorption, as assessed by albumin kinetics, had profound effects on net ultrafiltration.

Rubin and associates from Mississippi described disruption of stagnant fluid films in a rat model of peritoneal dialysis by vibrating the animals. This study emphasized the importance of stagnant fluid films in limiting peritoneal dialysis efficiency. No practical consistent way for disrupting these films in the clinical setting has evolved. Total-body vibration or shaking would not seem acceptable to most patients.

The Missouri group described experiences with tidal peritoneal dialysis. With this technique, a constant reserve volume of dialysis solution is left in the peritoneal cavity, on top of which a tidal volume is cycled. This increases fluid membrane contact throughout the procedure and enhances clearances. This is similar to the older technique of reciprocating peritoneal dialysis, but with that technique, high circulating volumes were reconstituted in an extracorporeal dialysis system. Tidal peritoneal dialysis uses prepared solutions in a single pass. Since this report, additional enthusiasm for tidal peritoneal dialysis as a more efficient cycler therapy has emerged.

1987

Based on a study by Ahrens and associates at the University of Wisconsin, CAPD patients with *Staphylococcus aureus* nasal carriage had significantly more exit-site infections than noncarrier CAPD patients (one episode per 13.6 patient months versus one episode per 50.6 patient months). Also, exit-site infections caused by *S. aureus* were more frequent in the nasal carriers of this organism. The role of nasal carriage of organisms and the importance of prevention thereof continue to receive attention.

Bell and colleagues from San Diego compared osmotically driven convective transport with hydraulically driven convective transport during peritoneal dialysis in rabbits. Sieving coefficients for a number of test solutes were less than one for all solutes tested with both hydraulically and osmotically driven convective transport. The authors thought these findings challenged the simple heterosporosity model of peritoneal transport, which is an attempt to explain open diffusive transport characteristics in association with tight osmotically driven convective transport. Definitive explanations for the sieving characteristics of the peritoneal membrane are still lacking after over 20 years of study.

Bargman and the group from Toronto administered 1–25-I-Human EPO (erythropoietin) into the peritoneal cavity of rabbits with and without dialysis solution. They observed that EPO is almost completely absorbed from the empty peritoneal cavity and is less efficiently absorbed when diluted in peritoneal dialysis solution. This study helped to stimulate the interest in subcutaneous administration of EPO to CAPD patients that has evolved in recent years.

Investigators from Baxter Laboratories, Deerfield, Ill. demonstrated synthesis of phosphatidylcholine by rat mesentery during in vitro incubation of tissue. Synthesis rates were equivalent to those of lung tissue from the rat. The production of phosphatidylcholine, a known surface active agent, by peritoneum was proposed to have important implications for the physiology of peritoneal dialysis. Studies have followed from numerous centers suggesting effects of phosphatidylcholine on peritoneal transport and membrane integrity.

1988

Churchill presented the results of a Canadian CAPD Clinical Trial Group study that examined the rates of peritonitis in a prospective randomized trial of Y-set connectors versus standard systems. Sixty-one new CAPD patients were allocated to the Y-set and 63 to the standard system in patients from eight CAPD programs in six Canadian cities. The peritonitis rate in patients on the Y-set was 1 every 21.5 patient months, and the peritonitis rate in patients on the standard system was 1 every 9.9 patient months. This careful study has a very important effect on confirming results from previous studies in Europe.

Okamoto and associates from San Diego showed that abdominal compression in rabbits leads to a fall in fluid absorption despite increased intraperitoneal pressure. The authors suggested that the effect was due to decreases in absorption into adjacent tissues rather than changes in lymphatic flow rate.

A report from Mexico City documented recovery of human immunodeficiency virus (HIV) Ag in dialysis fluid from two of three patients with positive serum HIV antibody. They concluded that the dialysis fluid of HIV-infected patients may contain the antigen and is therefore potentially infective.

Recombinant human growth hormone was instilled into the peritoneal cavity of six children undergoing continuous cyclic peritoneal dialysis at UCLA. Their data suggested that daily intraperitoneal growth hormone administration is a feasible approach to improve the growth velocity of children undergoing peritoneal dialysis. Long-term clinical studies have been initiated.

Flessner and colleagues at NIH studied the simultaneous bidirectional transport of monoclonal antibody between blood and the peritoneal cavity in rats. Of interest was the observation that 50 to 60% of the antibody absorbed from the peritoneal cavity was found in local tissues, with highest concentrations in the diaphragm and anterior abdominal wall. This group has emphasized here and elsewhere the importance of the movement of large-molecular-weight substances into abdominal wall tissues in the overall process of net absorption.

In rabbit studies, Fox and colleagues from San Diego concluded that the contribution of visceral peritoneum to peritoneal dialysis transport is small and that improved solute exchange following evisceration probably reflects improved dialysate-parietal peritoneum contact.

Studies from Cardiff, Wales, reported that the half-life of intravenous EPO in CAPD patients is similar to that reported for hemodialysis patients.

Floege summarized the results of several studies in Europe that looked at the possibility of tumor necrosis factor production in the peritoneal cavity of CAPD patients. Dialysate/plasma concentrations of tumor necrosis factor were near unity despite their relatively high molecular weight. This suggested local production.

Oreopoulos reported a multicenter collaborative study from North America and Europe. The nutritional status of 224 CAPD patients from six centers had been assessed. Of these patients, based on scientific criteria, 8% of patients were severely malnourished, 32.5% mildly malnourished, and 59.4% normal.

1989

Nolph and colleagues from Columbia, Missouri, compared tidal peritoneal dialysis in patients using an all L-lactate solution with dialysis using a solution containing a racemic mixture of D- and L-lactate. Absorption and metabolic rates for both isomers were found to be similar. Rates of metabolism kept up with rapid absorption rates, with the result that serum concentrations did not change significantly from control levels. The authors conclude that either type of solution is suitable for tidal peritoneal dialysis.

Zimmerman and the group from Wisconsin described a randomized controlled trial of prophylactic rifampin for peritoneal dialysis catheter-related infections and peritonitis. Baseline nasal or exit-site colonization with *S. aureus* was an independent risk factor, but rifampin decreased exit-site infections in both colonized and noncolonized patients. The catheter-related infection rate was 0.25 episodes per patient year in the rifampin group and 0.94 episodes per patient year in controls. Peritonitis rates were similar.

Chronic Viral Diseases in Dialysis Populations

1983

One of the first experiences with hemodialysis in patients with acquired immune deficiency syndrome (AIDS) was described at a joint session with the NKF in 1983. This report came from the group at Downstate Medical Center in Brooklyn. This group has continued to expand our knowledge about the problems of dialysis in HIV-positive patients and about the entity of AIDS nephropathy.

1984

From Suny at Buffalo, Cunningham and associates evaluated responses to hepatitis B vaccine in 111 hemodialysis patients. A total of 42 patients received three doses, and 18 responded by developing antibodies. Compared to the incidence of response in the dialysis unit employees, the hepatitis B vaccine appeared to be much less effective in hemodialysis patients (42% versus 92% conversion rate).

Aronoff and associates from Indianapolis presented a randomized double-blind controlled clinical trial of hepatitis B vaccine in 24 hemodialysis patients that evaluated the response to varying doses. A control group was also studied. Nonuremic subjects seroconverted more frequently than did either of the dialysis patient groups. Doubling the doses of the vaccine did not improve the response of the dialysis patients. The authors concluded that reducing the dose of the vaccine to half the recommended one did not decrease the response and did reduce cost.

1986

Arnow and colleagues from the University of Chicago undertook screening for human immunodeficiency virus (HIV) antigen and envelope and core antibodies using commercial enzyme immunoassay kits. Six patients had a positive assay for antigen, all of low reactivity, and none was positive for core or envelope antibody. They did not have clinical or T-cell studies suggesting AIDS infection. The authors considered the six patients to have false-positive results and warned that the frequency of false-positive screening in hemodialysis patients may be high.

1987

Ortiz and associates from Miami screened 81 chronic hemodialysis patients for HIV antibodies twice over a 2-year period. Nine patients were positive on the initial testing by both the enzyme-linked immunosorbent assay (ELISA) and Western blot, 2 were false positive (positive ELISA, negative Western blot), and 70 were negative. At follow-up 2 years later, five of these patients had died (two of AIDS) and four were alive. Only one seroconversion was documented in the 45 HIV-negative patients retested 2 years later. This patient was a Haitian woman who had received several blood transfusions. The authors concluded that the incidence of HIV infection in their dialysis population was very high; nevertheless, they found no evidence that the infection is highly transmittable in the dialysis unit.

1988

During the 1988 meeting, an entire free communication session was focused on AIDS and the nephrologist. The group from Brooklyn concluded that nosocomial transmission of HIV in a hemodialysis unit employing Centers for Disease Control (CDC) AIDS guidelines is unlikely. In all of the 27 positive patients, a known risk factor for HIV could be identified. No patient without a recognized risk factor for HIV infection initially was or subsequently became seropositive. Twenty-four of 25 staff members were tested, and all were found to be seronegative for HIV even though they were caring for 27 HIV-positive patients.

From the CDC in Atlanta, results from a multicenter study to estimate the prevalence and incidence of HIV antibody in chronic hemodialysis patients were reported. The seroprevalence rate in hemodialysis patients in the study was 0.77%. This represents 10 of 1291 patients tested who were positive to both ELISA and Western blot. All 10 infected patients had recognized risk factors for HIV infection.

Ortiz screened hemodialysis patients in Miami. Blood transfusion seemed a likely way of contamination for HTLV-1 in their population.

1989

Perez and colleagues from Miami assessed the prevalence of non-A, non-B hepatitis infection in two chronic hemodialysis units by testing sera from 92 patients and 35 staff using a recently developed assay for antibodies to hepatitis C virus. In the patients, 12% were positive for C antibodies, and of the 12%, 73% had antibodies to hepatitis B and 27% had antibodies to HIV as well. All staff members were negative. They concluded that hepatitis C is prevalent in hemodialysis units and is often associated with hepatitis B infection.

Complete seroconversion after intradermal administration of recombinant hepatitis B vaccine in hemodialysis patients was reported from Japan in a joint session with the NKF.

Hemodialysis patients with nasal carriage of *S. aureus* were treated intranasally with an ointment containing pseudomonic acid. The studies were conducted in Heidelberg, Germany. In 55 carriers, patients were randomized to receive placebo ointment or the antibacterial ointment. After 3 weeks, 50% of those treated with the antibacterial substance showed elimination of *S. aureus* on mucosa and skin. The authors state that longer studies will be needed to see if the overall incidence of *S. aureus* infections is reduced.

Anemia, Iron Overload, and Erythropoietin (EPO)

1969

By noting a fall of 45 to 55% in the hematocrit following bilateral nephrectomy in six hemodialysis patients, Goodwin et al. from Brooklyn made the important point that the renal remnants produced some erythropoietin, even though it was not detectable by their assay.

1976

The problem of detecting iron deficiency in hemodialysis patients was solved when Sarles and Remmers from Galveston and Rosen's group from the University of California, Irvine, independently reported an excellent correlation between serum ferritin levels and bone marrow iron stores.

1979

Ali et al. described the problem of severe iron overload. On the basis of autopsy findings in 45 hemodialysis patients, gross iron deposits were found in the liver and spleen in about half the patients. These findings correlated with markedly elevated serum ferritin levels.

1982

Eschbach and his associates from Seattle reported a study on uremic sheep maintained on hemodialysis, which was no small accomplishment, since sheep are much more difficult to dialyze than their human uremic counterparts. Eschbach et al. demonstrated that the anemia of these uremic sheep had a highly significant response to sheep erythropoietin, which was harvested from the serum of severely anemic sheep. This important observation proved that lack of the hormone rather than uremic blocking agents or lack of marrow responsiveness was responsible for the anemia of uremia. The work provided the stimulus for industry to try to synthesize human erythropoietin using genetic technology, a project that was to prove to be enormously successful.

1983

Fosburg and his colleagues from Harvard demonstrated that desferrioxamine could safely and effectively remove sufficient iron from hemodialysis patients to stabilize the overload. This problem was soon to be eliminated by the introduction of EPO.

1987

This was the year that EPO burst on the scene in dramatic fashion. The main event was a massive poster/discussion session chaired by Eschbach, who presented the results of the national multicenter study. In addition, there were posters and papers from numerous investigators on all aspects of the subject. The main conclusion was that curing the anemia had a much greater than expected effect on patient well-being, suggesting that uremia and anemia have a deleterious effect on well-being that is synergistic. One paper of particular significance was the report of Robertson et al. from Seattle that whereas the exercise tolerance was improved with the rising hematocrit, the limiting factor in hemodialysis patients was muscle dysfunction and not cardiac output as in normal individuals. Bergstrom had reported from Stockholm earlier that hemodialysis of normal individuals causes muscle catabolism, which can be prevented by dialyzing with biocompatible membranes. The implication of these two observations is that long-term hemodialysis patients may have sustained damage to their skeletal muscles that can be prevented in the future by the use of biocompatible membranes.

1988

Again, papers about EPO were too numerous to cover here. Sargent's group from San Francisco concluded that elevating the hematocrit (Hct) from the 20 range to the 35 range had no significant adverse effect on dialyzer performance. On the other hand, Bosch et al. from George Washington concluded that clearance was inversely proportional to Hct, while Besarab et al. found a significant change in phosphate clearance only. Following treatment of the anemia with EPO, Schaefer et al. from Wurtzburg reported improved sexual function in both sexes and found a marked fall in serum prolactin, while the Seattle group noted a rise in testosterone following treatment of the anemia with EPO.

1989

EPO again dominated the presentations. Now, however, the emphasis had shifted to dosage formats and routes of administration. This emphasis resulted in part from the very restrictive Medicare regulations that mandated administration IV in the center using a fixed dose. Hence, different dosage schedules and routes of administration such as subcutaneous and intramuscular were tried. Ways were also devised to let home dialysis patients administer the hormone at home, especially intraperitoneally for CAPD patients. Although results were encouraging, definite conclusions were premature.

Studies of Dialysis Populations

1971

Compty and Shapiro from Minneapolis summarized experiences with 20 patients with diabetic nephropathy treated for a total of 242 patient treatment months by chronic hemodialysis over a 4-year period. Rehabilitation was considered extremely poor compared to that in nondiabetics in the same age groups and was related primarily to the high incidence of blindness (43%). There was a 37.5% mortality during the first year. Myocardial infarction was the most frequent cause of death. This early paper was a preview of what was to come, since diabetic nephropathy is now the most common cause of renal disease in patients entering renal replacement programs.

1976

Pennisi reported results of cooperative studies at the University of Southern California and at Northwestern in children undergoing chronic hemodialysis. Somatomedin activity was reduced but improved with time on routine hemodialysis. The somatomedin activity did not correlate with nutritional intake.

Kirsch and colleagues from Boston analyzed information on 1163 consecutive patients begun on chronic dialysis in California during a 22-month period. Units located in more concentrated population areas selected older and more seriously ill patients and dialyzed patients in each functional capacity level less intensively than in less concentrated areas. Nonprofit units tended to recommend renal transplantation for patients in each functional category more readily than did for-profit units. This report was one of the early studies suggesting the presence of important relationships between the location and ownership of dialysis units and policies for patient selection and treatment.

1979

Haas and associates from Seattle monitored 392 hemodialysis patients enrolled in a prospective longitudinal evaluation of atherosclerotic risk factors. An association was found among serum triglyceride levels, systolic blood pressure, and cardiovascular events (myocardial infarction, stroke, and mesentery infarct). A possible role for high triglyceride levels and high systolic blood pressure in the development of atherosclerosis was suggested.

1981

Jain and associates from Rochester, New York, described morbidity, rehabilitation, and mortality in a population of hemodialysis patients over 60 years of age at a joint session with the Clinical Dialysis and Transplant Forum.

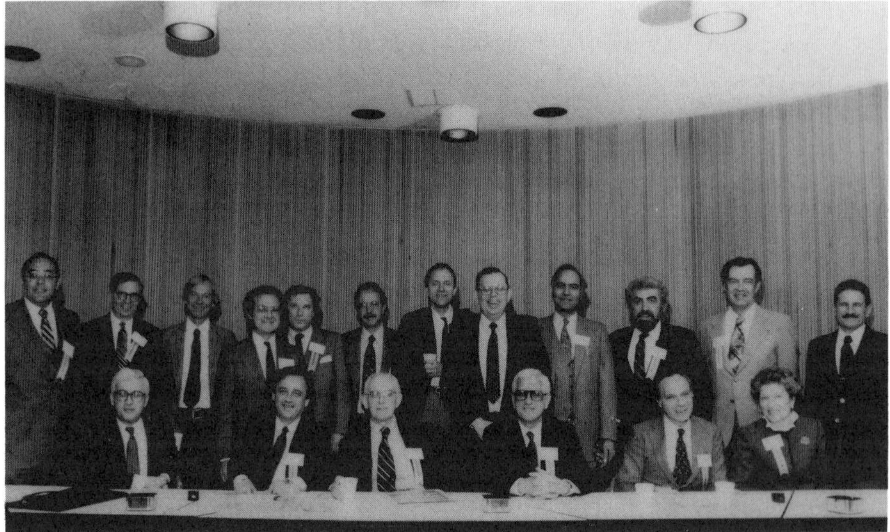

Figure 4.3. Faculty picture of a course entitled "Prevention of Kidney Disease and Survival Over 10 Years on Dialysis." The course was sponsored by The Long Island College Hospital and the National Kidney Foundation of New York. The picture was taken at the World Trade Center in New York City, Mar. 31, 1981. Standing, from left: Joseph Letteri, Joseph Schluger, Allen C. Alfrey, Sheldon Glabman, Alvin Goodman, Kurt Stenzel, Carl Kjellstrand, Eli Friedman, Khalid Butt, Norman Levy, John Maher, David Nelkin; seated, from left: Barry Brenner, M. M. Avram, Belding Scribner, David Baldwin, Carmelo Giordano, Nancy Cummings.

1982

Rikli and Kappel from Columbia, Missouri, studied the relationship of demographic characteristics to end-stage renal disease patient survival in the Missouri population. This study and the one in 1981 highlight the interest in dialysis population characteristics and outcomes as the experiences with chronic dialysis expanded.

1983

Wells and colleagues from Omaha assessed the relative risk of atherosclerosis in 28 undialyzed renal failure patients, in 35 CAPD patients, and in 37 hemodialysis patients. All were computed to 41 matched control subjects. Changes in plasma levels of triglycerides, total cholesterol, and other serum indicators suggested increasing risk of atherosclerosis with time on CAPD and decreasing risk with time on hemodialysis.

1986

Kjellstrand and Logan from Minneapolis calculated the fraction of patients treated by chronic dialysis in different population groups. The number of patients on dialysis was derived from statistics from the Health Care Financing Administration, and the risk of patients dying of uremia in each group was determined from United States Vital Statistics. The most favored group was the white male, age 25 to 44, in whom 76% received dialysis. The white female over age 65 was the least favored, with only 13% receiving dialysis. Patients over age 75 had 1/13th the chance of receiving dialysis of patients 15 to 24 years of age. Women had 80% the chance of men and, when age corrected, blacks always had less of a chance than whites, except in patients over age 64. The authors concluded that considerable discrimination exits in high-technology medicine.

Matteson and Kjellstrand from Minneapolis compared 5-year cumulative survivals in 769 age-matched diabetics after the patients started dialysis or underwent cadaver transplantation. They concluded that 5-year survival was no different between dialysis and cadaver transplantation.

Roberts and Kjellstrand reviewed records in 26 competent patients who died because they discontinued dialysis although there was no medical reason to do so. They were compared to 40 competent patients in whom medical complications triggered the decision to stop. More patients who stopped for no medical reason were on home dialysis (8/26) as compared with patients who stopped because complications developed (3/40). The authors suggest that home dialysis patients are at high risk to discontinue dialysis because of the stress of the dialysis procedure itself.

1987

A paper from Morgantown, West Virginia, had surveyed 51 in-center hemodialysis and 35 CAPD patients with a mean age of 57 years concerning their attitudes toward withholding cardiopulmonary resuscitation and withdrawal of dialysis. They found that most dialysis patients want to participate in decisions regarding life-supporting therapy, favor cardiopulmonary resuscitation, and have seldom considered stopping dialysis.

Port and associates from Ann Arbor reported that termination of life-sustaining dialysis therapy led to death in 282 of 5208 patients who started therapy for end-stage renal disease in Michigan during 1980 to 1985 with follow-up through 1986. Prior transplant failure or prior CAPD therapy did not significantly influence the percent of patients dying because of dialysis withdrawal. There was a 60% increase in overall withdrawals for the years 1980 to 1985. Withdrawal was more common in whites than in blacks (13% for whites and 4% for blacks). The authors state that increasing withdrawal and racial differences deserve further evaluation.

1988

Analysis of factors influencing the survival of dialysis patients was undertaken at the Henry Ford Hospital in Detroit, Michigan. The important predictors of reduced survival were found to be black race, diabetes mellitus, a low KT/V (less than 0.8), a high KT/V (greater than 1.2), a low protein intake (less than 0.8 g/kg/day), and a high-protein intake (greater than 1.2).

Lustig and his colleagues from Brooklyn showed that total cholesterol concentrations in serum fall more in hemodialysis than in CAPD patients. These findings were based on studies in 126 hemodialysis and 53 CAPD patients.

Collins and associates from Minneapolis and Kjellstrand from Stockholm analyzed results in Minneapolis in 2004 patients starting chronic dialysis since 1966. Cardiovascular diseases decreased from 50% of all deaths the first year to 15% beyond 9 years on dialysis. Infections increased from 10 to 25%. Stopping dialysis increased from 15 to 30%. Beyond 6 years of dialysis, infections were the most common cause of death.

1989

Churchill, representing a Canadian Hemodialysis Morbidity Study Group, reported on findings in 1439 patients of the Canadian hemodialysis population enrolled in a study focusing on a weekly census of morbid events. Probabilities of morbid events were then calculated for the population. By 1 year of follow-up, the probability of hospitalization was 66%, and hospitalization for myocardial infarction or angina was 9.5%. The probability of experiencing a seizure was 4.3%; a clinically important hypertensive problem 14.9%; pulmonary edema, 11.3%; significant clotting in grafts and fistulas 24.5% and 8.5%, respectively; and access infection in grafts and fistulas 19.2% and 3.9%, respectively.

Biocompatibility

1967

In 1967, the concept of biocompatibility as it related to hemodialysis was limited to the interaction between the clotting constituents of blood and the dialyzer blood path, in particular the hemodialysis membrane. The hemodialysis membrane in 1967 was exclusively cellulosic in nature and was dominated by the membrane from Wuppertal, Germany regenerated cellulose using the Cupraammonium process-Cuprophan).

1968/1969

In 1968, the landmark paper by Goffinet and Kaplow from Yale identified a phenomenon that had, incredibly, been overlooked by hemodialysis clinicians and whose explanation first drew attention to the interaction of the hemodialysis membrane with elements of the blood that were other than simply elements of the clotting cascade. They reported a profound neutropenia that occurred within the first 20 minutes of initiating blood flow through the dialyzer. Subsequent work was to reveal that polymorphonuclear leukocytes left the peripheral circulation and lodged in the capillaries of the lung only to return in the latter hours of dialysis. This proved to be a complement-mediated event. The paper by Nidus and Pineda from New York in 1969 identified a "neutropenic factor" in dog blood that had been exposed to a twin coil (cellulosic) dialyzer. They further identified that it was important to sustain calcium concentration in the blood or plasma, as citrated blood did not generate a neutropenic factor. Although they did not identify these events as complement related, they were nonetheless accurate in their observations.

1976/1977

In 1976, more evidence appeared that the interaction between elements in the blood and the dialysis membrane caused measurable changes to occur. The abstract by Nolph et al. from Missouri in collaboration with Siemsen from Hawaii identified significant quantities of circulating antibodies to nuclear antigens in patients who were on hemodialysis. The speculation was that cell elements broke up on contact with the dialysis membrane, releasing their nuclear material in a manner that resulted in the formation of autoantibodies. This work extended their preliminary observations from the year before (Husted et al.) in which an increased incidence of nuclear antibodies was found in patients with chronic renal failure treated by dialysis and/or by transplantation. The clinical consequences of these abnormalities have yet to be identified. In 1977, Bogue et al. from Salt Lake City, Utah, reported a lack of clinical cardiopulmonary dysfunction with use of a synthetic membrane (AN69-polyacrylonitrile) in contrast to the use of cellulosic membranes. At that time, the polyacrylonitrile membrane was the only noncellulosic membrane commercially available for hemodialysis. Subsequent work supports its lack of release of anaphylatoxins.

It should be noted that the important work of Craddock et al., establishing the relationship between pulmonary vascular leukosequestration and the activation of complement by cellulosic dialysis membranes, was published in 1977 in the *Journal of Clinical Investigation* and *New England Journal of Medicine* but was not presented to the ASN.

1978

The 1978 ASN program introduced the first concerns about a fall in arterial oxygen tension during dialysis and hemofiltration. The papers by Sherlock et al. Chronic Dialysis and Transplant Forum (CDTF Joint Session) from New York and by Kraut et al. from Los Angeles identified a reduction in partial pressure of oxygen during artificial kidney treatment. They went beyond the original hypothesis that the reduced oxygen tension was secondary to white cell damage to alveolar capillary membranes (i.e., complement activation due to bioincompatibility of the membrane) and pointed out that exposure to dialysis fluid, and in particular acetate containing dialysis fluid, could result in a reduction in minute ventilation secondary both to the loss of CO_2 across the artificial kidney membrane and to alteration of the respiratory quotient as a result of the metabolism of acetate.

In this same program year, joint work by Bernick and Port from Ann Arbor and Favero and Brown from Phoenix examined the transport of bacteria and pyrogens from dialysis fluid to blood and concluded that this did not occur. They postulated that the causes for fever in the hemodialysis unit population were related to breaks in the membrane that permitted passage of these large-molecular-weight and cellular structures into the blood or the presence of a *Limulus* lysate assay negative pyrogen that crossed the membrane. The accuracy of this latter hypothesis is only now being proved. Two additional papers addressed the concern about reduced oxygen tension. Work from Nissenson et al. from Los Angeles concluded that the artificial kidney membrane simply acted as a lung to arterial pCO_2 and reduced the minute ventilation, and that in turn caused the fall in pO_2. Wathen et al., however, concluded that acid-base changes moving serum pH to the alkaline side could account for a shift in affinity between oxygen and hemoglobin (Bohr effect) that could account for the reduced PO_2. Although this may occur, this latter mechanism has not proved to be a significant contributor.

1980

Hakim and Lowrie attempted to discern the relative effects of membrane biocompatibility and dialysis fluid composition on dialysis-associated hypoxemia and found that both had a significant role to play. Comparing Cuprophan with synthetic membrane (polymethylmethacrylate) and using a prospective crossover study format in which acetate and bicarbonate were alternately used in the bath produced the conclusion that hemodialysis hypoxemia is a multifactorial event.

Nakamura et al. from Tokyo presented an interesting paper at the CDTF in 1980 in conjunction with the ASN meeting. They noted a greater degree of leukopenia and complement activation when hemodialysis was carried out with a new as opposed to a reused membrane.

1982

This observation was not confirmed until 1982, when Cheung et al. from San Diego, using specific radioimmunoassays for the anaphylatoxins C3a and C5a and dialyzers undergoing reuse with a saline rinse formaldehyde storage protocol, showed comparable data. This work suggested that adsorption of plasma proteins to the membrane could modify the surface in such a way that it no longer activated complement. Work to be subsequently commented on showed that this concept was somewhat simplistic and that the binding of regulatory proteins of the complement systems such as factors H and B are very important in the overall impact on complement activation.

Additional information on biocompatibility surfaced in 1982 with a paper by Walker et al. from Ontario in which studies in a sheep model were carried out to assess the effects of the interaction between dialyzer membranes and blood. This proved to be an exceptionally sensitive model and later would sustain criticism that it might be too sensitive to be reflective of what actually happens in maintenance dialysis patients. The paper by Seton et al. from Kansas City showing a dissociation of hemodialysis leukopenia and hypoxemia when sodium citrate was used as a regional anticoagulant brought into focus the role of calcium as a cofactor in the complement activation pathways and lent understanding to the 1969 observation of Nidus and Pineda. With calcium removed, exposure of the blood to cellulosic membrane was unable to produce sufficient C5a to result in leukopenia.

In an interesting comparison of membranes, Marchant et al. from Cleveland identified differences between Cuprophan and polyacrylonitrile (PAN) membrane in terms of the plasma clearance of β-thromboglobulin. The PAN membrane was shown to remove greater quantities of β-thromboglobulin either by clearance or by adsorption of that protein. Interestingly, this occurred in spite of work by Chenoweth et al. showing absent complement activation by PAN membrane as contrasted with Cuprophan. The present studies on platelet activation show comparable levels of thromboxane B_2 production, pointing out that the presence or absence of biocompatibility depends on the assay used to examine for this phenomenon.

Tielemans et al. from Brussels examined the percentage of T3, T8, and T4–T8 ratio in two groups of patients on hemodialysis, one with eosinophilia and the second without. These studies showed different patterns with the eosinophilia group that were characterized by deficient suppressor function. The suppression appeared to be correlated with the number of years on maintenance dialysis. Last, Bommer et al. from Heidelberg, Germany, identified that spalation products (particles) from dialysis tubing could activate macrophages. The clinical impact of this observation has yet to be identified but is classed as a phenomenon showing bioincompatibility of another element in the extracorporeal circuit of hemodialyzers.

1983

In this program year, Walker et al. from the London, Ontario, group reported two important papers. The first was a patient study in which invasive methods were used to study hemodynamic responses in eight chronic renal failure patients during the first 30 minutes of hemodialysis with membranes of different composition and therefore biocompatibility. In addition, nine patients with acute renal failure were invasively studied during the course of hemodialysis with Cuprophan membrane. All showed a measurable rise in systolic pulmonary artery pressure. Chronic renal failure patients using Cuprophan and cellulose acetate membranes showed a reduction in right ventricular ejection fraction with no change in the left ventricular ejection fraction. This work has come to be widely cited in support of the presence of an increase in pulmonary artery pressure during the early phase of hemodialysis with complement-activating membranes in the human circumstance. The second presentation by Walker et al. using sheep showed not only that the rise in pulmonary artery pressure was significant, but that it likely was not attributable to physical blockade by polymorphs in the microcirculation of the lung. Direct biopsy observation identified a rise to peak values in pulmonary artery pressure prior to the arrival of the polymorphs. The rise could be blocked by pretreating the animals with indomethacin. These studies were not performed on-line. Rather, in vitro exposure of blood to membranes of different composition was performed and then injected IV into sheep who were monitored for cardiodynamic parameters.

Ing et al. from Chicago reported a series of 23 severe anaphylactoid reactions early in the course of hemodialysis using Cuprophan hollow-fiber dialyzers from five different manufacturers. At this time, this represented the largest series of these "first-use reactions" that had been reported. Although no etiology was determined, there was the strong implication from their clinical histories that inadequate rinsing of the dialyzer played a role. Work not reported at this meeting by Pearson et al. from Chicago subsequently confirmed Ing's speculations that residual material in the dialyzer (i.e., ethylene oxide) activates the classical pathway of complement, and the Cuprophan membrane activates the alternate pathway. It is likely that both pathways sum clinically to the major anaphylactoid reaction reported in those patients who have developed antibodies to the ethylene oxide (ETO) albumin haptene and also are exposed to Cuprophan.

Work by Rubin et al. from New Jersey supported observations initially made elsewhere that hemodialysis-associated hypotension could be ameliorated by reducing the temperature of the dialysis fluid by 2°. The mechanism for this reduction is not explored in the present study but likely reflects both an alteration in physiological reactivity and alterations in the tempo and degree of blood-membrane interaction.

Last, work by Cheung et al. from San Diego using Cuprophan, cellulose acetate, and PAN membrane showed not only that these membranes were different in their capacity to activate complement, but also that the adsorptive qualities differed, with the PAN membrane taking up large quantities of the anaphylatoxin C3a. This in vitro observation has been confirmed by in vivo studies in which the PAN membrane has been shown to be quantitatively significant in removing anaphylatoxins from the plasma during routine hemodialysis.

1984

Work by Maggiore from Reggio, Italy, in follow-up of his previous observation, and the work in 1984 reported elsewhere by Rubin et al. showed a reduction in complement activation and release of anaphylatoxins during cool hemodialysis.

A second paper by Walker from the Ontario group examined the sheep model. He was able to dissociate the effects of dialysate composition, that is, acetate or bicarbonate, from blood membrane interaction that caused anaphylatoxin release and the rise in pulmonary artery pressure and arterial hypoxemia.

1985

Work reported elsewhere by Henderson et al. identified a possible role for interleukin-1 (IL-1) in some of the signs and symptoms noted in the maintenance dialysis patient. The paper by Port et al. from Ann Arbor on the release of interleukin-1 during hemodialysis addressed whether dialysate composition could play a role rather than this release being purely the result of blood-membrane interaction and the generation of complement. Their study compared standard dialysis solution that contained both bacteria and pyrogens with sterile pyrogen-free saline solution. They used a cellulosic membrane in a hollow-fiber format. Measurement of IL-1 was by both a rabbit bioassay and a thymocyte proliferation assay. They determined that there was significantly more IL-1 released with dialysate than with sterile saline and concluded that in addition to the membrane effect, there were factors in the dialysis fluid responsible for interleukin release. Work by Lonnemann et al. from Hannover, West Germany, with the collaboration of Dinarello from Boston, compared the impact of endotoxin on interleukin-1 release during hemodialysis with Cuprophan hollow-fiber dialyzers. They also concluded that endotoxin in the dialysis fluid can induce monocyte interleukin release and speculated that undetectable leaks in the membrane may occur to permit passage of this large-molecular-weight substance from dialysis fluid to blood and hence stimulation of the monocyte.

Wayman and Cheung from Salt Lake City, using the swine rather than the sheep model, identified that thromboxane mediates the pulmonary hypertension seen when Cuprophan-activated plasma is infused and that the source of this thromboxane is the lung itself. This work supports the observation of Walker et al. in 1984, which argued against physical blockade by white cells as causing the hypertension noted in the sheep after exposure to the Cuprophan-activated plasma.

1986

In this year, an entire dialysis session and an invited lecture addressed problems of biocompatibility. It had become swiftly apparent that this matter of complement activation by hemodialysis membrane was more complicated than had initially been perceived. In a paper from New York and Boston by Schulman, follow-up work in the sheep model confirmed prior work by Cheung et al. that PAN membrane actively adsorbs the complement products of blood-membrane interaction from the blood. This was demonstrated by Cuprophan-activated plasma, which was then incubated in a PAN dialyzer and subsequently given intravenously to sheep. Incubation of the blood with the PAN dialyzer blocked the rise in pulmonary artery pressure and the other previously observed hemodynamic events that resulted from injection of Cuprophan-activated plasma alone. Parker et al. from Salt Lake City extended this theme of membrane binding to Cuprophan and cellulose acetate, pointing out that complement binding of C3b to the cellulosic membrane likely did not play a role in whether a membrane was active in triggering complement or not; it was rather whether the membrane had the ability to bind the regulatory proteins of the alternate complement pathway such as factors H and B.

Betz et al. from Heidelberg, in a complement-free in vitro system, identified that Cuprophan membrane itself, without the presence of complement-activation products, could trigger the release of interleukin-1 from monocytes. This theme was echoed and confirmed by Lonnemann et al. and the group from Hannover, West Germany, working in conjunction with Shaldon from Montpellier, France, and Dinarello from Boston.

Churchill et al. from Hamilton, Ontario, Canada, did a multiple crossover trial (with random allocation to treatment order) on whether the dialyzers were reused and could find no difference in patient's symptoms. Their reuse technique involved an automated system, and they did not identify which agents were used to clean the dialyzer. In an adjacent paper by Kuwahara et al. from Lausanne, Switzerland, it was noted that the hemodialyzer reprocessing technique could make striking differences in the degree of biocompatibility of the reused membrane when assessed by complement activation (leukopenia). In his hands, peracetic acid (4%) consistently reduced the degree of leukopenia and prevented neutrophil activation in the reused membrane.

Dr. R. M. Hakim from Boston gave the invited lecture on "Issue of Biocompatibility in Hemodialysis," suggesting that this topic had come of age. His survey of the literature concluded that this was an area that needed close attention by the dialysis world, albeit there was not at present strong evidence clinically as to the ill effects that complement activation over a long-term period would have in the patient.

Work by Cheung et al. from Salt Lake City examined sodium hypochlorite specifically and noted that when this agent was employed in the reuse protocol for Cuprophan membranes, the complement-activating potential was thoroughly restored and the membrane behaved as if it were unused.

Expanding the horizon of biocompatibility, Kay and Raij of Minneapolis, using a complement-free system in vitro, reported that natural killer cell function decreased in hemodialyzed patients when the membrane used was Cuprophan as contrasted with polycarbonate hemodialysis membrane, indicating that yet another cell element in the blood must be included when assessing biocompatibility. The function of natural killer cells in tumor surveillance was cited as a potential long-term problem for patients on Cuprophan hemodialysis. This work may be taken in conjunction with the work of Port from Ann Arbor, Michigan, who compared the incidence of neoplasms in dialysis patients using two computer-linked population base data systems: the Michigan Kidney Registry and the Michigan Cancer Foundation Registry. This study pointed out that a two- to fivefold higher incidence of tumors of the kidney, uterus, prostate, and bone marrow (multiple myeloma) occurs in patients on hemodialysis as contrasted with nonuremic patients. A fourfold increase in cancers of tongue, lung, and colon was also noted.

Dumler from Detroit raised an interesting possible link between biocompatibility and the generation of β-2 microglobulin. In five randomly selected patients, they used either new cellulosic dialyzers or dialyzers after reprocessing. They did not identify their mode of reprocessing. Significant differences were found in that the new dialyzers produced a much greater rise in β-2 microglobulin concentrations when contrasted with reprocessed dialyzers. This work has yet to be confirmed, and the complexity of assessing plasma concentration levels when total body water content changes leaves this observation in question but of high interest.

1987

In this program year, studies in the area of biocompatibility were focused more on mechanisms for the observations that had been made heretofore. Gerard et al. from Boston and Nashville examined complement receptors on the neutrophil and the monocyte during hemodialysis and identified that down-regulation did occur as had been reported elsewhere but that it did not persist long enough to be explanatory of the return of white blood cells from their peripheral margination in the lung.

Cheung et al. and Parker from Salt Lake City had a pair of papers following up on their previous observations in identifying the crucial role of membrane binding of the regulatory protein factors B and H to the membrane. The ratio in which they were bound determined the degree of complement activation produced by Cuprophan and/or cellulose acetate membranes. Parker, in a rather innovative study using two cobra venom factors in the swine model, was able to show that both C3a and C5a contributed to the pulmonary hypertension associated with this model. Heretofore, only C5a was considered to be active.

Last, in this program year, Kandus et al. from Chicago, by creatively sequencing Cuprophan membrane and PAN membrane during clinical hemodialysis, were able to show that PAN membrane could take up and block biological effects of the complement-activating products generated by Cuprophan membrane, an in vivo correlation of the in vitro studies previously reported by others.

1988

This was the year in which an interest in the possibility of backfiltration of dialysis fluid (from casing to blood path) appeared in the program. Schmidt of Frankfurt had earlier reported elsewhere that for membranes with high hydraulic permeability, significant quantities of backfiltration could occur under routine clinical operating conditions. Hyver and Peterson from Palo Alto, California, reported that backfiltration could in large measure be blocked by running blood and dialysis fluid in the cocurrent direction.

1989

Cheung et al. noted that heparin bonding to Cuprophan dialysis membranes reduced the amount of complement activation during hemodialysis. Hanser et al. from Vienna noted that the terminal attack complex of the complement system was measurably present in the blood of patients at the conclusion of dialysis with complement-activating membranes.

Papers showing significant perturbation of white cell function and the role of complement-activating membranes were presented by Himmelfarb et al. from Nashville, Horl et al. from Freiburg, Germany, and R. Vanholder from Ghent, Belgium, indicating intense interest in this manifestation of biocompatibility.

Adequacy of Dialysis

Disputation over what constitutes adequate therapy in the patients with end-stage renal disease is as old as the therapy itself. Introduction of this topic to the ASN program did not occur until 1971 in a paper by Millora et al. of Albany, in which a sophisticated electroencephalographic assessment of patients during maintenance dialysis and following renal transplantation showed differences suggesting that electroencephalogram (EEG) abnormalities were not restored to normal by maintenance dialysis.

1973

In 1973, a paper by Easterling et al. from Ann Arbor reported the results in 12 patients of halfing dialysis time and doubling membrane area (2 m^2) for an average of 13 months treatment at conventional blood and dialysis fluid flow rates. No clinical or biochemical deterioration was noted, and their nerve conduction velocity did not change. The authors concluded that treatment with 2 m^2 of membrane for 2 to 2½ hours three times per week is a satisfactory form of therapy. Papers such as this and such as that of Millora are reflective of the concerns expressed elsewhere (the American Society for Artificial Internal Organs), relating adequacy of treatment to the numbers of hours as well as to the membrane area employed in therapy (the square meter-hour hypothesis proposed by Babb and Scribner). This latter concept flowed from basic engineering principles and clinical observation of patients undergoing Cuprophan hemodialysis.

1976

Concurrent concerns about toxins other than simply urea, creatinine, phosphate, uric acid, and so on were ongoing in the dialysis community and were reflected in the 1976 invited lecture by Jonas Bergstrom from Stockholm on uremic toxicity. In particular, concern for middle molecules and the impact of their clearance or lack thereof on adequacy of therapy was presented in summary format, albeit much of the primary work in this area had been reported elsewhere.

1978

Dyck et al. from Rochester presented studies on comparing peripheral nerve function with serum chemistries as a means for assessing adequacy of hemodialysis. They were unable to show correlation of peripheral nerve function between patients on short (1½ to 2 hours, three times per week) versus long (2–3 hours, three times per week) treatment schedules; heretofore, peripheral nerve conduction velocities were considered a sensitive index of adequacy.

1979

An interesting paper by Mitch et al. from Baltimore raised the possibility that by manipulating dietary protein intake, adequacy of treatment could be accomplished in a shorter time. Essential amino acid supplementation was provided, and biochemical, nutritional, and nerve function parameters were found to be suitably maintained when the dialysis schedule was shifted from three times per week to twice weekly.

1980

A paper by Shaldon et al. from Montpellier introduced the concept that had been presented by others elsewhere of the potential for shorter treatment time with adequacy maintained by using hemofiltration as opposed to classical hemodialysis. In this same year, a paper by R. V. M. Cestero of Rochester reported the use of urea kinetic modeling to guide the patient dialysis prescription. Urea kinetic modeling had been explored elsewhere in considerable detail.

1982

In 1982, work by Kachel et al. from Frankfurt, Germany, identified amyloidosis of the carpal tunnel as a complication of long-term renal failure. This group subsequently identified that the amyloid was different in nature and composed of β-2 microglobulin subunits. This 12,800-dalton middle molecule would prove to be a uremic toxin.

1984

Urea kinetic modeling, which had been given prominence with the National Cooperative Dialysis Study, for assessing adequacy came under fire in a paper by Keshaviah et al. from Minneapolis in which one of the basic assumptions of urea kinetic modeling (i.e., single-pool status for urea) was questioned. This same group, with Collins as first author, presented their experience with short, efficient hemodialysis in which care was taken to model both urea and a middle molecule (Vitamin B_{12}) to ensure that comparable small- and middle-molecular-weight clearance was accomplished even though a shorter treatment time was offered. In an interesting companion paper from Baltimore, Weir et al. compared twice-weekly and three-times-weekly hemodialysis for morbidity and mortality over a 5-year period. Comparable weekly time on dialysis between the two groups was maintained. Comparable or somewhat improved morbidity and mortality figures were noted in the twice-weekly group, suggesting the importance of middle molecules to the pathogenesis of uremic complications.

1986

von Albertini et al. from Los Angeles reported on 1 year of experience in a limited number of patients being treated for 6 hours a week on hemodiafiltration. This combination of hemodialysis and hemofiltration with high blood and dialysis fluid flow rates (500 mL/minute and 700 mL/minute), using two high-flux membranes in a series, resulted in serum chemistries that were no different from control observations made with standard three-times-weekly 4-hour Cuprophan hemodialysis.

Continued experimentation with these ultraefficient dialysis techniques continued. In reports from Keshaviah et al. from Minneapolis on high-efficiency bicarbonate hemodialysis in which large surface area membranes and high blood and dialysis fluid flow rates were employed and from Shinaberger of Los Angeles, comparing conventional dialysis to high-efficiency dialysis and high-flux diafiltration, morbidity and mortality were considered comparable.

Also in 1986, two papers from France (Zingraff et al., Paris, and Y. Caverle et al., Rennes) addressed the importance of removing β-2 microglobulin. In this same program year, papers by Acchiardo et al. from Memphis and Gotch et al. from San Francisco described high-flux hemodialysis techniques for employing shorter treatment time but sustaining adequacy of therapy.

1987

An invited lecture by Drueke of Paris led a session with papers by Peterson of Palo Alto, Zingraff of Paris, and Kumano et al. of Kanagawa, Japan, all addressing the concern about β-2 microglobulin and dialysis-related amyloidosis and the implications for adequacy of its removal.

In this same program year, continued concern about the best way to assess adequacy of dialysis was noted in papers by Keshaviah et al. of Minneapolis and Vanholder et al. from Ghent, Belgium. The first paper reappraised the kinetic modeling in the National Cooperative Dialysis Study, and the second looked at three different methods for estimating urea kinetics in hemodialysis.

1988

Levin et al. from Detroit, in conjunction with Held of the Urban Institute and others, reported on the impact of shorter dialysis procedures on mortality in a large statistical sample of Medicare hemodialysis patients. It was shown that increased mortality was associated with shorter length of dialysis time using sophisticated statistical techniques; this once again points to the importance of poorly removed middle molecules as an explanation for this increased mortality.

Also in this program year were papers expressing concern about β-2 microglobulin and how best to remove it. See, for example, Tayeb et al. from Detroit.

1989

Two papers (Blake et al. from Toronto and Tayeb et al. from Detroit) expressed concern about routine application of urea kinetic modeling as it is employed with hemodialysis to the CAPD population. They pointed out that such application indicates that CAPD patients are grossly underdialyzed, which is at odds with the clinical findings in which CAPD compares favorably with hemodialysis for both mortality and morbidity.

In this same program year, a continued level of interest in urea kinetic modeling to quantify dialysis was expressed. See, for example, Flanigan et al. from Iowa.

A clinical symposium on high-efficiency hemodialysis was held in this program year, where concerns about prescription of high-efficiency treatments were brought forward by Parker from Dallas, and the risks and problems of this form of therapy were explored by Levin of Detroit.

Summary

Clearly, one of the most important developments of the late 1960s and early 1970s was the introduction of the capillary hemodialyzer. Most of the original presentations were given at the ASAIO. This configuration greatly facilitated the later development of a multitude of new, more versatile dialysis membranes. Another very important paper was that of Tenckhoff and Schecter in 1968 introducing the Tenckhoff catheter, which provided the access to the peritoneum that made possible the introduction of CAPD by Popovitch, Moncrief, and Nolph in 1977. The introduction of the concept of biocompatibility by the description of dialysis leukopenia by Goffinet and Kaplow from Yale in 1968 was another landmark.

In 1975, Alfrey solved the very threatening problem of dialysis dementia by identifying aluminum contamination of tap water as the cause.

In 1974, Novello described the problem of acetate intolerance with big dialyzers, and in 1976, Graefe clearly demonstrated that the answer was to return to dialysis with bicarbonate.

The key paper by Eschbach in 1982 showing that erythropoietin cured the anemia of uremic sheep led to the later development of synthetic EPO, which has had a profound impact on the well-being of dialysis patients.

As we look to the future, dialysis amyloidosis remains the greatest threat to the well-being of long-term survivors on dialysis. Otherwise, the future looks very bright indeed, especially because of the great improvement in well-being that results from the correction of anemia with EPO.

5

Immunology, Pathology, and Anatomy

Ramzi S. Cotran, Alfred L. Michael, C. Craig Tisher, and Robert L. Vernier

State of the Art in 1966[a]

A Quarter Century

The Proceedings, Volume 2 (Morphology, Immunology, Urology), and other volumes provide an overview of the research current at the time in the fields of immunology, pathology, and anatomy. The state of the art in experimental renal disease was well advanced and was summarized by the La Jolla group. In nephrotoxic nephritis in rats, the biphasic nature of the disease was recognized, and the nephrotoxic γ-globulin was appreciated as a "planted antigen" on the glomerular basement membrane (GBM) in the autologous phase. Both the acute and chronic "serum sickness" models, using primarily bovine serum albumin, were recognized as immune complex diseases. The role of serum complement fixation in both models was appreciated, as was the mediator role of C5b in stimulating the influx of polymorphonuclear leukocytes (PMN) as an important early event in the glomerular injury. The autologous autoimmune nephritis model of Heymann was recognized as a model of membranous glomerulonephritis. The relationship of NZB/NZW-F1 hybrid autoimmune nephritis in mice to human lupus nephritis was also appreciated.

Of the renal disease in human beings, acute poststreptococcal glomerulonephritis was appreciated as an immune complex disease. The classification of various forms of chronic glomerulonephritis was evolving but primitive. The syndrome of IgA nephropathy was appreciated (Berger), dense deposit disease was recognized, and there was great interest in analgesic-induced interstitial nephritis by our European colleagues. Dr. Kimmelstiel's group reported that "the most conspicuous glomerular changes" in early diabetic glomerulosclerosis were "an increase in the number and widening of the

[a] Review of the Proceedings of the Third International Congress of Nephrology, Washington, D.C., 1966

mesangial trabeculae. Thickening of the GBM does not precede but accompanies or follows the mesangial lesion."

Electron microscopy of the kidney had advanced. The "wire loop" lesion of systemic lupus erythematosus (SLE) nephropathy was well illustrated, as were the subepithelial deposits of membranous nephropathy. The normal renal tubule was described, but incomplete understanding of the cell types was revealed by statements such as "The collecting duct: the organization is simple with relatively sparse organelles. The basilar plasma membrane is unfolded to form shallow compartments which usually contain only cytoplasmic ground substance."

Technological Advances: 1967–1992

The improved understanding of kidney disease over the past 25 years has followed advances in research technology. Included in the field of immunology are improved protein separation techniques, radioimmunoassay and enzyme-linked immunosorbent assay (ELISA) methods for quantitation of antibody and antigen, and improved immunofluorescence and immunoelectron microscopic and cytochemical techniques. In the late 1970s, the application of monoclonal antibody technology permitted great advances in antigen and cell marker localization and identification, including delineation of complement components and receptors and recognition of the role of cytokines in cell activation and injury. The development of improved cell culture methods has also been remarkable, and the mesangial cell may be the most studied cell.

Organization of the Review

The Review Committee elected to organize the review of immunology, pathology, and anatomy in the subsections that follow:

- I. Immunology
  - A. Immune Mechanisms
  - B. In-Situ Mechanisms of Immune Glomerular Injury
  - C. Molecular Charge
  - D. Complement
  - E. Mediators of Glomerular Injury
  - F. Role of Macrophages, Lymphocytes, and Cell-Mediated Immunity in Glomerulonephritis
  - G. The Glomerular Mesangium
  - H. Tubulointerstitial Nephritis (TIN)
- II. Pathology
- III. Anatomy

Immunology

Immune Mechanisms

Review of the Proceedings of the Third International Congress (1966). Frank Dixon reviewed the experimental models of immunological renal diseases, including nephrotoxic serum nephritis (also called NTS, Masugi nephritis, anti-GBM nephritis), induced by antibody to glomerular basement membrane (GBM) antigens; the recognition of the heterologous and autologous phases of the response; the role of complement fixation and its chemotactic effect for polymorphonuclear leukocytes; and the presumed mediation of the immediate renal injury by complement. Immune complex induced renal injury was discussed as "one-shot" serum sickness; passive serum sickness, induced by injection of perfused complexes into animals; and chronic glomerulonephritis, induced in animals by repeated injections of foreign serum proteins.

The pathogenesis of the autoimmune glomerulonephritis that develops in NZB/NZW-F1 hybrid mice and the many similarities to human lupus were discussed.

Dr. Walter Heymann reviewed "Experimental Analogues of Human Nephropathies," including nephrotoxic nephritis, the foreign protein immune complex models, and the model he introduced in 1959 (subsequently called Heymann's nephritis). In the latter disease, rats injected with homogenates of kidney from either rats, guinea pigs, rabbits, or humans, developed glomerulonephritis and nephrotic syndrome, presumably by autoimmune mechanisms.

Review of Abstracts of the ASN (1967–1991). Abstracts submitted during the 25 years of the American Society of Nephrology (ASN) clarified many aspects of immune-mediated renal disease. The target antigen for human anti-GBM nephritis or Goodpasture syndrome was recognized as a component of type IV collagen [α3(IV) NC1], and a related chain (Alport antigen and/or α5(IV) was identified as the principal component missing in Alport syndrome. Immunologic studies using monoclonal antibody probes led to further dissection of the complex structure of renal basement membranes and cell surface antigens. The concept of in situ immune complex disease was developed with multiple studies of Heymann's nephritis and the recognition of the epithelial cell surface pit antigen and the sequence of events leading to membranous nephropathy. A variety of other model systems exploiting the use of charged antigens and other molecules in combination with antibodies and enzymes expanded the possibilities for addressing the pathogenesis of human renal disease. The roles of the complement system, humoral and cellular immunity, and biological active molecules and mediators were evaluated during this era. More recently, all the tools of cell biology, in vitro systems, and molecular biology have been brought to bear on the role of the immune system in renal disease.

Studies of the anti-GBM models of glomerulonephritis (GN) in animals were of great interest in 1967. It was shown that injection of homologous or autologous GBM antigens isolated from rabbit urine was capable of inducing antibodies to GBM and glomerulonephritis, with linear IgG distributed along the GBM. Autoimmune anti-GBM nephritis was also induced in monkeys by injection of human GBM and in sheep by injection of human lung (Steblay nephritis). It was shown that anti-GBM antibody obtained from serum or eluted from kidneys of patients with glomerulonephritis and linear IgG staining of the GBM caused nephritis and proteinuria when passively transferred by injection into unilaterally nephrectomized squirrel monkeys.

In 1969, anti-GBM nephritis in eight patients was described. These patients had rapidly progressive renal failure, pulmonary hemorrhage (5/8), and linear IgG on the GBM. The linear pattern of immunofluorescence had been first described in 1964–1965, but the significance of this pattern was not appreciated. Serum of patients contained antibody that fixed to human GBM in a linear pattern, as did renal eluates, and in 1970 quantitation by indirect immunofluorescence was described. These observations were confirmed by other studies, and in 1974 and 1978, quantitative immunoassays for anti-GBM antibodies in the circulation were documented. In 1979, 27 kD and 53 kD components of collagenous soluble GBM were shown to be reactive with Goodpasture antibodies. These are now recognized to be predominantly monomers and dimers of the noncollagenous domain of the $\alpha 3$ chain of type IV collagen [$\alpha 3$(IV) NC1].

A variety of other glomerular antigens were described in the glomerulus in 1973. The use of monoclonal antibodies in dissecting renal basement membrane antigens was described in 1981. Type IV collagen had been recognized as a constituent of basement membrane, and in 1988 Goodpasture's anti-GBM antibody was reported to recognize subunits of type IV collagen. At the 1985 meeting, a genetically discriminating antibody, identifying a 26 kD collagen peptide obtained from a transplanted patient with Alport's familial nephritis, was described.

In 1986 and at subsequent meetings, additional observations on the nature of the Goodpasture antibody and its relationship to the missing antigen(s) [$\alpha 3$(IV) NC1, $\alpha 4$(IV) NC1, Alport antigen] in Alport's syndrome were described. Studies from several laboratories characterized newly described chains of collagen IV $\alpha 3$(IV), $\alpha 4$(IV), and $\alpha 5$(IV) and speculated that the Goodpasture antigen was located in the $\alpha 3$(IV) NC1 chain of the noncollagen domain of collagen IV, whereas the Alport antigen identified another distinct collagen chain. In 1986, the NC1 domain of type IV collagen was implicated in the pathogenesis of Steblay nephritis.

Studies in experimental anti-GBM nephritis in 1980 demonstrated accentuation of the disease in experimental hypertension. Fixation of antibody to alveolar-capillary basement membrane occurred only after lung injury induced by oxygen toxicity. In 1982, the importance of macrophages in the autologous phase of the disease was discussed. Studies of the role of terminal complement components in the full expression of the disease yielded conflicting results, although there was some effect early in the disease (1983 and 1986). Administration of antiserum with specificity for other glomerular basement membrane components (e.g., heparan sulfate proteoglycan) was shown to induce proteinuria. The participation of other factors, including arachidonic acid metabolites in this experimental disease, was described at subsequent meetings. In 1986, essential fatty acid deficiency was shown to inhibit infiltration of macrophages, and this was associated with the inhibition of prostaglandin-E2 (PGE2). The role of enzymes from white cells in injury to the glomerular capillary wall was supported by the demonstration that elastase mediates glomerular injury in vivo (1987). In addition, certain metalloproteinases were shown to degrade GBM in vitro. At the same meeting, a rabbit model of anti-GBM nephritis was described in which there was a striking increase in T cells and macrophages in the interstitium and surrounding Bowman's capsule. In 1987, increased renal fibrosis and collagen synthesis were described in this model. The contribution of transforming growth factor-β (TGF-β) in this process was suggested.

The occurrence of anti-GBM antibody and other autoantibodies was observed after administration of mercuric chloride and was related to polyclonal B-cell activation. The latter—also observed after penicillamine and graft versus host disease—was associated with the development of membranous nephropathy (1989).

Immune complex mechanisms of glomerular injury also continued to be explored in annual meetings. In 1969, methods for evaluating antigen quantitation in experimental disease were described. In 1969 and 1970, the GN occurring in patients with bacterial endocarditis was shown to be associated with granular GBM fluorescence for IgG and complement and with electron-dense deposits in the glomerulus. Further studies in animal models included the demonstration in 1971 of the disappearance of immune deposits in the chronic "serum sickness" model, by daily injections of antigen in excess of the quantities of antibody measured, suggesting that solubilization had occurred. The immune deposits were shown to disappear within 5 to 6 days of repeated daily injections of large excesses of the antigen.

The essentiality of macrophages but not complement in the renal injury of acute serum sickness was also demonstrated in 1980 by depleting animals of macrophages or complement. Although experimental serum sickness nephritis was presumed to be principally a consequence of humoral immunity, the recognition of small numbers of glomerular T cells in addition to macrophages left open the issue for participation of cell-mediated immunity. Studies using cationized bovine albumen in C6-deficient rabbits to induce glomerulonephritis suggested a role of terminal complement components early in the disease even though there was no evidence for a pathogenic role of complement in classical serum sickness nephritis. In human disease, methods for measurement of circulating complexes were developed and compared in 1976–1978.

The role of electrostatic charge in the localization of immune complexes was addressed in 1979–1980 (see the next section). These studies demonstrated that cationic antigens (bovine serum albumin [BSA], IgG, ferritin, protamine), in contrast to neutral or anionic molecules, localized in the peripheral capillary wall.

The subsequent administration of antibody led to significant glomerulonephritis. The pathogenesis of various forms of immune complex nephritis was discussed in a symposium in 1981. A new mechanism of immune complex transport and clearance in primates involved binding to the complement receptors of erythrocytes and was first described in 1981 and extended in meetings held in 1984, 1987, and 1989. The multifactorial influences in immune injury to the glomerulus were summarized in a symposium in 1983, and reports in subsequent years implicated the participation of enzymes (e.g., elastase), complement components, reactive oxygen species, arachidonic acid metabolites, platelets, and cationic proteins. The importance of platelet activating factor (PAF) in the inflammatory injury seen in in situ immune complex injury (1986) and in a model of murine lupus nephritis (1990) injury was demonstrated using a specific receptor antagonist. Biotinylated proteases were administered in in situ disease and were targeted by localized avidin to immune deposits with a reduction in injury and proteinuria.

Other models of immune complex disease involved the "planting" of antigens (e.g., concanavalin A, cationized proteins) and subsequently administering antibody resulting in in situ immune complex disease. The manifestations of the injury and the clearance depended in part on the localization of the complexes in the capillary wall. Additional studies of the Heymann model in 1984 with antibody to the putative antigen (gp 330, gp 600) demonstrated fixation of the antibody on the surfaces of glomerular epithelial cells in vitro, followed by redistribution of the antigen and antibody to form patches and caps on the cell surfaces (see in situ mechanisms). The authors proposed that in this model the formation of subepithelial deposits resulted from shedding of immune complexes formed in situ on the plasma membranes of epithelial cells.

Another model of immune complex injury—an in situ interaction between antibody and mesangial cells—was described further in 1986. In this model, antithymocyte antibody induced an early complement-dependent lysis and subsequent proliferative glomerulonephritis. Later reports demonstrated an associated decrease in the ultrafiltration coefficient, the lack of platelet participation, and increased infiltration of macrophages as well as superoxide and eicosanoid production. In this disease, an increase in mRNA and expression of matrix components (laminin, type IV collagen) were observed.

An additional presumed but not proven antibody-mediated mechanism of renal and vascular injury was first described in Wegener's vasculitis in 1984. Antineutrophil cytoplasmic antibody (ANCA) was reported to be present in patients with Wegener's granulomatosus, polyarteritis nodosa, and other less well-defined vasculitic diseases with necrotizing glomerulitis associated with no or few immune deposits. Proceedings of subsequent meetings from 1985 to 1989 included observations on the role of ANCA in the stimulation and activation of neutrophils in vitro, the capacity of ANCA to damage endothelial cells in vitro, and studies demonstrating substrate-specificity of ANCA for proteinase 3 and myeloperoxidase and the specific disease associations. In 1989, an entire session was devoted to ANCA.

The role of cell-mediated immune renal injury is discussed in the section on macrophages and in the section on tubulointerstitial nephritis. Here it seems useful to describe several abstracts dealing with the putative cell (or cytokine) mediated mechanism for alterations in capillary wall permeability in the nephrotic syndrome. In 1975, three patients with Hodgkin's disease who developed a nephrotic syndrome were reviewed and compared with 32 previously reported patients. Of the 27 patients whose renal pathology could be evaluated, 11 had minimal changes with negative immunofluorescence. These authors concluded that the reversible nephrotic syndrome observed in association with Hodgkin's disease was probably due to an aberrant lymphoid cell or immune function. In 1976, supernatants from cells of a Hodgkin's tumor grown in culture were perfused into rats with appropriate control supernatants without changes in morphology or proteinuria. The search for the putative cytokine(s) or mechanisms responsible for this remarkable association continues. In 1984 and 1985, autoimmune glomerulonephritis in chickens induced by immunization with basement membrane could be transferred with sensitized cells in the absence of antibody (see the next section).

In-Situ Mechanisms of Immune Glomerular Injury

As indicated in the historical review, the Proceedings of the 1966 International Meeting included a review of the knowledge available concerning the mechanisms of glomerular injury by antibody to GBM (the nephrotoxic serum anti-GBM antibody model) and recognition of the fact that the primary anti-GBM γ-globulin served as a "planted" antigen for a secondary injury invoked when the recipient animal's immune system produced antibody to the localized foreign IgG.

Review of the ASN abstracts from 1967 to 1990 reveals several further contributions in this area of research in the late 1960s. The passive transfer to monkeys of eluted IgG from the kidney of two patients with rapidly progressive GN and linear GBM immunofluorescence was shown to result in (*1*) fixation of the IgG on the monkey's glomeruli and (*2*) proteinuria.

In 1976, the concept of "fixed glomerular antigens" was introduced by a study of the heterologous model of immune complex glomerulonephritis in rats (Heymann's GN, induced in rats by injection of antibody to FX1A, a partially purified antigen derived from proximal tubules). It was shown that perfusion of the rat kidney with anti-FX1A resulted in fixation of the antibody in a granular pattern on primarily the epithelial surfaces of the GBM. The authors proposed that the immune complexes formed in this locus arose not from the circulation, as had previously been thought, but from antibody binding to fixed antigens in the subepithelial region of the rat GBM.

The following year, another group of investigators evaluated the nephritogenic potential of a lectin, concanavalin A (ConA), which binds to glycoproteins of the GBM by nonimmune mechanisms. Perfusion of ConA, followed by antibody to ConA, resulted in "in situ" formation of immune complexes and proliferative glomerulonephritis in the perfused kidneys. In another study, the role of fixed glomerular antigens versus circulating immune complexes in the heterologous immune complex model of membranous nephropathy (Rab anti-FX1A) was investigated using the isolated perfused rat kidney. It was shown that kidneys perfused with anti-FX1A in a nonrecirculating system developed diffuse fine granular subepithelial deposits of rabbit IgG within 1 hour. The authors concluded that circulating immune complexes were not involved in this model but rather that the antibody bound to fixed glomerular antigens to form in situ complexes.

In 1981, the concept of a fixed subepithelial glomerular antigen in this experimental model of membranous GN was further explored and the mediation of the injury and proteinuria examined. Noncomplement fixing sheep γ-2, anti-FX1A was injected into rats as the "fixed" antigen. Kidneys containing this antigen were then transplanted into other rats that had been immunized with sheep IgG. These rats developed granular subepithelial deposits of sheep IgG, rat IgG, C3, and proteinuria. The proteinuria was abolished by depletion of C3 in the rats but not by depletion of circulating polymorphonuclear cells.

The "fixed antigen" of this model was subsequently shown to be large membrane glycoprotein with a molecular weight of 330 (gp 330), which resides in clathrin-coated pits of both the proximal tubular brush border and the glomerular epithelium and is generally recognized as the antigen of Heymann's nephritis. Many additional studies that further characterized this antigen and its possible role in membranous nephropathy in human beings were presented during meetings of the 1980s and in 1990.

Molecular Charge

It is now established that a great number of polyanionic molecules, including sialoglycoproteins and proteoglycans, are present in the glomerulus and that these molecules play significant roles in the maintenance of normal glomerular structure and permeability and in the pathogenesis of certain forms of glomerular injury. The history of this insight into glomerular function can be traced to two sets of early observations: whole-organ physiological studies that showed differences in the clearance of charged proteins compared to uncharged dextrans, and histochemical studies that demonstrated that glomeruli were rich in polyanionic sialic acid-containing residues. It was not, however, until the mid-1970s that the importance of glomerular charge was definitively formulated again by two sets of studies—one physiological and the other morphological. The physiological study showed differences in renal clearance among anionic, neutral, and cationic dextrans, and the morphological work demonstrated increasing penetration of the glomerular capillary wall by ferritin molecules of increasing isoelectric points. Results from these series of studies were read in the Renal Physiology session of the 1975 ASN meetings and eventually sparked the explosion of work onto the role of molecular charge, which predominated in the ASN programs of the late 1970s to mid 1980s.

Prior to 1975, there were occasional interesting preludes of what was to come. In the 1970 meeting, a paper on alterations in glomerular sialoglycoproteins during acute poststreptococcal glomerulonephritis was read, complementing other papers appearing in the literature showing reduction in stainable glomerular polyanion in experimental aminonucleoside nephrosis and human minimal change disease. In 1974, it was shown that polycations, such as protamine sulfate, induced reversible "fusion" of glomerular epithelial foot processes.

After the 1975 papers, molecular charge was prominently stressed in a symposium held in 1976 on the contributions of morphological techniques to the understanding of renal physiology. In 1978, papers were read on the modeling of glomerular capillary charges selectivity and the influence of molecular configuration on glomerular ultrafiltration. And for the first time, there was reference to proteoglycans as possibly important components of anionic sites in the glomerular basement membrane. By 1979, an entire platform session on glomerular permeability focused on issues of molecular charge, and a large number of abstracts on this topic were submitted through 1984. Some of the more critical discoveries reported in the meetings included the role of glycosaminoglycans, particularly heparan sulfate, in charge selectivity; the contribution of molecular charge to the glomerular localization of immune reactants and the development of experimental glomerulonephritis (an area that showed convergence of research on in situ immune complex disease with research on molecular charge); a description of alterations in charge and size selectivity in experimental models of glomerular injury and evidence for loss of polyanionic molecules in certain human disorders (such as lipoid nephrosis and the congenital nephrotic syndrome); a demonstration that cationic extracellular streptococcal antigens are present in human immune complex glomerulonephritis; and the identification of podocalyxin, the major glomerular sialoglycoprotein, which is defectively sialylated in experimental aminonucleoside nephrosis. The frenzy of research in this area abated in 1984, seemingly because conclusive experiments to define roles for the various anionic components were difficult to devise and because those interested in the glomerulus were increasingly preoccupied with the new mediators of glomerular injury and their molecular regulation.

In perspective, the research into molecular charge presented at ASN meetings between 1975 and 1984 draw the structural and biochemical map of many (but by no means all) of the polyanionic moieties within the glomerulus, established a role for a charged capillary wall in determining normal glomerular permeability, and also helped explain some of the determinants of immune reactant localization in the glomerulus. Research has not, as yet, provided definitive evidence of loss of charge selectivity as an important cause of proteinuria in human nephrotic syndrome. Recent ASN abstracts and related publications suggest that reductions in charge density do indeed occur in nephrotic states but that these lead to loss of protein through defects (shunts) in the capillary wall rather than diffuse loss of charge selectivity. The resolution of these issues must await further investigation.

Complement

Review of the Proceedings of the Third International Congress (1966). As mentioned in the historical review, the role of complement (C′), in both anti-GBM nephritis (nephrotoxic serum nephritis) and acute and chronic serum sickness models of glomerulonephritis, and the role of C5b as a chemotactic agent for polymorphonuclear leukocytes were appreciated as mediators of renal injury. It was also recognized that experimental disease was ameliorated by transiently decomplementing the host with either antibody to C′, aggregated IgG, or zymosan.

Review of the ASN Abstracts (1967–1990). In 1968, a serum factor (C3NeF) that specifically cleaved β1C (C3) was described in some patients with glomerulonephritis. Low levels of C3 were reported in acute and chronic glomerulonephritis and lupus nephritis. Breakdown products of C3 were recognized in glomerular deposits. Subsequently, C3NeF was detected in the serum of eight of nine patients with persistent hypocomplementemic glomerulonephritis and in some patients with SLE and acute glomerulonephritis; a decrease in the level was observed in patients treated with prednisone. In later years, C3NeF was shown to be an autoantibody to C3 convertase. In 1970 and 1971, membranoproliferative (MPGN) or mesangiocapillary glomerulonephritis (including MPGN associated with intramembranous deposits—currently called type II MPGN) was recognized as the pathological entity associated with reduction in serum C3. Evidence for participation of the alternative complement pathway was deduced from recognition of the presence of properdin in the glomerular deposits and the involvement of factors B and D. In 1973, a symposium on the role of the alternate complement pathway in glomerulonephritis was held. The recurrence of MPGN in the transplanted kidney was reported, and a year later differing complement profiles were noted in MPGN I and MPGN II. Immunohistochemical studies of the latter disease in 1977 demonstrated a characteristic glomerular deposition of C3 outlining dense deposits. In subsequent years, a variety of other complement components and regulatory proteins have been demonstrated in various forms of glomerulonephritis. In 1990, antiidiotypic antibodies to C3NeF in patients with MPGN were demonstrated, principally of the stimulating variety. These antibodies were shown to decrease after treatment with prednisone, and it was suggested that antiidiotypic antibodies may modulate autoantibody formation.

In 1975 and 1976, abstracts described the presence of complement receptors in human glomeruli, which were distributed on the surface of visceral epithelial cells. A decrease in the apparent number of receptors was observed in glomeruli with immune deposits containing complement components, while patients with no deposits or with mesangial deposits retained complement receptor activity. The precise role of these receptors has eluded explanation. Complement receptors on erythrocytes were shown to be important in the transport of immune complexes in the primate, as reported in abstracts from 1984 to 1989 (see Immune Mechanisms).

In 1978, the development of proteinuria in a model of in situ membranous nephropathy (passive Heymann's nephritis) was prevented by depletion of complement using cobra venom factor, whereas depletion of polymorphonuclear leukocytes (PMN) had no effect on protein excretion. These findings implicated a complement-dependent but PMN-independent mechanism for the glomerular capillary injury in this disease (see In situ Mechanisms).

In 1982, the renal distribution of poly C9, a neoantigen of the membrane attack complex of complement (MAC) was described, using a monoclonal antibody to this antigen. In glomerulonephritis, MAC was distributed in a pattern similar to that of C3, and in other renal diseases (diabetic nephropathy, hypertensive nephropathy), it was prominent in areas of glomerular sclerosis. These studies suggested a role for MAC in glomerulonephritis and other diseases. The urinary excretion of C5b-9 was increased in experimental membranous nephropathy (passive Heymann's nephritis) but not in other experimental renal diseases, including anti-GBM nephritis, ConA-anti-ConA disease, or cationized IgG-anti-IgG nephritis (1986). A similar increase was observed in human membranous nephropathy (1987). The localization of C5b-9 on the epithelial cell membrane and its intracellular transport were described in passive Heymann's nephritis. In 1990, the urinary concentration of MAC was evaluated in nephrotic syndrome by ELISA. Elevated levels were found in patients with membranous nephropathy (MN) and in some patients with other forms of the nephrotic syndrome. Immunosuppressive therapy was reported to result in a lower level of excretion. Other abstracts demonstrated high urinary levels, which were correlated with the severity of the disease and a progressive course. Other abstracts described the role of complement in mediating the synthesis of eicosanoids, oxygen metabolites, and the regulation of hemodynamic changes occurring in experimental immune models of glomerulonephritis. The participation of the terminal complement components in experimental disease was evaluated in C6 deficient rabbits—where a role was suggested in anti-GBM nephritis (1986).

Mediators of Glomerular Injury

In 1967, at the first ASN meeting, Dixon reviewed the immunological pathology of renal disease. The known mechanism of glomerular injury at that time was dependent on the activation of complement and the accumulation of neutrophils. It was realized then, however, that neither decomplementation nor depletion of neutrophils could abrogate the proteinuria in some models of GN (i.e., the homologous phase of nephrotoxic serum nephritis), and it was subsequently shown that proteinuria could occur in the absence of complement, neutrophils, or both complement and neutrophils. For these reasons, alternate mediators have been sought. A state-of-the-art lecture 22 years later summarized the enormous progress in dissecting the large variety of mediators of glomerular injury that were subsequently uncovered. Such mediators include oxygen-free radicals; arachidonic acid metabolites (including prostaglandins, leukotrienes, lipoxins); platelet factors; endothelial-derived vasoactive factors (endothelin, epidermal-derived growth factor [EDRF]); growth factors (e.g., platelet-derived growth factor [PDGF]; transforming growth factor [TGF]-β); cytokines (e.g., IL-1, tumor necrosis factor [TNF], IL-6, IL-8); and proteolytic enzymes. Review of the ASN abstracts reveals three important determinants for the proliferation of studies on these chemical mediators: (*1*) the discovery of these mediators and their role in nonrenal tissue injury (e.g., oxygen-free radicals in pulmonary injury and PDGF in the intimal hyperplasia of atherosclerosis); studies of these mediators in the kidney lagged behind studies in other organs, but models of glomerulonephritis have proved to be powerful for the study of the in vivo role of such mediators, since functional measurements of protein excretion and glomerular filtration rate (GFR) and quantitation of morphological alterations in the glomerulus are convenient end points for pharmacological interventions; (*2*) the realization that macrophages, lymphocytes, and platelets all infiltrate the glomerulus, and all can be stimulated to synthesize or secrete powerful biological active mediators; and (*3*) the discovery that intrinsic glomerular cells—endothelium, mesangium, Ia^+ resident macrophages, and epithelium—can all be induced to produce some of these mediators and that interactions between infiltrating and intrinsic glomerular cells may be critical to the progression of glomerular injury.

Role of Macrophages, Lymphocytes, and Cell-Mediated Immunity in Glomerulonephritis

Although earlier light and electron microscopic studies had noted the presence of monocytes in the glomeruli of patients and experimental animals with glomerulonephritis, the studies that eventually established an important role for macrophages in glomerular injury were sparked by the work of the Melbourne group, presented at the ASN meetings in 1975. In this study, cultures from outgrowths of crescents from four patients with rapidly progressive glomerulonephritis (RPGN) showed a very large number of highly motile cells that were avidly phagocytic and that had the "cinemicroscopic characteristics of macrophages." The authors suggested that "contrary to current belief, crescents in RPGN consist of macrophage-like cells, rather than proliferating epithelial cells." Although it is now clear that crescents are composed of both proliferating epithelium cells and macrophages, this work led directly to the first experimental studies, read at the 1977 ASN meetings, showing that monocytes infiltrate the glomerulus in an accelerated model of experimental glomerulonephritis and that prevention of monocyte influx by irradiation abrogates the proteinuria in this model. By 1978, studies from a number of laboratories justified a symposium lecture on the "role of monocytes in glomerulonephritis." Subsequently, histochemical marker studies in both experimental and human glomerulonephritis and intervention studies in various experimental models showed that monocytes infiltrated the glomerulus in a variety of glomerular diseases and that in certain instances, they were correlated with proteinuria.

In 1981, another original work was presented: in rat glomeruli, an Ia-positive resident glomerular cell with characteristics of a macrophage was present and could be differentiated from traditional resident mesangial cells. Although an Ia^+ resident macrophage-type cell has not yet been described in *normal* human glomeruli, the studies pointed to cellular interactions within the glomerulus as possible determinants in the pathogenesis of immune glomerular injury. In subsequent years, monoclonal antibodies against antigenic markers of leukocytes were introduced, and from these it is now apparent that macrophages are present in glomeruli in many forms of proliferative glomerulonephritis, particularly in crescentic disease of various etiologies and in postinfectious, cryoglobulinemic, and diffuse lupus nephritis, but that small number of monocytes are also found in noninflammatory glomerular diseases.

Research since 1983 has focused on the role of the large number of inflammatory and fibrogenic mediators produced by macrophages and their role in the acute hemodynamic changes, the genesis of proteinuria, the proliferation of mesangial cells, and the ensuring fibrosis. Studies have been done on reactive oxygen species, products of arachidonic acid metabolites, cytokines (such as interleukin-1 and TNF), growth factors (such as the platelet-derived growth factor), and a variety of enzymes. In addition, the role of activated macrophages in fibrin deposition was shown in experimental renal disease.

Lymphocytes are also present in certain forms of glomerulonephritis, and recent studies using monoclonal antibodies have shown accumulation of T cells in the glomerulus in experimental anti-GBM disease, preceding monocyte infiltration and glomerular injury. These T cells express interleukin-2 receptors, suggesting that they are functionally activated. The presence of activated T cells and macrophages suggests involvement of cell-mediated immune (CMI) reactions in glomerulonephritis, and such involvement is currently reasonably well accepted. Historically, however, early ASN meetings were dominated by studies on humoral mechanisms and, indeed, the rare studies suggesting glomerular delayed hypersensitivity were (sometimes publicly) derided. Although evidence for cell-mediated immunity in human glomerulonephritis is still difficult to pin down, several experimental models have strongly suggested CMI, and almost all first made their appearance at ASN meetings. It was first shown that in both anti-GBM and immune complex models of GN, mild proliferative GN resulted from the transfer of sensitized T lymphocytes. A model of experimental autoimmune glomerulopathy in chickens was introduced in an abstract, which was not accepted for either a poster or a platform session in 1977. But subsequent studies of this model, employing bursectomy, adoptive transfer of T cells, and intraglomerular localization of T cells, represent evidence that the lesions in the model are caused by sensitized T cells. More recently (1989, 1990), a convincing model of cell-mediated immune crescentic glomerulonephritis with marked interstitial involvement was reported in rats in which a hapten was infused into the renal artery after sensitization of these rats with a hapten-KLH conjugate. Transfer of sensitized T cells to naive recipients, followed by antigen injection into the renal artery, induced a focal crescentic glomerulonephritis. Exploitation of such models in rats will allow further dissection of the role of CMI and humoral immunity in glomerulonephritis.

The Glomerular Mesangium

Introduction. Although Zimmerman described a "fibroblast-like cell" in the mammalian glomerulus in 1933, it was not until the early 1960s that application of electron microscopy to studies of the kidney allowed a precise localization and description of these cells and their matrix. There followed a rapid expansion of knowledge regarding their phagocytic activity, smooth muscle contractility, and proliferative response to injury.

Review of the Proceedings of the Third International Congress of Nephrology (Washington, D.C.) in 1966 serves in part to establish a baseline for the state of knowledge regarding the mesangial cell at that time. At that meeting, the late Dr. Paul Kimmelstiel discussed "some glomerular changes by electron microscopy with predominant mesangial reaction" and stressed the importance of mesangial cell proliferation, the "expansion of the mesangium at the expense of the capillary lumen" in various glomerular diseases, and the "increase in number and widening of the mesangial trabeculae" in diabetic glomerulosclerosis. He speculated that the "mucopolysaccharides of the mesangial matrix are presumably deposited from the blood, but we have not ruled out the possibility that they are locally produced by mesangial cells."

Frank Dixon reviewed "the pathogenesis of immunologically induced nephritis" and mentioned "mesangial cell swelling and proliferation" as a feature of antigen-antibody induced acute serum sickness glomerulonephritis.

Jean Berger et al. described "the dépôts fibrinodes intercapillaires," shown by immunofluorescence to be primarily mesangial IgA, which was later to be recognized as that common kidney disease, IgA nephropathy.

The American Society of Nephrology Abstracts 1967–1990. The expansion of interest and knowledge regarding the mesangial cell over these 25 years is illustrated by the fact that the 1967 abstracts contain a single clinical paper describing focal glomerulonephritis with mesangial proliferation, whereas the 1989 and 1990 abstracts include at least 50 studies, each describing mesangial cells in culture. One could conclude that the mesangial cell has become the most intensively cultured of all cell types.

In 1973, a symposium on "The Mesangium in Renal Disease" updated the state of the art with regard to structural and functional considerations, the uptake and handling of immunoaggregates by the mesangium in experimental models of disease, and alterations of the mesangium in human renal diseases. A single paper reported the presence of myocin in the glomerular mesangium, described by immunofluorescence (IF), supporting the contractile property of that cell system that had been proposed and its probable relationship to arterial smooth muscle cells.

In 1975, the growth of "stellate" cells, presumably mesangial cells from glomeruli in culture, was described. As indicated earlier, the improved techniques for isolation and culture of mesangial cells have led to an enormous interest in this methodology.

During the 1970s and 1980s, interest in the function of mesangial cells increased with multiple studies of the uptake and clearance of intravenously injected substances such as aggregated proteins, immune complexes, and ferritin. The capacity of the mesangial cells (or infiltrating cells) to degrade endocytosed substances was documented. The movement of macromolecular substances taken up by the mesangial cells toward the vascular pole and the extraglomerular lasis cell system was observed. Interest in the contractile function of mesangial cells persisted in the late 1970s and 1980s with several descriptions of receptors for angiotensin II and arginine vasopressin on mesangial cells and speculation that the contractile response of mesangial cells could play an important role in the regulation of glomerular blood flow and/or glomerular filtration rate.

In the 1980s, further developments regarding mesangial cell structure evolved, including recognition of fibronectin as a secretory product of the cells and a prominent constituent of the normal mesangial matrix. The concept of mesangial expansion as an early and important characteristic of diabetic nephropathy, recognized earlier by Kimmelsteil, was confirmed by quantitative structural-functional studies in humans with diabetic nephropathy, relating the expansion of the mesangium inversely to GFR. In experimental animals (rats), expansion of the mesangium following injection of polyvinyl alcohol (PVA) also resulted in decreased GFR but unchanged renal blood flow (RBF) until arterial pressure (AP) was incrementally lowered. With progressive lowering of AP, the PVA rats appropriately failed to autoregulate RBF, suggesting that mesangial expansion interfered with afferent arteriolar dilation and/or other hemodynamic determinants of autoregulation.

Additional important structural-functional concepts introduced in the 1980s included the recognition of bone-marrow-derived resident Ia-bearing monocytes within the mesangium. Depletion of these cells from the glomerulus and the interstitium was shown to occur following the feeding of rats a diet deficient in essential fatty acids (EFAD diets). Rats fed an EFAD diet and subsequently injected with nephrotoxic serum demonstrated striking amelioration of glomerular inflammation and proteinuria, suggesting that kidney monocytes played an important role in the mediation of the glomerulonephritis of this standard experimental model.

In the late 1970s and early 1980s, improved understanding of mesangial IgA nephropathy evolved through the development of several experimental models with similar morphological and immunological characteristics. In one of these models, 60% of mice who were fed several proteins (ovalbumin, ferritin, or bovine γ-G) for 14 weeks developed mesangial IgA deposits, as compared with 12% of control mice. Presumably, mucosal antigenic stimulation can generate a specific IgA immune response that can result in deposition of IgA in the mesangium.

The transgenic mouse model was introduced to the meetings in 1985 as a model of glomerular sclerosis. In 1990, application of this technique with human immunodeficiency virus (HIV) proviral DNA injected into mouse eggs resulted in mice with mesangial expansion and proteinuria by 25 days of age, which eventually developed into focal segmental glomerulosclerosis, said to resemble the lesion seen in patients with HIV infection.

As mentioned earlier, studies of both human and rat mesangial cells in culture involved more than 100 papers submitted during the late 1980s and the 1990 meeting. The synthesis of several cytokines (IL-1, 2, 6, 8) and prostaglandins and the effects of several growth factors, endothelin, endothelial relaxing factor (nitric oxide), hormones, and many other substances too numerous to mention, on mesangial cell growth, proliferation, and synthesis were evaluated. Of special note were studies of transforming growth factor beta (TGF-β) which was shown both in vitro and in vivo (in a model of glomerulonephritis) to mediate the up-regulation of proteoglycan production and mesangial expansion in rats. Obviously, the complex interplay of the large number of factors that apparently participate in the regulation of mesangial cell function and structure will require some time for sorting and integration before the true significance and potential implications for human renal diseases can be realized. It is an exciting time in the evolution of knowledge regarding the mesangial cells.

Tubulointerstitial Nephritis (TIN)

Review of the Proceedings of the Third International Congress (1966). The proceedings relevant to this section include discussions of microdissection of nephrons from patients with nephronophthisis, a description of 21 patients with the recently described condition termed oligomeganephronia, and several chapters on the toxic nephropathies and analgesic nephropathy. Included in the discussions of the mediation of the toxic nephropathies were the heavy metals, solvents, antibiotics, and others drugs and their potentials for inducing tubulointerstitial nephritis. The accumulated clinical reports of renal injury caused by analgesic abuse were largely from European centers. Recognition of the high incidence of analgesic abuse in 10 watchmaking factories in northwestern Switzerland in 1965 and recommendations presented regarding elimination of phenacetin-containing medications in this population likely contributed to the reduction in the incidence of this problem worldwide.

Review of the Abstracts of the ASN (1967–1990). The pathological renal lesions present in 26 patients who had each taken mixed analgesics totaling at least 3 kg of phenacetin were reviewed in 1968. The initial lesion was described as an increase in collagen around vasa recta and tubules in the medulla. These lesions were present in some patients without a loss of renal function. Progressive changes, including interstitial and periglomerular fibrosis, tubular atrophy and dilation, basement membrane thickening, and medullary necrosis, were described in patients with reduced renal function. The clinical and pathological findings in seven patients with renal failure and interstitial nephritis associated with large doses of penicillin or methacillin were also described by another group. Penicillin hapten bound to renal tissue in the same sites as IgG was described in one patient by immunofluorescence microscopy, suggesting a hypersensitivity mechanism for this nephropathy. This immunopathological association is now recognized to be extremely rare.

An early description and comparison of the clinical findings and pathological lesions of medullary cystic disease and nephronophthisis, presented by the late Dr. Maurice Straass in 1969, suggested that the pathological lesions in both diseases were "indistinguishable," although different mechanisms might be involved.

In 1973, a model of autoimmune tubulointerstitial nephritis (TIN) was induced in C4-deficient guinea pigs by injection of tubular antigens. Activation of the complement system was presumed to have occurred via the alternative pathway of complement. In the same year, interstitial and tubular basement membrane (TBM) deposits of immune complexes were described in chronic serum sickness nephritis in rabbits. In 1978, a model of TIN was described in guinea pigs that were sensitized to tubular antigens. Lymphocytes from spleen, lymph nodes, and peritoneal exudate were shown to be cytotoxic for fetal guinea pig kidney cells in culture. TIN with in situ deposition of immune deposits on the ascending limb of the loop of Henle was also described in rats following the administration of rabbit antirat Tamm Horsfall protein. Subsequently, antibody to Tamm Horsfall protein was described in pigs with reflux nephropathy. In 1979, a symposium on tubulointerstitial disease dealt with intrarenal reflux, antiidiotypic antibodies in the treatment of anti-TBM disease, the association of glomerular lesions, and connective tissue responses. Studies of a model of TIN in Brown-Norway rats in 1980 described suppression of the disease by autologous antiidiotypic immunity. In 1982, the spontaneous interstitial nephritis that developed in Kd mice was considered to have an autoimmune cell-mediated basis.

In another study in 1980, interstitial nephritis developed in SJL mice by adoptive transfer of lymphoid cells or serum from mice with TBM antigen-induced TIN. Subsequently, adoptive transfer of an antigen-specific, Ia-restricted T-cell line for nephrotic mice induced disease in normal mice. In the Brown-Norway rat, a similar form of TIN could be induced after immunization with bovine TBM.

A number of studies using the mouse system were reported in subsequent years, including the induction of effector T cells by L3T4 helper cells in vitro (1984); the interaction of suppressor and countersuppressor T cells (1985); the inhibition of effector cells by administration of long-term suppressor T cells (1986); the demonstration of idiotypic network (1989); the cloning of the nephritogenic antigens (1988); the transcriptional regulation of MHC class II expression; and the characterization of an antigen-specific cytotoxic line (1989). In 1990, other studies further explored different aspects of the TIN model using the techniques of molecular biology to evaluate cytokine expression and production by cloned T cells, the mRNA of a resident T-cell receptor, and the modulation of $\alpha 1$(IV) collagen gene expression by murine tubular cells. Early gene expression (c-*fos*, c-*jun*, epidermal growth factor [EGR], c-*myc*, JE) was noted to be increased in the Brown-Norway rat model of TIN (1991).

The isolation of a target antigen implicated in human antitubular basement membrane nephritis was also described in 1990. A 54-Kd, noncollagenous glycoprotein was isolated from human TBM and partially characterized. Injection of 50 μg of this antigen into guinea pigs resulted in a severe TIN associated with IgG and C3 deposits along the tubular basement membrane. In 1986, interstitial nephritis was identified as an important pathological feature of aminonucleoside nephrosis. There was also recognition of TIN and fibrosis as a prominent part of a disease in rabbits induced by anti-GBM antibody (1986, 1987). In the human, TIN was reported to be associated with nonsteroidal antiinflammatory drugs.

Pathology

The initial ASN meeting served as a forum for several clinicopathological studies in which renal biopsies were the source of the pathological material. Papers on focal glomerulonephritis, poststreptococcal glomerulonephritis, rapidly progressive glomerulonephritis, lupus nephritis, and an immunofluorescence study of biopsies from human renal allografts found favor with the program committee. The natural history of focal proliferative, diffuse proliferative, and membranous lupus glomerulonephritis was described, and the poor prognosis with corticosteroid therapy alone was documented in diffuse proliferative lupus nephritis. The ultrastructural appearance of the lesions of lupus nephritis was also presented. Immunofluorescence evaluation of human allograft biopsies established that extensive early arterial deposition of IgG, C3, and fibrinogen was associated with accelerated rejection; heavy linear glomerular IgG deposition could forecast progressive glomerular lesions (? recurrence); acute rejection was relatively free of immunoglobulin localization in the kidney; and long-term allografts with impaired renal function had mesangial fibrinogen deposits and linear deposition of IgG, C3, and fibrinogen in the glomerular capillaries. The relationship between medullary cystic disease and familial juvenile nephronophthisis was also described at the 1967 meeting. The histopathology of a variety of intrinsic and extrinsic lesions producing renal artery stenosis was also discussed.

Curiously, only one abstract describing diabetic nephropathy was submitted to the first meeting, and it was not presented on the program. The pure nephrotic as well as the nephritic-nephrotic pediatric patient was described in abstract only, and the generally poor prognosis in the heterogeneous nephritic-nephrotic group of individuals was noted.

The following year, pathological descriptions of analgesic nephropathy, the hemolytic-uremic syndrome, and so-called familial thrombocytopenia were presented. The interstitial nephritis occurring with heavy exposure to penicillin and methicillin was also described and thought quite likely to represent a hypersensitivity reaction. An abstract not selected for presentation provided one of the earliest descriptions of the ultrastructure of the obsolescent human glomerulus. Another abstract not presented documented the nonresponsive character of membranous glomerulonephritis to corticosteroid therapy in contrast to lipoid nephrosis.

The 1969 meeting saw no significant increase in the number of abstracts submitted or presented that described the pathology of the human kidney. Evidence was presented that Goodpasture's syndrome and rapidly progressive glomerulonephritis with anti-GBM antibodies were part of the same clinical spectrum. Additional evidence was presented that in the childhood nephrotic syndrome, the presence of abnormal glomerular pathology was generally associated with a poorer prognosis.

Again, papers describing the pathology of diabetic nephropathy were scarce. A single abstract not presented on the program noted the similarity between lesions in monkey, rat, and dog kidneys in animals with experimental diabetes and the lesion of diffuse intercapillary glomerulonephritis in humans. Abstracts were also submitted but not presented that documented the natural history of idiopathic membranous glomerulonephritis (one of the earliest published reports) and substantiated that lobular and membranoproliferative glomerulonephritis were similar but were not a stage in the evolution of idiopathic membranous glomerulonephritis as previously thought by many pathologists. An interesting abstract not presented documented the fact that the majority of biopsies from patients with nonstreptococcal acute oliguria glomerulonephritis have crescentic lesions but lack subepithelial immune complex deposits.

At the 1970 meeting, additional evidence was provided that certain penicillin derivatives including methicillin and ampicillin, the latter in association with furosemide administration, caused a hypersensitivity reaction resulting in tubulointerstitial nephritis and acute renal failure. This meeting also saw the first description of dense deposit disease, a variant of membranoproliferative glomerulonephritis, now called type II MPGN. Evidence was also presented that subacute bacterial endocarditis was capable of producing an immune complex form of glomerulonephritis.

Descriptions of several pathological renal lesions including the adult form of Henoch-Schonlein purpura and the intraendothelial myxovirus-like structures in systemic lupus erythematosus appeared in abstract only.

The fifth meeting of the Society in 1971 saw the first communications describing a possible relationship between the intravenous use of heroin and renal disease manifested clinically by the nephrotic syndrome and renal failure and pathologically by focal membranoproliferative glomerulonephritis and interstitial nephritis as well as end-stage disease. Additional experience with the dense deposit form of membranoproliferative glomerulonephritis, a lesion originally described by Berger in 1968, was presented. Other pathological reports that appeared on the program included descriptions of the Nail-Patella syndrome, the membranoproliferative lesion of sickle cell anemia, the "virus-like" particles located within the endothelial cells in kidneys of patients with viral hepatitis, and a "membranoproliferative" lesion observed in patients with alcoholic cirrhosis. This meeting saw the first reports in humans and animals of a possible relationship between exposure to hydrocarbons and the development of so-called Goodpasture's syndrome. An important abstract not presented at the annual meeting emphasized the frequent finding of histological and immunofluorescence abnormalities in the kidney biopsies of patients with so-called "benign hematuria."

At the sixth annual meeting of the Society in 1973, a study of adult lipoid nephrosis documented the poor therapeutic response to corticosteroids of individuals with focal segmental glomerulosclerosis. Attendees at this meeting saw for the first time in two separate symposia the inclusion of morphological data to provide structural-functional correlations in the kidney. The symposia were entitled, "The Mesangium in Glomerular Disease" and

"Mechanisms of Acute Renal Failure." Recurrence in renal allografts of Henoch-Schonlein purpura and membranoproliferative glomerulonephritis was also described.

An abstract not presented described several patients with nonalcoholic liver disease who had immune complex renal disease in the form of either membranous or membranoproliferative glomerulonephritis. Interestingly, only one abstract that dealt with diabetic nephropathy was submitted, and it was not presented. It described significant early renal lesions in symptomatic diabetic patients who were normotensive but proteinuric. Another interesting abstract not presented described reversible clinical and pathological abnormalities in the kidneys of infants with congenital syphilis following penicillin treatment.

In 1974, several abstracts appeared on the program describing various forms of renal injury. Occupational lead nephropathy with vascular, mesangial, and tubular damage was reported. In a large prospective study of adult patients with the nephrotic syndrome, one-third were found to have renal vein thrombosis, which was thought to be a complication of the underlying disease rather than the primary cause of the nephrotic syndrome. Additional evidence of recurrence of lupus nephritis in a renal allograft was also presented. An abstract was also presented that demonstrated significant differences in the immunopathological complement profile between type I and type II membranoproliferative glomerulonephritis.

At the 1975 meeting, an important observation on diabetic patients receiving renal allografts was presented. Hyalin degenerative lesions were observed within arteriole walls of the allograft as early as 2 years after transplantation. An early report was also presented describing the suspected role of macrophages in glomerular crescent formation. The proposed "third type" of membranoproliferative glomerulonephritis was also discussed.

The 1976 meeting saw an early description of the ultrastructural findings in glomerulonephritis associated with cryoglobulinemia. The fibrillar character of the deposits, probably representing circulating cryoglobulins, was emphasized.

The first real interest in diabetic nephropathy was underscored when an entire symposium was dedicated to the subject at the 1976 meeting. At this same meeting, the presence of diffuse lupus nephritis was reported in the absence of obvious clinical renal involvement. Data were also presented documenting the presence of the nephrotic syndrome in renal allograft recipients with chronic rejection alone. An early report of de novo membranous glomerulonephritis in the renal allograft was also presented.

The 1977 meeting of the Society saw the initial demonstration of enhanced renal injury in hypertensive rats made hyperglycemic with administration of streptozotocin, thus supporting the theory that changes in the characteristics of renal perfusion are pathogenetically important in the development of diabetic renal disease. Other presentations described the apparent relationship between the charge characteristics of Bence-Jones proteins and renal injury, the relationship between cyst fluid composition and lining epithelium ultrastructure in human polycystic kidney disease, and the absence of a relationship between physiological findings in acute tubular necrosis (ATN) and the renal histopathology. A detailed description of C3 localization in type II MPGN was also presented. The lesion of acute crescentic glomerulonephritis without anti-GBM antibodies or immune complex deposits was also described at the meeting.

At the 1979 meeting, evidence from kidney biopsy material was presented that identified the presence of a C3 activating factor in patients with MPGN that allows continued activation of complement via the alternative pathway. Studies were described that provided evidence for localization of the so-called "Goodpasture" antigen along the lamina rara interna of the GBM in human biopsy specimens. It was also reported that children with steroid-sensitive and frequently relapsing nephrotic syndrome can have three types of glomerular lesions: minimal change histology, focal and segmental glomerulosclerosis, and mesangial proliferation. It was found that, following prolonged therapy with cyclophosphamide, most patients who continue to relapse have focal segmental glomerulosclerosis or mesangial proliferation.

At the 1980 meeting, data were presented that in IgA nephropathy, Henoch-Schonlein purpura, and lupus nephritis, the glomerular IgA deposits consist predominately of IgA_1 monomers of polyclonal origin rather than secretory IgA. Data were also presented on patients with unilateral renal agenesis for accelerated focal glomerulosclerosis in the absence of reflux nephropathy. An excellent paper reviewed the carefully documented incidence of various forms of recurrent glomerulonephritis in renal allografts in a large transplant population.

Diabetic nephropathy was the focus of a symposium at the 1980 meeting. Topics that were discussed included the relationship between glucose homeostasis and glomerular lesions, physiological alterations in the diabetic kidney, the natural history of the glomerular lesions in humans, and the problems of uremia in the diabetic patient.

In the 1981 meeting, the spotlight was focused on glomerulonephritis in the form of a state-of-the-art lecture and the presentation of a large number of free communications. The latter included a report from the International Study of Kidney Disease in Children that emphasized the importance of specific histological variants of minimal change disease and diffuse mesangial cellularity on outcome. Also included was a study describing the outcome of the nephrotic syndrome in children with focal segmental glomerular sclerosis. Other diseases that received attention included IgA nephropathy, dense deposit disease, and the congenital nephrotic syndrome. In the latter entity, the absence of glomerular basement membrane heparan sulfate was described. This meeting also saw the initial description of so-called "IgM nephropathy." Another first was the report of the presence of bone-marrow-derived Ia-bearing cells in the rat glomerular mesangium.

In 1981 there was a great deal of interest in the effect of the electrical charge of antigens and immune complexes and the GBM on the pathogenesis of renal disease. An introductory lecture entitled "The Role of Immune Complex Electrical Charge in Immune Nephritis" was followed by several abstracts that examined the effects of altered GBM electrical charge and the charge of immune complexes in the initiation and progression of several forms of kidney disease.

In 1982, several clinicopathologic studies in various forms of primary and secondary renal diseases were presented. For instance, in lupus nephritis, an excellent correlation was reported between the more severe and active forms of glomerular disease and the presence of immune complex deposits along the tubular basement membranes. Renal lesions were also described in sickle cell nephropathy, type II diabetes mellitus, and glomerulosclerosis. Renal allograft failure was described and attributed to recurrent dense intramembranous deposit disease. Interest also focused on characterizing the extrinsic cellular components of the glomerulus in several forms of renal disease by employing monoclonal antibodies to cell surface markers. It was also demonstrated in diabetes mellitus that the characteristic linear staining pattern of the GBM observed with immunofluorescence macroscopy was confined to those proteins with an iso-electric point (pI) of 6.0 or lower. This suggested that positive charge sites are present in the altered GBM of humans with diabetes mellitus.

Mesangial IgA nephropathy was reviewed in a minilecture, and two reports described examples of so-called IgM nephropathy. In the latter, evidence was presented that the underlying histopathology, that is, minimal change disease versus focal glomerulosclerosis and not the presence of mesangial IgM, determined the prognosis.

In 1983, the concept of HIV-associated nephropathy was presented in three abstracts. Pathological findings included focal and segmental glomerular sclerosis, mesangial proliferation, and tubulointerstitial nephritis. Other glomerular lesions were less common. Structural-functional studies were described in patients with insulin-dependent diabetes mellitus who were biopsies when the GFR ranged between 40 and 120 mL/min/1.73 m^2. Quantitative examination demonstrated an excellent correlation between mesangial thickening and the decline in GFR. Furthermore, it was concluded that in the absence of clinical nephropathy it was not possible to estimate the risk for diabetic renal disease without a kidney biopsy.

The interest in diabetic nephropathy, both experimentally and clinically in the early and mid-1980s, was clearly evident at the 1984 meeting. Included was an invited lecture, "Structure-Function Relationships in Diabetic Nephropathy" along with numerous abstracts presented on the subject. Evidence was presented from kidney biopsies of insulin-dependent diabetic patients that the best direct structure-function correlation existed between the creatinine clearance and the capillary filtering surface. At this same meeting, evidence was presented that in patients with steroid-responsive minimal change nephrotic syndrome there was a 35% reduction in the number of anionic sites in the lamina rara interna of the GBM of renal biopsies. It was suggested that this alteration might help explain the proteinuria in these patients.

The results of a review of a large group of renal biopsies from patients with focal segmental glomerular sclerosis suggested that the earliest lesion that actually precedes sclerosis may be visceral epithelial cell necrosis.

After the introduction of so-called AIDS-associated nephropathy at the 1984 meeting, a minilecture on the subject and additional reports were presented at the 1985 meeting. One state-of-the-art lecture looked in detail at rapidly progressive glomerulonephritis.

At the 1986 meeting there was growing interest in the diagnostic significance of autoantibodies against neutrophil cytoplasm (ANCA) in patients with renal disease. The best correlations were reported between their presence and biopsy evidence of Wegener's granulomatosis and polyarteritis nodosa.

At this meeting, there was continued reporting of the gamut of renal lesions in patients infected with HIV. Tubuloreticular inclusions were described in the endothelial and interstitial cells in renal biopsies from both symptomatic and asymptomatic patients. In a detailed study employing light, electron, and immunofluorescence microscopy of renal biopsies from patients with AIDS and nephropathy, heroin nephropathy, and idiopathic focal segmental glomerulosclerosis (FSGS), it was concluded that histological and clinical features of AIDS-associated nephropathy indicate a more rapidly progressive form of FSGS with distinguishing ultrastructural characteristics. At these same meetings, an interesting case report was presented that described extreme GBM and TBM disorganization in association with profound glomerular alterations and renal failure in two infant siblings.

A year later at the 1987 meeting, ANCA-positive vasculitis and AIDS-related complex (ARC) and AIDS-associated nephropathy were the subjects of several abstracts. However, significant new features associated with these entities were not described. Data were presented from patients with myeloma cast nephropathy that confirmed the currently held opinion that the syncytial cells surrounding the myeloma casts are not derived from tubular epithelium.

The interest in ANCA-positive glomerulonephritis (ANCA-GN) continued at the 1988 meeting. A detailed clinicopathologic study involving 48 patients demonstrated that ANCA-GN is characterized by very few immune deposits and segmental necrosis and crescent formation and is frequently accompanied by a variety of extraglomerular necrotizing vasculitides. Now included in the ANCA-GN category are patients with pauci-immune crescentic glomerulonephritis, microscopic polyarteritis, and Wegener's granulomatosis.

Several interesting pathological observations in the human kidney were described at the 1989 meeting. A retrospective study of minimal change disease (MCD) in children revealed that the mean glomerular tuft area in those patients who subsequently went on to develop focal glomerular sclerosis was significantly greater than that in patients with clinical and pathological findings characteristic of MCD. Additional information was provided on fibrillary glomerulonephritis. Although this is an ultrastructurally distinctive form of immune complex glomerulonephritis, there is considerable diversity in both the clinical presentation and the light microscopic histopathology from patient to patient. Also, attention was called to the fact that in patients with acute tubular necrosis, cellular damage is often more severe in the medulla than in the cortex.

The 1989 and 1990 meetings also witnessed intense interest in the significance of ANCA antibodies in patients with renal disease. Interestingly, evidence was presented suggesting the presence of these antibodies in most forms of vasculitis, not just the microscopic form of polyarteritis.

Anatomy

At the inaugural meeting of the Society no pure morphological papers describing the anatomy of the kidney were presented, although a single abstract detailing the ultrastructure of the distal tubule of the nondiseased human kidney was submitted. Likewise, the single structural-functional abstract describing the morphology of Henle's loop and its relation to urinary concentration in the kidney of humans and monkeys also was not included on the program.

A year later a structural-functional investigation employing isolated rabbit collecting tubules demonstrated that widened lateral intercellular spaces were functionally an extension of the extracellular space and that water exited the cell by osmosis across both the lateral cell walls and the cell surface in contact with the basement membrane. The lateral intracellular space dilated because of hydraulic resistance to outflow affected by the slit at the base of the intercellular space. This paper was followed a year later by similar observations obtained in vivo in the collecting duct of rats with hypothalamic diabetes insipidus.

In the mid-1970s the first reports describing intramembranous particle aggregates in toad urinary bladders exposed to vasopressin and an osmotic gradient were presented. Early reports describing the ultrastructural appearance of tight junctions in normal and volume-expanded animals appeared in abstract only. These were followed by freeze-fracture studies demonstrating that with volume expansion in the rat, there was a significant increase in the number of discontinuities in the tight junction of the proximal tubule, suggesting that these sites may relate to increased permeability of the intercellular channel.

The 1976 meeting represented a true milestone for morphologists when an entire symposium entitled, "Contributions of Morphological Techniques to Understanding of Renal Physiology" and part of a poster session, "Renal Morphology and Physiology," were presented.

In 1977, additional attention was focused on the formation of intramembranous particle aggregates in toad urinary bladder, namely the time course in relation to exposure to vasopressin and the possible role of microfilaments in the aggregation phenomenon. Interesting data were also presented using thick sections (0.5 μm to 1.5 μm) and standard transmission electron microscopy to document the apparent existence of a very limited number of ramifying mitochondria in mammalian proximal and distal tubule cells; these data were contrary to widely held opinions.

At the 1980 meeting, the importance of molecular charge in the kidney received considerable emphasis. One state-of-the-art address dealt with the organization, nature, and function of fixed negative charges in the glomerular basement membrane. A free communication was presented that described enhanced uptake of cationic versus anionic ferritin by cells of the distal convoluted tubule.

A year later the detailed ultrastructural appearance of the glomerular endothelium was described using a combination of scanning and transmission electron microscopy.

In 1982, the first structural-functional data were reported from the rat outer medullary collecting duct that suggested the presence of hydrogen ion secretion by intercalated cells via insertion of proton pumps into the apical cell membrane during acute respiratory acidosis. Data were also presented from turtle bladder that suggested control of proton secretion was, at least in part, due to endocytosis and recycling of the proton pumps.

At the same meeting, abstracts were presented that defined more precisely the pathway of ADH-induced osmotic water flow across the rabbit cortical collecting duct and the role of prostaglandins and aggrephores in ADH-induced osmotic water flow in the toad urinary bladder.

At the 1983 meeting, there was a considerable interest in the apparent relationship between certain ultrastructural changes and functional characteristics in various hydrogen ion transporting epithelia. In addition to several abstracts that were presented on the subject, a minilecture was devoted to the topic.

A pure morphological paper described the heterogeneity of the ultrastructural features of the cells of the thick ascending limb of Henle and for the first time identified two histological cell types in this region of the nephron.

At the 1984 meeting, an entire symposium was devoted to the subject of morphological insights into transport mechanisms. Topics that were covered included potassium, water, and proton transport. At this same meeting, evidence was first presented in the turtle urinary bladder that two types of carbonic anhydrase-rich cells appeared to be present.

At the 1985 meeting, vasopressin-induced intramembranous particle aggregation was quantified in isolated rabbit cortical collecting tubules using freeze-fracture electron microscopy. A dose-dependent relationship was demonstrated between vasopressin and the number of aggregates as well as the number of particles per aggregate inserted into the luminal membrane of principal cells. Data were also presented from turtle urinary bladder that intracellular pH regulation in mitochondria-rich cells is the consequence of exocytic insertion of proton pumps into the apical cell membrane.

At the 1987 meeting, attention was called to the structural heterogeneity of the cells that form the inner medullary collecting duct (IMCD) in rat kidney. Intercalated cells were described with principal cells in the initial one-third of the IMCD, while the distal two-thirds of this tubular structure was formed by IMCD cells with histological features that were distinct from the principal cell.

At the 1988 meeting, there was continued interest in proton and bicarbonate secretion by the collecting duct. In a structural-functional study, induction of acute metabolic alkalosis in the rat caused intercalated cells (IC) in the outer medullary collecting duct and type A IC in the cortical collecting duct that are involved in proton secretion to decrease in both volume and luminal surface area. In contrast, type B cells that are believed to secrete bicarbonate underwent hypertrophy in association with an increase in the basolateral membrane compartment. These morphological findings suggested that proton secretion by type A and outer medullary collecting duct IC is suppressed, while bicarbonate secretion on type B IC is enhanced in acute metabolic alkalosis.

Localization of carbonic anhydrase-positive intercalated cells in the rat collecting duct was described using light and electron microscopic immunocytochemistry and employing both a monoclonal and a polyclonal antibody against carbonic anhydrase II. Cytoplasmic immunoreactivity was limited to intercalated cells only in the collecting duct, and there was no evidence for the presence of this enzyme in inner medullary collecting duct cells.

At the 1989 meeting, considerable interest was shown in the structure and function of water channels in various transport epithelia. Evidence was presented that separated the recycling mechanism for water channels in the collecting duct principal cell and the toad bladder granular cell from the conventional endocytic pathway present in most types of cells. Interest in structural-functional studies of proton and bicarbonates transport by intercalated cells in the collecting duct remained high. Observations were presented in the rabbit cortical collecting duct that with the induction of acute metabolic acidosis in vivo, the activity of bicarbonate-secreting type B intercalated cells was greatly diminished in concert with a decrease in cell size.

At the 1990 meeting, intercalated cell structure and function was discussed intensely. Evidence was presented suggesting that intercalated cells isolated from cortical collecting ducts and grown in culture gradually acquire structural and functional characteristics of principal cells. Other data presented suggested that bicarbonate loading could influence the early appearance of type B intercalated cells in the neonatal rat cortical collecting tubule. It was also reported that enhanced chloride delivery to the rat cortical collecting duct stimulated type B intercalated cells, while acute alkalosis caused atrophy of type A cells and withdrawal of H^+-ATPase from the apical plasma membrane and storage in apical cytoplasmic vesicles.

6

Acute Renal Failure

Jay H. Stein, Norman G. Levinsky, and Franklin H. Epstein

Acute renal failure (ARF) has been a topic of considerable interest to the membership of the American Society of Nephrology (ASN) since the society's initial meeting in 1967. These scientific contributions have been subdivided in this chapter into Pathophysiology of Acute Renal Failure (written by J. Stein), Clinical Aspects of Acute Renal Failure (written by N. G. Levinsky), and Toxic Nephropathy (written by F. H. Epstein).

Pathophysiology of Acute Renal Failure

Mechanisms

One can appreciate the flavor of the field of ARF from the initial meeting of the American Society of Nephrology in 1967. At that time, studies were phenomenologic, and there was very little synthesis of the pathophysiology. At that meeting, McDonald and associates showed that chronic salt loading had a substantial protective effect on the glycerol model of acute renal failure. The authors suggested that the renin-angiotensin system was a major pathophysiologic factor in the glycerol model. Cirksena evaluated the effect of intravenous injection of methemoglobin-ferrocyanide in the rat. Although there was a slight increase in intratubular pressure, the studies were not definitive. Barenberg and associates, again using micropuncture techniques in the rat, showed a marked fall in glomerular filtration rate in a mercuric chloride model. Last, Hollenberg and associates showed preferential renal cortical ischemia in human beings by angiography and krypton washout techniques. Thus, it was suggested that a number of factors play a role in the pathophysiology of acute renal failure in animals and in humans, but the intricacies are far from clear.

Flamenbaum et al evaluated another nephrotoxic model of acute renal failure, uranyl nitrate, in the 1971 meeting and demonstrated marked cortical ischemia and an alteration in the intrarenal distribution of blood flow as measured by radioactive microspheres. The emphasis at that time was on renal hemodynamics, but there was still no clearcut delineation of more specific mechanisms.

The issue was clearer by the 1973 meeting. In fact, acute renal failure was becoming so important that a symposium was held. Carl Gottschalk presented important papers on the pathophysiological events, Norman Hollenberg stressed hemodynamics, Donald Oken continued his emphasis on the renin-angiotensin system, and Michael Kashgarian discussed morphological correlations. Arendshorst, Finn, and Gottschalk presented a classic study evaluating proximal intratubular pressure prior to, 2 to 3 hours after, and 24 hours after renal artery ischemia in the rat. The studies unequivocally demonstrated that tubular obstruction was present in this model of acute renal failure. It is of interest that obstruction was present 24 hours after ischemia but that this was masked to some extent by severe afferent arterial vasoconstriction. At this same meeting, a study was presented that for the first time suggested that an alteration in the glomerular ultrafiltration coefficient may also participate in the renal functional impairment seen in ARF. Using the unilateral infusion of norepinephrine into the renal artery, Baehler et al. presented physiological and morphological evidence that the glomerulus may indeed be involved in this model. Subsequent studies presented at a number of ASN sessions confirmed this finding. At the 1973 meeting, Torres and his associates also presented the first suggestion that the prostaglandins may be involved in acute renal failure. They used the glycerol model in the rabbit to demonstrate that the administration of indomethacin accentuated the renal functional impairment.

This time period served as a landmark for the synthesis of the general pathophysiological events that occur in acute renal failure. By that point it was clear that multiple factors were involved in the reduction of renal function seen with various models of acute renal failure. These included renal vasoconstriction, tubular obstruction, leakage of filtrate across damaged tubular epithelium, and a reduction in the glomerular ultrafiltration coefficient.

In subsequent meetings, many papers were presented that amplified these findings. For example, in 1983, Cushner and associates delineated the effect of volume expansion to protect against the development of glycerol-induced acute renal failure. Using morphological and physiological measurements, the studies clearly indicated the role of cast formation in this model. Further, at the 1984 meeting, Tanner et al. studied the morphological effects of chronic obstruction at the single tubule level. One day after obstruction, the entire length of the proximal tubules downstream from a paraffin block showed cellular injury. By 1 week, less-differentiated cells lined the collapsed lumen of the tubule. At 1 month, there was severe proximal tubular atrophy and extensive interstitial fibrosis. At the 1976 meeting, Donohoe and associates unambiguously demonstrated the role of tubular back leak in acute ischemic renal failure. Horseradish peroxidase (HRP) was microinjected into proximal tubules, and there was leakage through the cytoplasm of necrotic proximal tubular cells into the interstitium. A similar abnormal permeability to HRP was seen following intravenous injection, demonstrating once and for all that the findings with the microinjection technique were not a pressure artifact.

With this understanding of the phenomena involved, the emphasis on acute renal failure shifted to studying various nephron segments and eventually the basic biochemical aspects involved.

Segmental Differences in Response to Injury

The various segments of the nephron have different metabolic capabilities. Proximal tubules use aerobic metabolism, while the loop of Henle and other medullary segments function primarily by anaerobic means. Further, the pO_2 in the medulla is extremely low; thus, the various nephron segments may respond quite differently to ischemic and nephrotoxic injury. Hanley showed some of the functional alterations in individual nephron segments after ischemia. Using the isolated tubular perfusion method in an ischemia model in the rabbit, he found a marked decrease in fluid resorption in the proximal convoluted and straight tubules, a marked reduction in the ability to reduce the chloride concentration along the ascending limb, and a reduction in the hydroosmotic effect of vasopressin in the cortical collecting segment. These studies clearly explain a number of the events that occur in acute renal failure, including the inability to concentrate the urine and the high fractional excretion of sodium seen in most of these models. At the 1980 meeting, Hanley found similar changes in models of ureteral obstruction. In 1981, Epstein, Balaban, and Ross presented a paper on mitochondrial anoxia in the isolated perfused rat kidney. This presentation initiated a series of studies and presentations at subsequent ASN meetings that evolved into a concept that the outer medulla, existing in hypoxic environment, is extremely susceptible to ischemic injury. From these studies it was first hypothesized and then demonstrated that a reduction of work in the thick ascending limb, by administration of either ouabain or furosemide, would protect the thick ascending limb from hypoxic damage as well as attenuating a reduction in glomerular filtration rate (GFR).

Protection

From the first meeting in 1967, the effects of various protective agents in acute renal failure have been emphasized. As noted previously, McDonald and his associates showed that chronic volume expansion protected the kidney in the glycerol model of acute renal failure. There have been numerous clinical papers, even as early as the 1968 and 1969 meetings, on the effects of diuretics, including mannitol, furosemide, and ethacrynic acid, in the prevention of acute renal failure. The studies indicate that when administered prophylactically these agents may prevent renal functional impairment, but once fixed acute renal failure occurs, their only value may be in converting an oliguric to a nonoliguric form of acute renal failure.

In the last 10 years, a number of experimental studies have further delineated the mechanism whereby these agents protect against various forms of acute renal failure. Hanley, in presentations to the ASN in 1979 and in 1980, presented studies that indicated that mannitol and furosemide had a protective effect in acute renal failure. In this same 1979 meeting, Johnston, Bernard, and Levinsky were the first to demonstrate that the vasodilatory effect of mannitol was mediated to a large extent by increased prostaglandin synthesis. In 1989, Sheridan and Lieberthal demonstrated that atrial natriuretic peptide combined with mannitol had a marked protective effect against ischemia in the rat. Experimental studies to evaluate the effect of mannitol continue, although we are still not certain how it works and still have not clearly demonstrated that it has definite effects clinically superior to volume expansion alone.

As mentioned previously, atrial natriuretic peptide has been shown to have a protective effect in experimental acute renal failure. Prostaglandin E_2, bradykinin, and converting enzyme inhibitors are three other potentially vasodilatory substances that also seem to exert a protective effect in at least some experimental models of acute renal failure.

The effect of free oxygen radicals and other related antioxidants has been studied in a number of organ systems and has generally been found to play a role in cellular injury and death. This concept and its effects on renal function were first presented at the 1983 meeting in a paper by Paller on an ischemic model in the rat. Paller gave superoxide dismutase, a free oxygen radical scavenger, prior to clamping and before release of the renal artery, as well as a dissimilar scavenger, dimethyl thiourea. Both of these agents, as well as the xanthine oxidase inhibitor allopurinol, protected against functional impairment as measured by changes in the serum creatinine. Subsequent papers have used deferoxamine, glutathione administration, and sodium benzoate in various models. All these agents presumably are antioxidants. Interestingly, Mandel and his group, in 1989, demonstrated that glutathione protected against anoxic injury to proximal tubules in vitro. Yest they were not certain that the effects were related to an antioxidant effect. Rather, glutathione was shown to increase the production of glycine, which apparently exerts a separate effect on prevention of cellular injury. Thus, while much evidence suggests that the presence of free oxygen radicals plays a role in the production of cellular injury in acute renal failure, the protective effect of antioxidants is far from clear.

In the 1978 meeting, a symposium was held on enhancement of recovery from acute renal failure. Vasoactive agents were discussed, as were the use of amino acids during recovery from acute renal failure and the role of osmotically active agents, such as mannitol. In addition, Norman Siegel at Yale presented the first studies on the use of adenine nucleotides in various models of acute renal failure. This seemed like mysterious business because it was not clear how adenosine triphosphate (ATP) would get into the cells and why magnesium was necessary as a carrier. Subsequently the authors found that ADP or AMP had the same effect. In 1985, studies from the laboratories of Weinberg and of Mandel demonstrated that ATP was degraded to adenosine, which then entered the cells and provided substrate for new adenine nucleotide production. This hypothesis was buttressed in 1988 by a study from the Yale group, indicating that inhibition of adenosine deaminase would enhance recovery from ischemia.

Other protective models have included complement depletion, the administration of amino acids, and manipulations that reduce outer medullary congestion. At the 1987 meeting, Weinberg demonstrated the surprising protective effect of glycine. In this study he demonstrated that the protection was not accompanied by improvement of cellular ATP and thus was not limited to hypoxic injury. These studies were amplified by another study from Weinberg's group in 1988. In 1989 Epstein showed that glycine attenuated *cis*-platinum–induced acute renal failure in intact rats.

Cell Biology

The major focus in acute renal failure in the past several years has related to the cellular events that occur with ischemic injury. A search through the archives of the American Society of Nephrology shows that cellular mechanisms in this disease were first mentioned in studies from the laboratory of the late Leah Lowenstein. Her group evaluated membrane turnover in normal states, renal hypertrophy, and acute renal failure. In 1981, Matthys, Patel, and Venkatachalam described a membrane phospholipid defect in ischemic renal damage. They suggested that the selective brush border damage may have been due to phospholipase activation, which started a vicious cycle toward cellular injury and eventual cell death. In 1982, Siegel and his collaborators used nuclear magnetic resonance to study alterations in adenine nucleotide concentration during renal ischemia. The study indicated that the technique could be used to determine in vivo metabolism of adenine nucleotides, that tissue ATP and tissue pH fell rapidly during ischemia, and that the recovery of ATP levels was incomplete for as long as 3 hours after an ischemic renal insult. In this same meeting, a number of other papers evaluated adenine nucleotide profile during ischemic injury and mitochondrial function during nephrotoxic and ischemic acute renal failure. As alluded to earlier, Paller presented data on the role of free oxygen radicals at the 1983 meeting, and Humes and the Denver group continued studies on the role of calcium in altered mitochondrial function during ischemic and nephrotoxic injury. By the 1987 meeting, active interest in the role of calcium in ischemic injury had begun to wane. LeFurgey and associates from Duke demonstrated that calcium did accumulate in the cytoplasm of proximal cells during anoxia, but the mitochondria did not show calcium accumulation. Further, they could dissociate the accumulation of calcium in the cytoplasm from cellular damage. Humes and his group also had concluded from other in vitro studies that cellular calcium did not seem to be a major determinant of cell injury in the proximal tubule.

1988 was obviously a year for growth factors. Using molecular biological techniques, Ouellett and his associates demonstrated expression of early growth response genes, which may be important determinants of functional tissue recovery after renal ischemia. Safirstein demonstrated that ischemic injury reduced a precursor of epidermal growth factor mRNA as well as urinary epidermal growth factor (EGF) levels, while at the same time the kidney expressed an increased number of EGF receptors. Similarly, Fine and his group found that EGF enhanced renal regeneration and accelerated recovery from ischemic acute renal failure in an ischemic model in the rat. Also noted was up-regulation of EGF receptor binding, which contributed to the regenerative response. Similar studies were continued at the 1989 meeting, and excitement about this important area of renal research continues.

Clinical Aspects of Acute Renal Failure

The state of knowledge about clinical acute renal failure (ARF) at the time of the first ASN meeting in 1967 can be inferred from the two major textbooks of nephrology of the time. Each had been published within 5 years of that meeting. The chapter on ARF in Strauss and Welt's *Diseases of the Kidney*, the first comprehensive textbook of nephrology, was written by the late John P. Merrill. In the first edition, published in 1963, the scheme for clinical classification is similar to that now in use. The distinction among prerenal failure, postrenal failure, and parenchymal renal failure begins the chapter. Merrill draws on Oliver's famous nephron dissection studies to divide the causes of acute parenchymal renal failure into ischemic and nephrotoxic categories. The list of nephrotoxins shows a preponderance of environmental over medicinal toxins. In considering the mechanism of renal insufficiency in humans, Merrill emphasizes the importance of persistent reduction of renal blood flow (RBF) due to vasoconstriction. The possibility that renal interstitial edema causes oliguria is still under active discussion. Merrill himself believes that "the evidence to date indicates that edema plays a major role in the causation of acute renal failure." Although decapsulation of the kidney to reduce pressure caused by interstitial edema is not effective after ARF is established, Merrill notes recent evidence that early decapsulation may be beneficial. The value of urinary sodium and osmolality is denigrated for differential diagnosis between prerenal and parenchymal renal failure. Of greater value in Merrill's opinion is a therapeutic trial with intravenous fluids. In a separate chapter, Merrill reviews the use of hemodialysis in the management of acute renal failure. Although conservative management by restriction of fluids, sodium, and potassium is emphasized, Merrill supports treatment of patients "clinically sick with uremia" by dialysis. He lauds the impressive results of Teschan with prophylactic daily dialysis in a military hospital but cautions that prophylactic dialysis would be difficult in less efficiently organized civilian hospitals.

Nephrology, written by Hamburger and associates, was published in French in 1966. Acute renal failure is positioned in a spectrum of acute tubular and interstitial nephritis that includes toxic acute tubular necrosis, ischemic (ATN), acute hematogenous interstitial nephritis, and acute ascending pyelonephritis. The authors note that in "very exceptional cases" ATN may be nonoliguric. These authors, like Merrill, draw on Oliver's studies to classify the pathology of human ARF as toxic or postischemic. Again there is emphasis on the pathophysiological significance of persistent reduction of renal blood flow, determined by various techniques suitable for use in humans. Arguments for and against the importance of intrarenal shunts in human disease are reviewed without firm conclusions. Merrill had noted initial studies suggesting that mannitol given early in the course of renal failure may prevent persistent renal insufficiency. Writing a few years later, Hamburger et al. review additional clinical studies but are unimpressed. They recommend a limited trial of mannitol but emphasize the need to stop if one dose does not produce a "frank diuretic response." These authors give less emphasis to conservative treatment and more to early dialysis in order "to keep the patient in satisfactory physical condition, to preserve an adequate margin for safety, to diminish the frequency of complications, and to shorten convalescence."

Causes

A major theme of ASN abstracts over the past 25 years has been the identification and description of new clinical types and causes of ARF. The advent of new pharmaceuticals has led to a series of new toxic causes of ATN. Thirteen abstracts from 1976 through 1986 dealt with radiocontrast nephropathy. Other "medicinal nephrotoxins" that received attention at ASN meetings include nonsteroidal antiinflammatory drugs, captopril, various antiinfectives, and penthrane. The importance of the burgeoning area of pharmacological nephrotoxins was emphasized by a symposium in 1979, "Acute Renal Failure due to Pharmacologic Agents." Aminoglycosides and radiographic contrast media were emphasized.

Earlier papers on contrast nephropathy reviewed its incidence and identified factors such as prior chronic renal failure and diabetes mellitus, which enhance the incidence of ARF. Beginning in 1983, a number of papers began to question the frequency of the phenomenon. Controlled studies by a group at McGill indicated that ARF was not more frequent in patients receiving computed tomography (CT) scans with contrast than in a control group. A controlled study in 1987 concluded that the incidence of ARF was low even in patients with chronic renal failure who receive contrast. In that year a paper took note of the advent of nonionic contrast media, putatively less nephrotoxic than standard media. This study indicated that the advantage of nonionic media might in fact be minimal.

Two papers in 1982, one from two collaborating hospitals in Boston and the other from the Cleveland Clinic, described a new entity. Both groups had observed that captopril may induce acute renal failure in patients with bilateral renal artery stenosis or with stenosis of the artery to a solitary kidney.

Newly recognized infections such as toxic shock syndrome (1980) and AIDS (1983) were identified as precursors of ARF. Old standbys as causes of ATN, such as postoperative ARF and prerenal failure, continued to receive some attention at ASN meetings. The phenomenon of nonoliguric renal failure, hinted at in pre-ASN texts, was well established by the mid-1970s. The prevalence and clinical features of this type of ARF were well delineated in an abstract in 1976 by the group at the University of Colorado. The relatively better prognosis of nonoliguric ARF was emphasized.

Diagnosis

By the first ASN meeting, the key diagnostic features of ARF were reasonably well established. However, over the years there has been some attention to urinary indices in the differential diagnosis among prerenal failure, acute parenchymal renal failure, and other kidney diseases. For example, in 1976 the group at the University of Colorado evaluated urinary osmolality, urinary sodium, and various derivatives thereof (fractional excretion of sodium, "renal failure index" [urinary sodium divided by u/p creatinine]). They concluded that the renal failure index and fractional excretion of sodium are the best urinary tests for separating the various categories of acute renal failure. A group at the University of Alabama (1983) devised a bedside technique (single injection of radiolabeled hippurate) for estimating renal plasma flow and indicated that the level of renal plasma flow (RPF) is a useful index of outcome in severe ARF. Although the idea seems of interest, it has received no further attention at ASN meetings.

Outcome

A major concern of nephrologists during the past two decades has been the persistently high mortality of patients with ARF, despite greater understanding of techniques for conservative management and the advent of efficient, easily delivered dialytic therapy. This topic has received attention at

ASN meetings from the very first one in 1967 and throughout the next two decades. A paper from the Mayo Clinic at the first meeting in 1967 assessed the factors affecting survival and the effect of earlier and more frequent dialysis. Familiar prognostic features such as patient age, severity of underlying disease, and complications influenced the outcome in this study. Frequent dialysis affected morbidity favorably but did not improve mortality. A paper from the nephrology group at Downstate Medical Center in 1978 challenged the general view that nonoliguric ARF has a better prognosis than oliguric ARF. They found that although nonoliguric patients required dialysis later than oliguric patients, survival was equally poor in all postoperative patients who required hemodialysis, regardless of urine output. In a paper presented in 1981, a group at the Hennepin County Medical Center reported that 8 to 16% of patients with ATN developed severe chronic renal failure. Of these, half required chronic hemodialysis. Prognostic factors for this unfavorable outcome were advanced age of the patient, preexisting renal disease, and additional acute renal diseases other than ATN. However, fully one-third of the patients who developed chronic renal failure after ATN had none of these prognostic factors. A group at the Massachusetts General Hospital reported in 1984 that sepsis, respiratory failure, and oliguria were the major factors predicting nonrecovery of renal function in ATN. Age, sex, cause of ATN, and other complications were less important prognostic indices. A group at Walter Reed Army Medical Center (1984) also emphasized sepsis and oliguria as bad prognostic factors. Hypotension also predicted high mortality. The authors emphasized that aggressive therapy including dialysis had not been associated with a substantial decline in mortality.

Prevention and Enhanced Recovery

Given the poor prognosis of established ATN, nephrologists have studied various methods to prevent or speed recovery from ARF. During the first decade of ASN meetings, a number of papers reviewed the efficacy of mannitol and loop diuretics as prophylactic and therapeutic agents. In 1968, the second year of ASN meetings, two papers noted apparent efficacy of ethacrynic acid in "reversing" acute renal failure. Another suggested that a response to mannitol can be predicted from the u/p osmolality and the duration of oliguria. Abstracts suggesting efficacy of ethacrynic acid early in the course of ATN were published the following year. Also noted was a now familiar and still controversial suggestion that even if diuretics do not reverse ARF, those patients who can be "converted" to nonoliguric ARF have better prognosis than those who remain persistently oliguric. A logical place to look for a beneficial effect of mannitol is radiocontrast nephropathy, since treatment can be prophylactic. A controlled study presented in 1981 demonstrated that mannitol is in fact protective against radiocontrast-induced acute renal failure in patients with preexisting chronic renal failure. By 1978, interest in enhancing recovery from acute renal failure was sufficient for a symposium on the topic to be organized. Mannitol, vasoactive agents, adenine nucleotides, and amino acids were reviewed at that conference. The latter two continue to be under active investigation in experimental disease. The value of amino acids in human disease was questioned in an abstract presented by a group in Los Angeles in 1978. In more recent years, other agents have been proposed as beneficial in reversing or preventing ATN. For example, in 1984, a study suggested that calcium channel blockers are useful to minimize the severity and duration of ARF in humans. In 1988, atrial natriuretic peptide was found to reduce the severity of ARF in patients at high risk for contrast-induced ATN.

Pathology

Surprisingly little attention has been paid at ASN meetings to the pathology of human ARF. A paper in 1970 noted difficulty in distinguishing the severity of functional impairment in ARF from renal cellular morphology. A study in 1976 reported that cytoplasmic changes in the proximal tubule regularly followed gentamicin therapy in humans. These included tightly packed laminated membranes, or "myeloid bodies," which are characteristic but have an uncertain relation to nephrotoxicity.

Pathophysiology

It has been difficult to analyze the pathophysiology of human ARF because of limitations in techniques suitable for use in humans. Two of the most important studies have been presented at ASN meetings. At the very first meeting in 1967, Hollenberg, Epstein, Basch, and Merrill reported that there is renal cortical ischemia in human acute oliguric renal failure. Using the then novel technique of radioactive xenon washout, these investigators demonstrated that there was drastic reduction in cortical blood flow in patients with ARF due to a number of toxic and ischemic causes. Confirmation of the xenon technique was obtained by noting failure of the kidney cortex to bleed on open renal biopsy in several patients and failure of selective angiograms to demonstrate cortical vascular filling in any patients. This paper demonstrated the utility of xenon washout and confirmed in humans the evidence from studies in animals that persistent cortical ischemia may be a mechanism causing renal insufficiency and oliguria.

Brian Meyers and his associates at Stanford have developed ingenious clearance and infusion methods to evaluate the pathophysiology of ARF in humans. They reported their results in a series of ASN abstracts between 1977 and 1984. The first two (1977 and 1979) were not chosen for presentation. By 1980, the importance of these studies had become evident to reviewers, and subsequent abstracts were reported at ASN meetings (1980, 1983, 1984). The investigative methods combined standard inulin and para-aminohippurate (PAH) clearances, excretion studies of dextrans of graded molecular size relative to inulin, and estimates of renal inulin spaces. The data provided evidence that in human ARF, as in animal models, backleak of tubular fluid and intranephronal obstruction are important causes of renal insufficiency. Despite certain limitations of the indirect methods, these ASN abstracts describe the most comprehensive and successful evaluation of the pathophysiology of human ARF to date.

Hepatorenal Syndrome

Relatively little has been presented at ASN meetings about this cause of acute renal failure. However, at the second meeting in 1968, the nephrology group at the Peter Bent Brigham Hospital in Boston presented their important observations on the pathogenesis of the hepatorenal syndrome. Using the xenon washout method, they compared the hepatorenal syndrome to other kinds of acute renal insufficiency (as presented at the 1967 ASN meeting). A specific feature of the renal circulation in the hepatorenal syndrome was extreme variability in moment-to-moment renal blood flow. This was superimposed on the profound reduction in cortical blood flow typical of other kinds of ARF. Angiography revealed constriction of intrarenal vessels in living patients with the hepatorenal syndrome, which disappeared postmortem. The investigators concluded that a major pathophysiological mechanism in hepatorenal syndrome is "a functional element acting upon the vessels." Intraarterial infusion of phentolamine failed to reverse the vasoconstriction, suggesting that it was not due to enhanced sympathetic nervous activity.

In 1976, Schroeder and associates reported that either portocaval or peritoneal-jugular shunts significantly improved renal function in the hepatorenal syndrome. They cautioned that initial functional improvement was not tantamount to long-term clinical benefit and called for a carefully controlled study to determine clinical utility. This was provided in an abstract presented by Linas and associates at the ASN meeting in 1985. They confirmed prior observations that peritoneal-venous shunts acutely improve renal function. However, only 1 of 10 patients treated with a shunt survived for more than a few days. The authors concluded that the shunt often stabilizes renal function but does not prolong life in patients with the hepatorenal syndrome.

Therapy

Remarkably little has been presented at ASN meetings on treatment for acute renal failure. As noted previously, a paper from Mayo Clinic presented at the first ASN meeting in 1967 reported that frequent dialysis improved morbidity but not mortality in patients with ARF. In 1974, a contrary conclusion was reached in a controlled evaluation of daily dialysis in posttraumatic ARF. Survival was found to be improved. As mentioned earlier, a 1984 abstract from Walter Reed reported that aggressive therapy including dialysis did not reduce mortality.

Toxic Nephropathy

Renal failure from toxic chemicals was well known early in this century. The 1910 edition of Osler's *Textbook of Medicine* mentions phosphorus, mercury, lead, and turpentine poisoning as causes of urinary suppression. Arthur M. Fishberg's 5th edition (1954) of *Hypertension and Nephritis* devoted a chapter to "The Necrotizing Nephroses" as a result of bichloride of mercury (frequently used for suicide attempts), carbon tetrachloride (widely employed at that time as a cleaning fluid and in industry), and obstruction by sulfonamide crystals, hemoglobinuria, myoglobinuria, and Bence-Jones proteinuria. Ethylene glycol, arsphenamine, and uranium nitrate (for the production of experimental renal failure) were also cited. In John Merrill's chapter on acute renal failure in the 1963 edition of Strauss and Welt's *Diseases of the Kidney*, the most important toxins reported to cause acute renal failure were said to be carbon tetrachloride, ethylene glycol, and bichloride of mercury. The initial cause of oliguria in "chemical nephrosis" was believed to be augmented back diffusion of glomerular filtrate through necrotic proximal tubules, followed by a decrease in renal blood flow due to swelling of the kidney. A. N. Richards, in 1929, had demonstrated back diffusion by direct observation on frogs poisoned with mercury. Consonant with this mechanism, Hayman found in 1939 that inulin and creatinine clearances were greatly depressed in dogs poisoned by uranium salts, although renal blood flow was only negligibly changed. The oliguria of sulfonamides was generally ascribed to intratubular crystallization, although the possibility of hypersensitivity nephritis producing renal shutdown without intratubular obstruction was also appreciated.

For the first 10 years of the American Society of Nephrology, the few abstracts on toxic nephropathy presented at the National Meeting reflected this classical interest. Mercury poisoning was shown, not unexpectedly, to reduce glomerular filtration rate (in the rat) and to be associated (in the dog) with a redistribution of renal blood flow from superficial to juxtamedullary nephrons. Uranyl nitrate, a classical tubular toxin, was used to demonstrate redistribution of renal blood flow and a decrease in glomerular filtration rate. This was associated with an increase in fractional excretion of sodium and distal tubular chloride concentration and an increase in renal renin content and secretion. Methoxyfluorane injury, increasingly encountered on surgical wards as a complication of anesthesia, was shown to be caused by the deposition of oxalate crystals in the kidney.

By 1975, members of the Society were beginning to report their investigations in animals of the nephrotoxicity of newer therapeutic agents like amphotericin and gentamicin. Lithium and *cis*-platinum joined this group during the next 2 years, followed by radiocontrast agents. During the 1980s, cyclosporine, acyclovir, and pentamidine attracted attention. Not surprisingly, all of the nephrotoxic compounds described at annual meetings of the Society since its inception (with the exception of uranyl nitrate) appear to have first aroused interest because of clinical observations of nephrotoxicity in patients. Sessions on toxic nephropathy have also been punctuated by occasional studies of the nephropathy of Bence-Jones proteinuria and of pigment nephropathy caused by hemoglobin or myoglobin.

Throughout the past 25 years, certain common themes have been sounded repeatedly in the application of general principles to the study of toxic nephropathy. These have included the physiological mechanisms invoked to explain renal failure; the potentiation of toxicity by ischemia, hypoxia, or dehydration; the effects of volume expansion, mannitol, and loop diuretics; the interaction of renal toxins with paracrine mediators of vasomotor tone and with calcium; the effects on renal cell biology of oxygen free radicals, mitochondrial toxicity, and enzyme inhibition; and the discovery of the distinctive role of anionic binding sites in renal brush border membranes for the toxicity of certain organic and metallic cations.

Mechanisms of Toxic Nephropathy: Redistribution of Blood Flow

The demonstration by Hollenberg and Merrill that acute renal failure in human subjects was accompanied by a redistribution of renal blood flow, with a relatively greater reduction of blood flow to the superficial cortex than to deeper portions of the kidney, was followed by an examination of this phenomenon in animal models of toxic nephropathy. A radioactive microsphere technique was generally used, abetted in some cases by the technique described by Hansen using lissamine green. In 1971, uranium nitrate nephropathy was found to be associated with a redistribution of renal blood flow from the outer to the inner cortex, and this was confirmed in 1975. The decrease in outer cortical flow was partially reversed when dopamine and furosemide were given within 15 minutes after the intravenous dose of uranium salt. Redistribution of renal blood flow after mercuric chloride administration in the dog was documented in 1982, and in the rat, mercuric chloride was shown to cause an increase in glomerulocapillary resistance to blood flow in the superficial cortex. Oxygen tension in the superficial renal cortex was also reduced by mercuric chloride administration (1983), as might be expected from local vasoconstriction, and this was reversed by concomitant administration of furosemide (1984). Somewhat surprisingly, the distribution of glomerular filtrate between superficial and deep nephrons was *not* found to be abnormal in *cis*-platinum nephropathy when Safirstein's group at New York's Mt. Sinai Hospital studied this by Hansen's technique in 1985.

Mechanisms of Toxic Nephropathy: Tubular Obstruction

Evidence for tubular obstruction in toxic nephropathy has been sought by several investigators, primarily by measuring proximal tubular pressure in superficial nephrons by micropuncture. In 1979, *cis*-platinum toxicity in rats was found to be associated with normal proximal tubular pressure in the presence of a diminished single nephron glomerular filtration rate, suggesting increased resistance to the tubular flow of urine. Similar observations implicating tubular obstruction were made in gentamicin toxicity (1981), and an increase in proximal tubular pressure was also observed in the experimental acute renal failure produced by lysine infusions (1983). Hemoglobin, myoglobin, and Bence-Jones protein were shown in 1976 to coprecipitate with Tamm-Horsfall protein to produce casts that, it was reasoned, were likely to contribute to intratubular obstruction. Irrefutable direct demonstration of tubular obstruction due to Bence-Jones protein was accomplished in 1989 when a human lambda protein injected by micropuncture into early proximal segments of perfused rat nephrons produced obstructing casts and greatly elevated resistance to tubular perfusion. The role of urinary pH was investigated by Zager, who in 1988 demonstrated that an acid urine converts hemoglobin to methemoglobin, which is less soluble than hemoglobin and was therefore likely to produce obstructing casts that contributed to oliguria. Intraluminal obstruction was also suggested in experimental cyclosporine A nephropathy and radiocontrast nephropathy, not through direct measurement but because intraluminal deposits of spherical or oval microliths were seen in cyclosporine-treated rats, and the radiocontrast agent diatrizoate was found to precipitate proteins derived from renal tubular suspensions (1985).

While it now seems likely that intratubular obstruction plays a role in many forms of toxic nephropathy, it has in general been difficult to interpret the evidence derived from simple micropuncture measurements of proximal tubular pressures, since these may fall as a result of a primary diminution in glomerular filtration rate and might also be lowered, even if obstruction is present, in the presence of significant tubular backleak.

Mechanisms of Toxic Nephropathy: Tubular Backleak

As already noted, back diffusion of glomerular filtrate was observed in the earliest micropuncture observations in frogs poisoned with mercury. The quantitative importance of backleak in various toxic nephropathies has, however, remained controversial. Blantz and his coworkers found considerable backleak in uranium nephrotoxicity, but Flamenbaum concluded in 1975 that backleak played a minor role in renal failure caused in rats by uranyl nitrate. On the other hand, in 1977, substantial backleak was demonstrated in rats with gentamicin nephropathy; only 63% of radioactive inulin injected into the proximal tubule was recovered in the urine, compared with 96%

recovery in control rats. Backleak was also demonstrated in 1979 in rats with *cis*-platinum nephrotoxicity.

Mechanisms of Toxic Nephropathy: Tubuloglomerular Feedback and Decreased K_f

A decline in glomerular ultrafiltration coefficient (K_f) in uranyl nitrate toxicity was described by Blantz in 1975, and subsequent studies revealed similar findings in other toxic nephropathies, including those caused by gentamicin, mercury, and *cis*-platinum. These were ascribed (1979) to morphological changes in glomerular endothelial cells as well as to reductions in the filtering area of the glomerular capillary bed. Both afferent arteriolar constriction resulting in a drop in glomerular capillary pressure and glomerular capillary constriction causing a fall in K_f have commonly been ascribed to tubuloglomerular feedback. Thus, in 1980, *cis*-platinum was shown to cause early afferent arteriolar constriction and (in 1982) to be associated with a decrease in proximal tubular stop flow pressure; however, the concentration of sodium in early surface distal tubular urine was normal rather than increased, as predicted by the tubuloglomerular feedback hypothesis. Because adenosine (as later demonstrated in 1988) potentiates tubuloglomerular feedback, it is of interest to note that theophylline, an adenosine antagonist, attenuated radiocontrast-induced intrarenal vasoconstriction (1984) and appeared to protect against myoglobinuric renal damage (1985). Theophylline also is protective in amphotericin B nephrotoxicity, even though the involvement of tubuloglomerular feedback in this condition was not clearly shown in stop-flow studies by Briggs and Schnerman (1989). The precise role of tubuloglomerular feedback in mediating renal failure due to nephrotoxins thus remains controversial.

Nephrotoxins Are Potentiated by Ischemia or Dehydration and Are Synergistic with Hypoxia

This general principle, familiar to renal clinicians and physiologists for at least 25 years before the first meeting of the American Society of Nephrology, has been amply confirmed by presentations at the Annual Meeting over the subsequent 25 years. In 1971, an abstract demonstrated clearly that acidosis and hypoxia potentiated the deleterious effects of methemoglobin. Dehydration (1980) and hemorrhage (1984) were similarly shown to enhance the toxic effects of myoglobin in animals. The deleterious effects of dehydration on the nephropathy of Bence-Jones protein in multiple myeloma had, of course, been observed frequently by clinicians. A brisk mannitol diuresis was shown in 1975 to blunt amphotericin B toxicity in dogs. At about the same time, the toxicity of gentamicin was clearly shown to be enhanced by a low-salt diet and ameliorated by increasing salt intake or

(1980) by mannitol diuresis. Subsequent studies confirmed the key influence of contraction of the plasma volume on gentamicin toxicity. Interestingly, furosemide, often given clinically in an attempt to ward off nephrotoxicity, was found in 1977 to enhance the toxicity of gentamicin if urinary losses of salt were not replaced. Such findings emphasize the importance of hydration and its effects on the systemic circulation in modulating nephrotoxicity. The circulatory effects of gram-negative toxins were presumably responsible for the marked synergy between gram-negative bacteremia and gentamicin toxicity, noted in 1985. Analogous effects of volume depletion and volume expansion were noted for uranyl nitrate, *cis*-platinum, and mercury in abstracts submitted between 1979 and 1983. The rule is as useful for newer nephrotoxins as for old ones; pentamidine toxicity in rats was noted in 1989 to be greatly enhanced by indomethacin and salt restriction, while in the same year radiocontrast nephrotoxicity was found to be potentiated by experimental congestive heart failure produced in dogs.

A mechanism for the synergy between certain nephrotoxins and hypoxia was suggested by the report in 1983 that the cellular injury produced by amphotericin in medullary thick ascending limbs of the isolated rat kidney could be completely eliminated by blocking active transport with ouabain. Amphotericin, a sodium ionophore, was postulated to increase cellular consumption of oxygen by medullary cells already operating in a hypoxic milieu. Other examples of synergy were also described. Gentamicin was shown to convert a sublethal ischemic cell insult in the proximal straight tubule (S_3) into a severe necrotic event. Hypercalcemia is synergistic with hypoxia in producing injury in medullary thick ascending limb cells. Lowering the calcium level in the perfusate protected against this injury.

Interaction with Hormones, Neurotransmitters, Paracrine Mediators, and Calcium

An increased production of renin characterizes many forms of renal injury, and it seems reasonable that this might contribute to renal vasoconstriction in toxic nephropathy. Converting enzyme inhibition was found to ameliorate uranyl nitrate toxicity (1981). However, Klotman and his associates (1982) found that captopril paradoxically exacerbated gentamicin toxicity, apparently because the disposal of bradykinin by its kininase was inhibited, and the production of thromboxane by the kidney was thereby stimulated. The angiotensin II antagonist, saralasin, did not prevent renal vasoconstriction caused by amphotericin (1986). Inhibiting sympathetic renal vasoconstriction with clonidine was found to protect against gentamicin toxicity (1982) as well as mercury poisoning (1981).

During the past decade, considerable attention has been paid to the interaction between prostaglandins and nephrotoxins. In general, prostaglandin formation by the kidney is increased early in renal injury, and inhibition of prostaglandin formation exacerbates the injury. An increase in prostaglandin formation was thought to contribute to the early concentrating defect induced by *cis*-platinum (1983) and to ameliorate the later fall in glomerular filtration rate seen in this form of toxic nephropathy. Similarly, glomerular production of prostacyclin and prostacyclin metabolites appears to be increased in early gentamycin toxicity, but subsequently, glomerular production of all prostaglandins diminishes (1985). On the other hand, cyclosporine clearly reduces the production of vasodilatory prostaglandins by aortic strips, isolated glomeruli, and mesangial cells, while increasing the production of thromboxane as reflected in the urinary excretion of thromboxane metabolites. Interestingly, the increase in thromboxane excretion stimulated by cyclosporine was eliminated by feeding rats fish oil, which also ameliorated cyclosporine nephrotoxicity in these animals. Thromboxane was also implicated in amphotericin toxicity in 1989 when Badr and coworkers found that a thromboxane A_2 receptor antagonist reversed renal vasoconstriction produced by amphotericin in the rat.

Just as calcium tends to potentiate hypoxic injury, as mentioned earlier, so hypercalcemia appears to worsen almost any kind of toxic renal injury. Starting in 1984, work presented at the Annual Meeting indicated that hypercalcemia enhances the toxicity of Bence-Jones proteins, that the administration of parathyroid hormone worsens gentamicin toxicity, and that parathyroidectomy attenuates renal injury due to gentamicin. Gentamicin toxicity is also increased by large doses of vitamin D (1986) and, interestingly, by the increase in circulating parathyroid hormone secondary to dietary calcium restriction, even though this is not associated with hypercalcemia. The calcium channel blocker nitrendipine decreased gentamicin toxicity (but verapamil did not) (1986). In cultured renal tubules, the direct toxicity of cyclosporine A was attenuated by reducing the ambient calcium in the medium (1987). An apparent exception to the general rule is that dietary calcium loading seems to inhibit gentamicin toxicity in intact rats (1982). This might be because of the effect of calcium loading to decrease circulating parathyroid hormone or conceivably because of an effect of hypercalciuria on the brush border binding and renal cell uptake of gentamicin.

Large doses of thyroid hormone (T_3) have been shown to be protective in ischemic nephropathy in the rat, and similar doses also appear to have a protective action in the nephrotoxicity caused by *cis*-platinum and by cyclosporine (1986). The mechanism is obscure, since many cell processes, including those of anabolism, catabolism, and active transport, are accelerated by triiodothyronine.

In the wake of several demonstrations that atrial natriuretic peptide could blunt or prevent the decline in renal function caused by experimental ischemic nephropathy, ANF was shown in 1987 to be capable of at least partially reversing acute cyclosporine toxicity and to protect against gentamicin toxicity in rats.

Finally, the discovery of endothelin predictably stimulated investigations into its possible implication in toxic nephropathy, particularly that caused by cyclosporine. Antiendothelin antibodies were shown in 1988 and 1989 to reverse renal vasoconstriction and acute renal failure caused by acute administration of cyclosporine, thus firmly implicating this new endogenous vasoconstrictor in the pathogenesis of cyclosporine nephropathy.

The Impact of Cell Biology on Studies of Toxic Nephropathy

Starting about 1980, and particularly after 1985, investigators interested in nephrotoxic renal failure turned their attention to studies of cellular biology and metabolism, using freshly prepared separated cells and tubules as well as renal cells in culture. Interest in free radicals as a mechanism of cell injury surfaced at the meetings of the Society in 1984, when gentamicin was shown to increase lipid peroxidation in the renal cortex and to accelerate the production of hydrogen peroxide by renal mitochondria. Disappointingly, inhibition of renal peroxidation by the administration of vitamin E did not appear to diminish the functional effects of gentamicin toxicity. Subsequently, free oxygen radical damage was implicated in cyclosporine A toxicity and *cis*-platinum damage to the kidney. *Cis*-platinum toxicity was diminished by a free radical scavenger (1985) and by pretreatment with superoxide dismutase or glutathione (1988). Adriamicin, known to produce cardiac damage through a free radical mechanism, was shown to increase lipid peroxidation in the kidney as well (1988). An explanation for the toxic effects of hemoglobin and myoglobin was also sought in oxygen free radical formation, it being reasoned that ferrous iron supplied by these compounds might catalyze the Haber-Weiss reaction, providing a source of hydroxyl free radicals within the kidney. The toxicity of hemoglobin-induced acute renal failure in rats appeared to be diminished by desferrioxamine, given to produce cellular iron depletion (1988).

Not unexpectedly, mitochondrial function, usually tested in proximal tubular cells, appeared to be disrupted by almost all toxic compounds tested. These included gentamicin, mercury, calcium, cyclosporine (with some exceptions), cephalosporin, *cis*-platinum, and radiocontrast agents.

A widely postulated mechanism of cell death in toxic as well as anoxic cell injury was postulated to be cell swelling, contributed to by *depletion of cellular ATP and failure of the sodium pump* in plasma cell membranes. In theory, therefore, the maintenance or repletion of cellular ATP together with enhancement of Na-K-ATPase activity might protect against toxic cell damage. The administration of magnesium ATP did indeed provide protection against gentamicin toxicity in rats (1986). Under these circumstances, extracellular ATP is probably broken down to form adenosine, which can be transported into the cell to serve there as an ATP precursor. Preliminary treatment of rats so as to increase the specific activity of Na-K-ATPase in the kidney was also found in some instances to diminish nephrotoxicity. Potassium loading, which increases renal Na-K-ATPase, protected against uranium toxicity (1986). Pretreatment with thyroxine also appeared to provide protection against gentamicin toxicity (1987) as well as acute toxicity produced by cyclosporine A (1986). Dexamethasone pretreatment provided some protection against gentamicin toxicity (1988). Vanadate, which inhibits Na-K-ATPase (as well as poisoning other cellular enzymes), potentiates gentamicin toxicity.

It might be predicted that renal toxins would affect new expression of a host of genes related to cell injury and repair, and exploration of this field is now beginning. In 1987, *cis*-platinum was shown to decrease total renal DNA turnover and to increase the expression of various growth factor genes in the kidney.

An important paper dealing with the mechanism of toxic cell injury was presented in 1988 as a poster by Dr. Patricia Wilson, who showed that in cultured proximal straight tubular cells, gentamicin and cyclosporine toxicity was mediated by a calcium-activated protease. Inhibition of the protease greatly diminished toxicity.

Lessons from Gentamicin Toxicity

More than any other nephrotoxin, aminoglycosides, and especially gentamicin, have been the subject of exhaustive study by members of the Society, particularly during the decade beginning in 1979. Not only is this form of iatrogenic renal failure commonly encountered in the clinic, but gentamicin produces a reproducible form of renal failure that is easily studied in the rat. Prior to 1979 it had been reported that gentamicin toxicity was, as indicated earlier, exacerbated by a low-salt diet and diminished by high salt intake. Under carefully controlled conditions, tobramicin appeared somewhat less toxic than gentamicin or neomycin.

During the 1980s, the cellular actions of gentamicin were explored. Gentamicin inhibits cell phospholipases, and as a result, the phosphoinositol cascade so important in cell signaling is disrupted in cultured proximal tubular cells. Because lipid hydrolysis is inhibited, the "myeloid bodies" characteristically seen on microscopic examination of kidneys poisoned with gentamicin are greatly enriched in phospholipids. In addition to decreasing the degradation of phosphoinositol, gentamicin apparently also increases its synthesis. Gentamicin also decreases proteinase activity in cellular lysosomes, diminishes protein synthesis in cultured cells, decreases Na/H countertransport and phosphate transport in brush border membranes of rat proximal tubules, and inhibits the translocation of protein and phospholipid to the apical brush border of cultured cells.

A symposium on gentamicin and radiocontrast nephropathy at the Annual Meeting of 1979 ushered in a series of especially interesting studies with important implications. In that year, Carlos Vaamonde and his colleagues reported that, unexpectedly, experimental diabetes produced in rats by streptozotocin effectively prevented renal toxicity from gentamicin. Subsequently it was discovered that experimental diabetes also protected against renal injury due to *cis*-platinum, uranium nitrate, radiocontrast agents, and mercuric chloride. Although at first it was hypothesized that the protection was afforded by glucose diuresis, it soon became apparent that this was not the case, since phlorizin, which produces glucose diuresis by interfering with its reabsorption in proximal tubules, did not protect against any of these nephrotoxic agents.

The key to this surprising finding was supplied rapidly by the work of several investigators, including Vaamonde, Kaloyanides, Humes, and Weinberg. Gentamicin gains access to proximal tubular cells by binding to the acidic phospholipids of brush border membranes (1980). In addition to cationic aminoglycosides, it is likely that other cationic renal toxins also bind to the negatively charged groups provided by phospholipids in apical brush border membranes. These probably include polyamines, uranium, and mercury. An excess of calcium in proximal tubular urine might conceivably be protective by competing for binding on acidic phospholipid sites. Streptozotocin diabetes is accompanied by a striking reduction in the phosphoinositol content of tubular cells, resulting in a reduction of gentamicin uptake. Phlorizin glycosuria, on the other hand, does not reduce renal phosphoinositol content and presumably because of this is ineffective in reducing aminoglycoside toxicity.

The hypothesis generated by these findings is that alterations in the binding of toxic substances by cell membranes (particularly but not exclusively the apical brush borders) might modulate nephrotoxicity. It seems possible, for example, that the protection against gentamicin toxicity afforded by a high-protein diet and partial renal ablation (1986), and the long-appreciated resistance to nephrotoxins exhibited by kidneys in the recovery phase of acute renal failure, could be explained by a decrease in specific binding sites for nephrotoxic molecules. It is conceivable that the protection against certain nephrotoxins induced by agents that increase cortical Na-K-ATPase (like streptozotocin diabetes) might be explained by concomitant changes in phospholipid content and brush border binding rather than by changes in the sodium pump per se.

Prevention of Renal Injury by Glycine

In 1987, Weinberg found that the aminoacid glycine exerted a cytoprotective action in proximal renal tubules exposed to anoxia, and this protective effect was soon found to extend to certain forms of toxic injury as well. Glycine prevented the damage to medullary thick limbs produced by amphotericin and radiocontrast agents in perfused rat kidneys. Glycine blunted proximal tubular injury caused by uranium nitrate and greatly ameliorated *cis*-platinum damage in intact rats, if the amino acid concentration in plasma was elevated by its infusion at the time *cis*-platinum was given. The protective action in some systems was shared by alanine. The mechanism of this unexpected effect remains to be elucidated.

7

Chronic Renal Failure

Leon G. Fine, Jared J. Grantham, and Joel D. Kopple

The American Society of Nephrology

The problem of chronic renal failure most likely justified the development of the field of nephrology. It was evident from the very first meetings of the American Society of Nephrology (ASN) that the pathophysiologists would follow closely in the footsteps of the physiologists in unraveling the adaptive mechanisms employed by the diseased kidney to maintain homeostasis and in defining the organ system derangements that result when the imperfections and inadequacies of such adaptations become manifest.

Three general trends in the direction of research within the field of chronic renal failure emerge. These are (*1*) altered homeostatic mechanisms and functional adaptations of the diseased kidney, (*2*) organ-system derangements and uremic toxicity, and (*3*) mechanisms of progression of chronic renal disease. Not considered in this section is the topic of therapy that sometimes intertwines logically with an in-depth understanding of mechanisms of disease and, equally often, starts out empirically and later acquires scientific rationale.

Figure 7.1 illustrates the approximate percent of abstracts submitted to the annual meeting of the Society in the three categories mentioned above. It may be seen that the first 5 years were characterized by a predominance of interest in pathophysiology and altered homeostasis with less emphasis on organ system derangements and uremic toxicity, whereas during the following 5 years these areas received roughly equal attention. Other than in the isolated abstract, the concept of there being a logical basis for understanding why renal diseases progress was not raised until the beginning of the 1980s, when interest in this field surged to assume primacy of importance, largely in studies of animal models. The decline in activity in this area since 1985 does not reflect a declining interest in the problem but rather a switch from studies of animals to evaluation of therapeutic options in patients. Thus, in the last few years, more and more abstracts in this area appeared in the clinical nephrology sections of the ASN meetings.

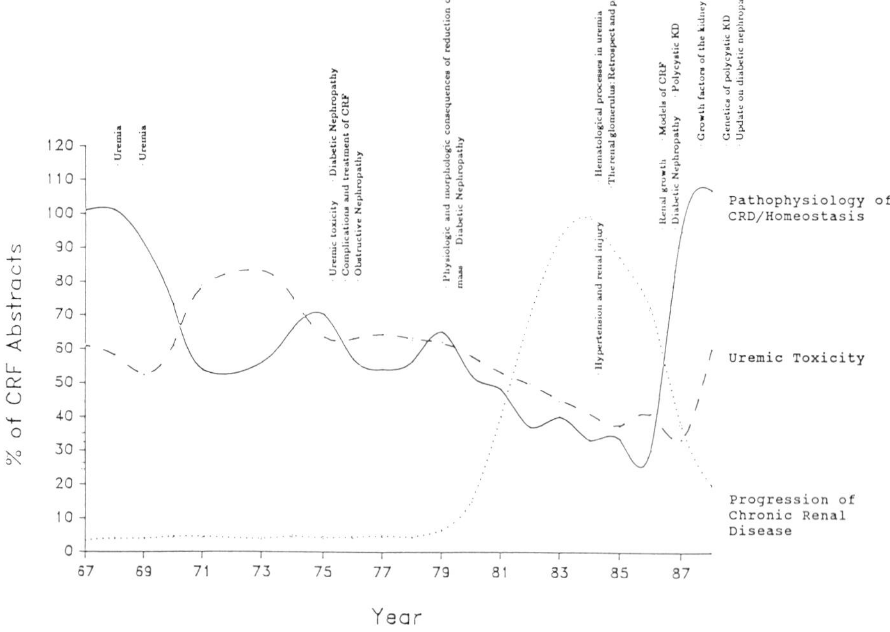

Figure 7.1. Trends in the subject matter of abstracts submitted to the annual meeting of the American Society of Nephrology in the general area of chronic renal failure (CRF). Abstracts were arbitrarily assigned to the categories: pathophysiology of chronic renal disease (CRD)/homeostasis (· · · · ·), uremic toxicity (– – –) and progression of chronic renal disease (——). A sharp increase in the latter category is shown for the early 1980s. The decline was not due to declining interest in the topic but rather to the fact that clinical studies started to predominate over animal studies and hence were presented in sessions dealing with clinical nephrology.

The topics of symposia and workshops are shown to illustrate changing emphasis over the years.

In the last 5 years, there has been a resurgence of interest in pathophysiology, spurred by the availability of new molecular biological techniques to study cell growth, gene expression, and cellular injury. Genetic diseases of the kidney, especially polycystic kidney disease, have assumed increasing importance.

The following sections discuss the three main areas of investigation delineated above, including the evolving patterns of investigation in each.

Pathophysiology of the Diseased Kidney and Altered Homeostasis

At the inception of the ASN in 1967, a few basic ideas were extant. Platt in England has shown that the function of the diseased kidney is not as haphazard as was previously thought and that there are elements of predictability about how nephrons in chronically diseased kidneys adapt their filtration, reabsorptive, and secretory functions. The concept of fractional excretion was central to discussions of this topic. Gottshalk, Oliver, and coworkers had pointed out that surviving nephrons in nephritis are not always "intact," whereas Bricker and colleagues amplified Platt's ideas, emphasizing that such nephrons either appear to be well preserved and continuously adapting or do not function at all, that is, the "intact nephron hypothesis." The demonstration by De Wardener that factors other than glomerular filtration rate (GFR) and mineralocorticoids modulate sodium excretion raised the hope that a humoral factor would be isolated to explain how changes in extracellular fluid volume result in changes in sodium excretion by the kidney.

With this as background, the first 5 years of the ASN witnessed a direct spillover into pathophysiology of the intense interest in micropuncture that had come to dominate renal physiology. This was the era of localizing *where* things happened along the nephron rather than *how* they happened. Micropuncturists enthusiastically attacked disease models too, with the remnant kidney bearing the brunt of the onslaught. The first indications that single nephron GFR differed in glomerular and nonglomerular disease emerged at the first few ASN meetings, and the consistent relationship between single nephron GFR and proximal tubular reabsorption in the same kidney, that is, GT balance, was highlighted.

Because natriuretic "hormone" was a topic of interest, the possibility that it regulates tubular function in disease came under study during these early years. No convincing evidence emerged despite early findings that supported the concept. The vogue at the time was to study organic anions, and because their transport was known to be sodium dependent, the relationships were found between putative inhibitors of Na^+ transport and organic anion transport. In 1969 and 1970 there were symposia devoted to the topic of uremia. These highlighted advances in the pathophysiology of nephron function and organ derangements in uremia.

The first 5 years of the 1970s saw further sophistication of micropuncture methods with studies of collecting duct function and a delineation of the contributions of different nephron subpopulations to sodium and water excretion in the remnant kidney. The pathophysiology of obstructive uropathy at a single nephron level was first addressed during this period.

A slow and progressive reduction in sodium intake was shown to reduce the "salt-losing" tendency of patients with diseased kidneys, further supporting the existence of extrarenal regulation of excretion. The search for humoral factors therefore continued, both for those that were thought to control renal hypertrophy ("renotropins") and for those that regulate sodium excretion by the kidney. In neither category was any substance isolated in a pure state, and most investigators were forced to elucidate their putative mechanisms of actions using impure preparations. Aldosterone was investigated as the principal regulator of potassium excretion by diseased kidneys but was found to account for only part of the regulation. Parathyroid hormone and its control by phosphorus intake became the focus of studies of divalent ion metabolism in uremia.

Reports of the nephron adaptations that occur in experimental glomerulonephritis were first presented in 1974, and the relationship between glomerular and proximal tubular function described above was ascribed to "physical factors."

In 1976, symposia were held on diabetic nephropathy and obstructive uropathy.

Around this time the first studies emerged that attempted to separate intrinsic nephron adaptations from those that are dependent on humoral factors. The use of the in vitro isolated perfused tubule technique was applied to the remnant nephrons. Adaptations in intrinsic proximal tubular function and potassium and water transport by the collecting duct were described in 1977 and 1978.

The use of new disease models proliferated around this time with the introduction of methods for inducing cystic disease and medullary necrosis and for modification of various forms of experimental glomerular injury. The suggestion that a hypolipidemic diet could modify glomerular injury was first presented in 1978. Further sophistication allowed glomerular hemodynamic studies to be extended to models of diabetic nephropathy and nephrotoxic serum nephritis. The nephropathy of potassium depletion and its link to altered cell growth was also pointed out.

In 1979, studies that addressed the mechanisms of macromolecular sieving by the diseased glomerular were presented, and it was pointed out that both molecular charge and size are determinants of importance. The accumulated wisdom of the previous decade prompted a symposium on "Physiologic and Morphologic Consequence of Reduction of Renal Mass" as well as a second one on "Diabetic Nephropathy."

The first half of the 1980s witnessed the emergence of new methods for studying nephron adaptations. The isolated perfused renal tubule was extended to different models of disease, isolated brush border membranes were used to identify intrinsic adaptations of transport systems, receptor physiology was applied to the glomerulus in diabetes, and a cell culture model of tubular cell hypertrophy was described. It emerged that many of the adaptations in the surviving nephrons of diseased kidneys are achieved by a "reprogramming" of tubular cell function, which can be manifested in vitro even in the absence of putative local and systemic humoral regulators.

At the same time as this work on tubular function was proceeding, interest in cystic disease was on the rise. In 1983, the existence of multicystic transformation of kidneys with chronic renal disease was first recognized, and new experimental models appeared. The first evidence that polycystic kidney epithelial cells could be grown in primary culture appeared in 1984. The interest in this area was sufficiently broad to call for an invited lecture on "Pathogenetic Mechanisms of Cystic Renal Diseases" in 1985. At the same meeting it was also reported that the gene for polycystic kidney disease (PKD) is located on the short arm of chromosome 16.

The glomerular afficionados continued to make headway, both in defining the glomerular hemodynamic response patterns in different disease states and in applying analyses of the determinants of glomerular filtration to the understanding of human glomerular function.

The latter half of the 1980s saw the blossoming of a new interest in renal growth control. To some extent this was a logical consequence of the general excitement in growth factors and growth control that was extant, but in a sense it also followed the realization that many renal diseases involve abnormalities of cell growth in one form or another and that the tools for studying the cellular and molecular mechanisms for these were now available. In 1986, a symposium on the "Biology of Renal Growth" was held together with one that dealt with advances that were being made in the area of polycystic kidney disease.

The tools of molecular biology were being avidly adopted to probe patterns of growth in renal disease. Oncogene expression, which was presumed to be involved in the initiation of hypertrophy, could not be demonstrated, whereas in a mouse model of polycystic kidney disease, abnormal expression of at least one oncogene was demonstrated. Insights into the pathogenesis of renal injury in chronic renal diseases were broadened by emerging observations that remnant nephrons are exposed to oxidant stress and that adaptations of tubular function, such as increased ammoniagenesis, could be involved in the genesis of renal failure by inducing tubulointerstitial injury.

On the clinical front, a symposium of "Diabetic Nephropathy: Current Status of Early Intervention" highlighted the growing concern of American nephrologists that diabetes was emerging as a major cause of end-stage renal disease (ESRD) and that early prevention was a logical goal for the future. The role of inositol metabolism emerged as a new focus of interest in this area.

In 1988, polycystic kidney disease was again in the forefront of clinical advances with a symposium dedicated to "The Genetics of Polycystic Kidney Disease." The ever-pressing problem of diabetes in the ESRD population sparked yet another formal "update" lecture on diabetic nephropathy. It became obvious that hereditary diseases of the kidney, including polycystic kidney disease and Alport's syndrome, would shortly yield to the advances in molecular genetics. The search for the culprit genes continued.

During the last few years of the 1980s, increasing knowledge of growth factor biology and growth processes continued to be of increasing interest to nephrologists. Symposia on growth factors and the kidney were held in 1988 and 1990, and the effects of specific growth factors on different renal cell types, including mesangial endothelial and epithelial cells, were described by a number of investigators. Not surprisingly, virtually all of the polypeptide growth factors were found to have effects on renal cells, and many were found to be produced by the kidney itself. Much of the research initially focused on signal transduction mechanisms, but, not surprisingly, very few novel mechanisms emerged. Most investigators found that renal cells possess signaling pathways that are very similar to those described in other cell systems. A minority of investigators in the field devoted their efforts to an understanding of the roles of growth factors and growth patterns in the processes of injury and regeneration that occur in a variety of acute and chronic diseases. These early studies also began to point to the importance of growth factors in controlling extracellular matrix deposition in glomerular and interstitial injury. Thus, the pathophysiology, pathogenesis, and progression of diabetic nephropathy was extensively discussed in both 1988 and 1989, with new emphasis on collagen synthesis by the glomerulus.

When viewed as a whole, the field of renal pathophysiology made significant headway over the last decade. The majority of investigators, however, were looking at what causes diseases to progress rather than at what causes them in the first place. This emphasis continues to be of concern in view of the limited headway that has been made in understanding the processes that initiate most of the common forms of chronic renal disease.

Organ System Derangements and Uremic Toxicity

The development and widespread employment of maintenance hemodialysis and renal transplantation in the early and mid-1960s led to a great surge in interest concerning the pathogenesis and clinical manifestation of the uremic syndrome. Uremia was no longer viewed as a terminal, essentially untreatable, disease but rather as an array of metabolic and biochemical derangements and toxicities that could be partly (with dialysis) or completely (with renal transplantation) repaired. Hence, it became more important than ever to understand the causes and manifestations of this syndrome so that patients could be maintained in better clinical condition prior to, as well as during, renal replacement therapy. Many of the papers on organ system derangements and uremic toxicity presented at the American Society of Nephrology meetings are discussed in the chapters on dialysis, mineral metabolism, or transplantation.

Papers presented at the meetings examined specific organ derangements, metabolic or biochemical disorders, and uremic toxins in chronic renal failure. In general, there were more descriptions of abnormalities in the physiology, biochemistry, metabolism, or clinical functioning of organs and organ systems than of increased concentrations of potentially toxic compounds. The organs and organ systems for which altered function and metabolism were described included the heart, pericardium, skeletal muscle, gastrointestinal tract (including pancreas), reproductive system, thyroid glands, parathyroid glands, central and peripheral nervous system, autonomic nervous system, adrenergic hormones, and coagulation system. Disorders in the physiology or metabolism of erythrocytes and leukocytes were also described. Papers addressed abnormalities in carbohydrate, amino acid, protein, and lipid metabolism in chronic renal failure. Data concerning parathyroid hormone toxicity, deficiency of vitamin D, other potential vitamin deficiencies, and elevated circulating levels of peptide hormones were presented. There were many papers on altered nutritional status and its causes in patients with chronic renal failure. The effects of uremia on cell transport were examined. An association between renal failure and cancer was described, and a debate was inaugurated as to whether chronic renal failure predisposes a patient to atherosclerosis.

From 1967 to 1970, most of the papers on organ dysfunction and uremic toxicity addressed glucose intolerance, peripheral neuropathy, bleeding disorders, impaired erythropoiesis, abnormal lymphocyte function, and altered calcium and phosphorus metabolism. From 1971 to 1975, there were, in addition, papers describing abnormalities of cellular metabolism, the effect of hyperparathyroidism on divalent ion metabolism and bone disease (including body mineral content and disordered growth in children), elevated concentrations of a variety of circulating peptide hormones, gastrointestinal disorders, encephalopathy, and abnormal amino acid metabolism in chronic renal failure. Abnormal thyroid tests were described, and ultimately it was shown that many patients with end-stage renal disease have a euthyroid sick syndrome. The positive relationship between the incidence of cancer and chronic renal failure continued to be addressed. In none of these disorders associated with uremia was a definitive toxin clearly defined as being solely responsible for a given derangement.

From 1976 to 1980, descriptions were reported of abnormal skeletal muscle physiology, increased skeletal muscle protein degradation, and abnormal fatty acid metabolism in the heart in uremia, as well as a high incidence of malnutrition in end-stage renal disease. The first of a series of reports of extraskeletal toxicity of elevated parathyroid hormone concentrations was presented. Findings related to autonomic nervous system dysfunction, abnormal lipid metabolism, and altered cellular transport of minerals were reported. The actions and potential therapeutic role for vitamin D analogues in renal osteodystrophy were examined.

From 1981 to 1989, papers continued to be presented on these same topics with, perhaps, greater refinement in the methods of investigation and in the understanding of mechanisms. The risk of cancer in chronic renal failure and the interactions between nutritional intake and altered biochemistry and metabolism both in chronic renal insufficiency and in the nephrotic syndrome were addressed. A number of diverse extraskeletal toxic effects of parathyroid hormone were added to the spectrum of toxicities in uremia, and the ability of acidosis to enhance protein catabolism in skeletal muscle provided some insight into the mechanism of muscle wasting in some patients with chronic renal failure.

Progression of Renal Disease

Until the 1980s, interest in and new thinking about the pathogenesis of the "end-stage kidney" had hit a dead end. Nephropathologists had taught for years about the "limited ways in which the kidney responds to injury" and had left it at that. Sclerosis was an unquestioned process that accompanied the progressive demise of renal function consequent to a variety of primary etiologies. Even the ⅚ nephrectomy rat model used by Bricker's group in the pre-ASN area to fashion the "intact nephron hypothesis" was criticized because the animals developed hypertension, glomerular sclerosis, and uremic syndrome and died. As a consequence, they were too unstable to allow the chronic uremic state to be studied. It is ironic that the renal ablation model and its relentless functional decline later became the cornerstone for ESRD progression studies.

In the 1970s, there were a few "hints" that the progression of renal diseases might be more interesting than previously appreciated. It was noted that, after subsidence of the acute inflammatory phase of poststreptococcal glomerulonephritis, some patients progressed, nonetheless, to renal insufficiency. Feeding diets low in protein content to azotemic patients was associated with subjective improvement in symptoms and a change in the rate of increase in serum creatinine levels. Malnutrition was also associated with changes in intrarenal hemodynamics and GFR in rats.

The soon-to-be frenetic pace of research in this field was ignited at the 1981 ASN meeting in a symposium on nutritional and metabolic factors contributing to the progression of renal failure, where the notion that glomerular hyperfiltration preceded glomerular sclerosis was introduced. By the following year, studies of the influence of protein intake on renal functional decline in both ablation and diabetic animal models had entered a stage in which mechanisms were being considered. In the early 1980s, the ASN meetings viewed dietary protein with suspicion. Animal meats were assiduously avoided at buffets and banquets out of fear of squeezing a few harmful extra drops of glomerular filtrate from the kidneys. Through a combination of excellent science and wide publication, a moribund field of study became the "hot stuff" of nephrology. The inexorable process known as ESRD progression was shown not to be invincible after all.

Early work focused on the role of glomerular hypertension in mediating sclerosis. Thromboxane synthesis was implicated in the pathogenetic sequence at an early stage of inquiry. The effect of nephron ablation sent transplant physicians scurrying to examine uninephrectomized kidney donors, and after a brief scare it was generally conceded that donors with absolutely normal kidneys and blood pressure were not at increased risk for developing clinically important glomerular sclerosis.

By 1985, over half of the abstracts in the chronic renal failure section of the ASN meeting dealt with some aspect of renal disease progression. The

Homer Smith Award lecture addressed "The Renal Glomerulus: Retrospect and Prospect." Diets were manipulated every which way. Rats were fed on alternate days, protein levels were varied in normotensive and hypertensive animals, and dietary lipids became suspects in the process of ESRD progression.

No sooner had the effect of angiotensin converting enzyme inhibition and calcium blockers been shown to improve glomerular hypertension and disease progression in 1985 and 1986, than a chink developed in the central dogma of glomerular hypertension. In 1987, hypertrophy of glomerular cells was held to be the basis of sclerosis rather than hyperfiltration, hyperperfusion, or hypertension, thus igniting a new path in the study of progression.

In the midst of the contentious NIH-sponsored "Modification of Diet in Renal Disease" (MDRD) study, several ASN reports in 1988 indicated that dietary protein levels alter the progression rate of some, but not all, renal diseases in humans and experimental animals. Male sex was touted as a risk factor for disease progression, and endogenous and dietary lipids were found to affect the progression rate in certain disease states.

By 1989, the cadence of "progression" abstracts had declined precipitously as researchers sought new ways to explore the mechanisms of ESRD in humans and to test whether patients with kidney disease respond to diets and drugs the same way as rats do. The legacy of the exciting 9-year surge in laboratory and clinical activity in this field is the almost routine adoption of low-protein diets for patients in the late stages of progressive renal diseases, and use of ACE inhibitors and calcium channel blocking antihypertensive agents in the early stages of disease. We should know by the end of the next decade if the preceding period was merely an intellectual exercise or a momentous step forward.

8

Renal Metabolism

Maurice B. Burg, Saulo Klahr, and Richard L. Tannen

A Quarter Century

The interest of nephrologists in renal metabolism was initially focused on renal ammonia and glucose metabolism and to a lesser degree on the coupling between renal metabolism and ion transport. These topics along with an interest in renal peptide hormone metabolism, fueled by the discovery of immunoassay techniques in 1960, predominated the nephrology metabolism presentations during the early years of the American Society of Nephrology (ASN). However, metabolism per se occupied only a minor role in the ASN program until the 1980s. At that time, the introduction of new technologies including nuclear magnetic resonance methods, cell culture capabilities, and molecular biology innovations catapulted the study of metabolism into an ever-expanding role at the ASN. A historical overview of advances in renal metabolism as presented at ASN meetings is given in the following sections, along with a discussion of two additional topics that have generated more recent interest: the regulation of cell volume and the metabolism of organic osmolytes.

Ammonia Metabolism

A role for ammonia in urinary acid excretion was recognized slightly more than one century ago; ammonia formation by the kidney was delineated approximately 70 years ago; and glutamine was identified as the primary precursor of urinary ammoniagenesis in 1943. This historical perspective along with the state of the field was presented in a classic review by Robert F. Pitts (in *Handbook of Renal Physiology*, p. 455, 1973), who gave a state-of-the-art address to the ASN on this topic in 1971 and in whose memory a symposium on ammonia metabolism in the kidney was dedicated in 1977, the year of his death.

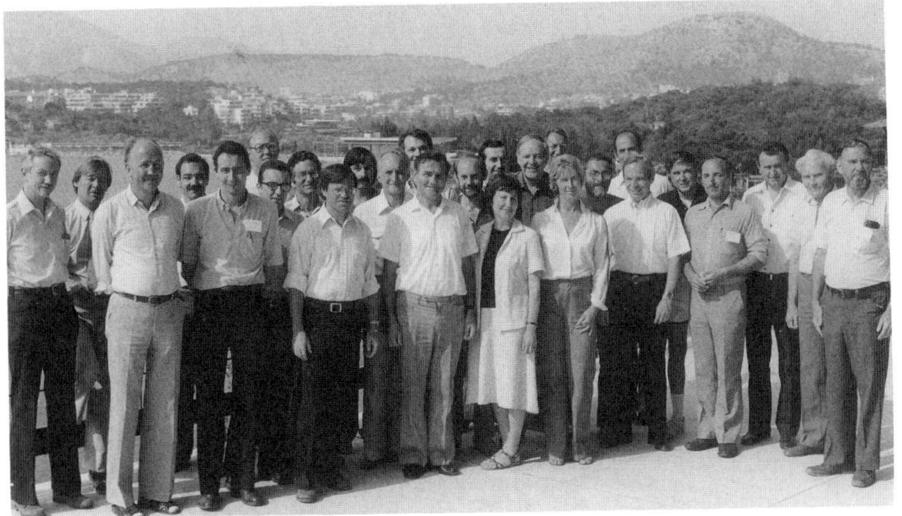

Figure 8.1. Participants in a workshop on Ammoniagenesis held in Greece in 1981. Many of the major contributors to this field are pictured.

Pitts's review provided an assessment of the state of this field at approximately the time of the first ASN meeting. At this juncture, a variety of potential enzymatic pathways for ammonia formation from glutamine had been delineated. Adaptation of ammonia production in response to chronic metabolic acidosis was well characterized, but its mechanism was uncertain. Inhibition of phosphate-dependent glutaminase activity by glutamate had been discovered, and a potential linkage with increased renal glucose production had just been proposed. The concepts of diffusion equilibrium for NH_3 in dictating ammonium excretion and even the possibility of NH_3 shunting from the loop of Henle to the collecting duct had been entertained. Studies using enzymology, whole animal arteriovenous (AV) gradients across organ beds, renal slices, micropuncture, and even ^{15}N methodology had been used to address these issues.

Since 1967, refinements of these techniques and the introduction of several new methodological approaches have helped advance our understanding of ammonia metabolism, although the mysteries of the adaptation to chronic metabolic acidosis still have not been completely unraveled.

The important trends in technological approaches were well reflected in presentations at the ASN meetings. In 1968 the use of isolated renal cortical mitochondria appeared on the program; in 1987 the refinement of submitochondrial particles appeared; in 1973 use of the isolated perfused rat kidney appeared; and in 1983 reports of ammoniagenesis by cultured renal papillary cells began a trend toward using cultured epithelium, which spread quickly to the use of the established proximal tubular cell lines (LLC PK_1 cells) in 1984 and primary cultures of human renal cells by 1987. New fluorescent dye techniques for measuring intracellular pH led to simultaneous measurements of cytosolic and intramitochondrial pH in 1986, and refinements in

^{15}N methodology began more widespread use of this technology as indicated initially in 1984 and 1985. Technological advances in the measurements of organ extraction and an increased interest in interorgan glutamine metabolism began to appear in 1980, although isolated reports had originally appeared as early as 1969. Surprisingly, the replacement of renal slices with renal cortical tubules, which began in the mid-1970s, is not reflected by presentations of ammonia metabolism at the ASN meetings. However, the development of a macromethodological procedure for obtaining relatively purified preparations of proximal and distal renal tubules was described at the 1980 ASN meeting.

The dramatic advances in micromethodological approaches to investigation of renal phenomena led to an explosive increase in knowledge concerning ammonia production and transport at a segmental level as well as the overall process of renal ammonium excretion. The application of micropuncture to the investigation of ammonia metabolism appeared on the ASN program in 1977, but widespread interest in the technique began in 1980 with reports of micropuncture of deep nephrons, followed in 1982 by the description of ammonia production by individual segments of the nephron and in 1983 by studies of both production and transport by isolated perfused nephron segments. Minilectures encompassing this topic appeared on the program in 1983 and 1987, and an entire symposium was conducted at the 1990 meetings.

It had been assumed that the increase in urinary ammonium excretion in response to an acute acid load resulted entirely from ammonia trapping in acidified urine rather than an alteration in renal ammonia production. Consistent with this view, most studies involving either renal cortical slices or isolated mitochondria could not demonstrate increased ammonia formation

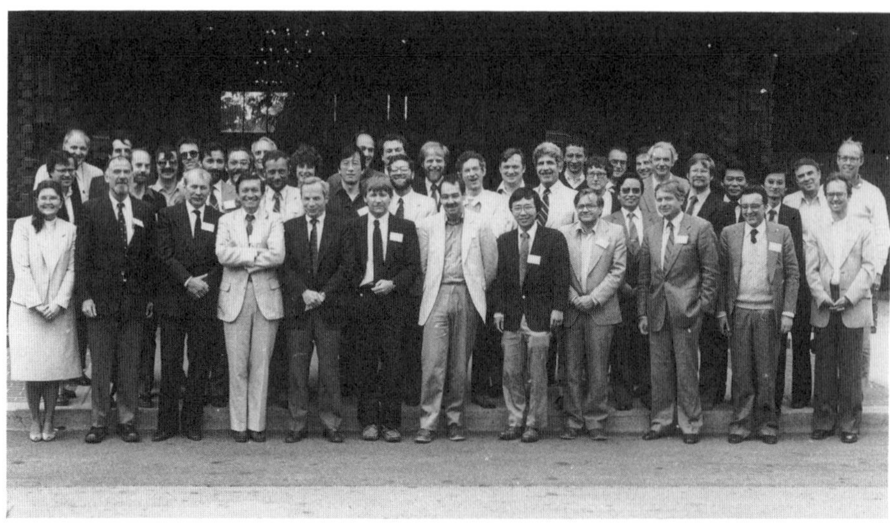

Figure 8.2. Participants in a workshop on Ammoniagenesis held in Monterey, California, in 1984.

on exposure of samples to an acidified medium. A landmark abstract in 1976 by Emmett et al. demonstrated increased ammonia production in response to acute acidosis by the rat kidney in vivo, and this finding was confirmed in vitro in 1977 by Tannen and Ross in the isolated perfused rat kidney. Subsequent reports showing a simultaneous decrease in intracellular pH and an increase in ammonia formation both by renal tubules and by cultured cells appeared in 1986 and 1987. A 1984 presentation demonstrated that in contrast to chronic metabolic acidosis, chronic respiratory acidosis does not result in an adaptive increase in the capacity for renal ammonia production.

Mechanisms accounting for both the adaptive and acute pH effects on glutamine metabolism have been a focus of study throughout the first 25 years of the Society. In 1968 and several subsequent years, Preuss and coworkers developed the concept that the redox state regulates glutamate deamination; also in 1968, Simpson reported studies of glutamine metabolism regulation by isolated renal mitochondria, which led in subsequent years to the suggestion that glutamine transport into mitochondria is the critical step altered in the adaptive process.

The 1977 meeting was particularly eventful with regard to the scrutiny of ammonia metabolism. There was a symposium on the topic, and Schoolworth and LaNoue presented the first studies addressing glutamate metabolism by isolated mitochondria and proposed that flux through glutamate dehydrogenase (GLDH) might be critical for the adaptation to metabolic acidosis. Hager and Simpson proposed that bicarbonate modulates mitochondrial anion transport, and Halperin and Cheema Dahdli reported on the

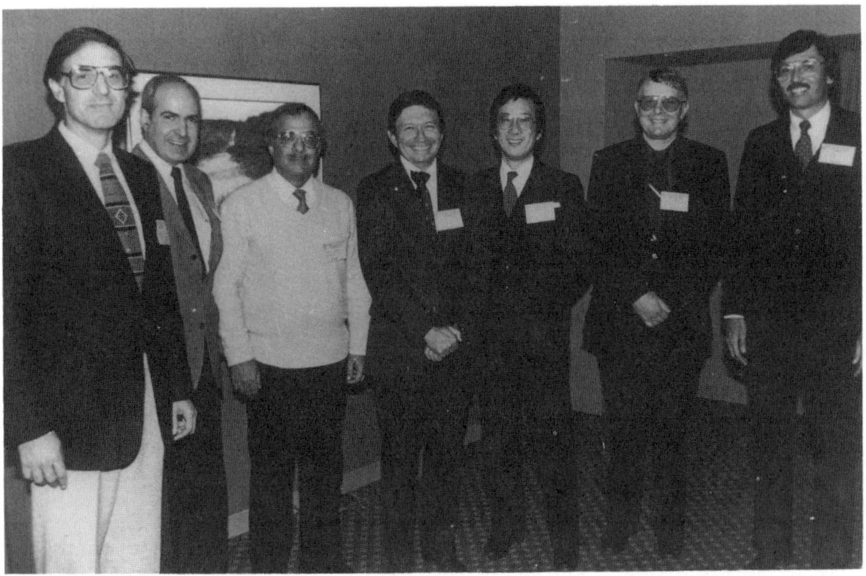

Figure 8.3. Founding members of the American Society of Renal Biochemistry and Metabolism pictured at the 1983 ASN meeting: From the left, Lazaro Mandel, Patricio Silva, Shaul Massry, Saulo Klahr, Kyoshi Kurakawa, Thomas Dousa, David Humes.

potential role of the mitochondrial dicarboxylate transporter in the response to acidosis. Reports of pH regulation of α-ketoglutarate dehydrogenase and succinic dehydrogenase appeared in the program in 1980 and 1984, respectively. The role of GLDH in the response to acute pH was addressed in 1984 using ^{15}N methodology in the perfused rat kidney and in 1989 using LLC-PK_1 cells in culture.

In addition to the phosphate-dependent glutaminase pathway, several other potential ammoniagenic pathways have attracted interest. The role of the glutaminase II pathway first appeared on the program in 1969 and resurfaced again in the late 1980s. In 1990, studies in cultured cells suggested that this pathway did not necessarily proceed through the omega amidase step and thereby produce ammonia. The purine nucleotide cycle was described as a potential ammoniagenic pathway by Bogusky and the Lownensteins in 1974, and additional reports by this group appeared in subsequent meetings. Although interest in the role of γ-glutamyl transpeptidase and its characterization as the previously described phosphate independent glutaminase developed in the early and mid-1970s, the potential role of this pathway in ammonia metabolism was not presented at the ASN meetings until 1987 and 1988.

Modulation of ammonia production by factors other than pH has been an area of ongoing investigative interest. During the late 1960s and 1970s, studies focused predominantly on metabolites that could modify ammonia production, based in part on the view that these alterations might explain certain features of the adaptive response to pH. Abstracts exploring the roles of α-ketoglutarate, ketones, and fatty acids appeared in the program. The emerging interest in signal transduction affected the study of ammoniagenesis in the 1980s, with reports that prostaglandins, phorbol esters, angiotensin II, and growth hormone could influence renal ammonia production and with a growing interest in the mechanism of action of these substances. In 1983 the surprising observation that perfusion of the proximal tubule lumen enhanced ammonia production was reported by Nagami and Kurokawa, and studies attempting to elucidate the mechanism subsequently appeared.

The influence of potassium on ammonia metabolism and, conversely, the influence of ammonia metabolism on potassium excretion received sporadic interest throughout the 1970s and 1980s. The reduction in potassium excretion by enhanced ammonia secretion and the localization of this phenomenon to a site in the renal tubule beyond the distal convoluted tubule was reported in the late 1970s. Inhibition of ammonia production as well as inhibition of thick ascending limb ammonium absorption by a high potassium level were the topics of several presentations in the 1980s. Other studies expanded further on the stimulation of ammonia production by a low potassium level.

Only a single abstract in 1973 and another in 1980 dealt with the role of extrarenal glutamine metabolism and its potential effects on renal ammoniagenesis. This topic, however, attracted considerable interest in the later

1980s, when it was suggested that pH regulation of ureagenesis by the liver rather than glutamine regulation by the kidney was primarily responsible for acid-base homeostasis. Indeed, a heated debate of this topic occurred in a 1988 Basic Science Controversy session with Daniel Atkinson presenting the "liver" and Mark Knepper the "kidney" view.

Other "ammonia topics" that received intermittent attention were the regulation of ammoniagenesis by the kidney with reduced renal mass, a topic of interest in the late 1970s and 1980s, and also the role of ammonia inhibiting energy metabolism, stimulating glycolysis and producing hypertrophy, a subject addressed in the late 1980s.

The micromethodological revolution in the assay of ammonia had a substantial impact on the study of renal ammonia excretion during the 1980s. Abstracts early in the decade, which focused on the role of deep nephrons, clearly demonstrated that ammonia was shunted from the ascending limb to the collecting duct for ultimate excretion. Studies of isolated perfused thick ascending limbs by Burg, Good, Knepper, and their colleagues demonstrated the presence of an active NH_4^+ transport mechanism by this nephron segment. Meticulous studies of isolated proximal tubules and collecting ducts confirmed that transport at these sites was primarily accounted for by passive diffusion of NH_3; such studies also characterized in detail the permeability characteristics of these segments to both NH_4^+ and NH_3 and demonstrated an acid disequilibrium pH in the collecting duct. The enormous interest in the topic of renal ammonia transport was reflected by minilectures devoted to this topic on the program in both 1983 and 1987 and by a consideration of this issue and its relationship to renal tubular acidosis at a symposium in 1990.

Glucose Metabolism

The kidney and the liver are the two gluconeogenic organs in the body. The nephrologic interest in gluconeogenesis was heightened by the suggestion that this process played a crucial role in the regulation of ammonia production, and 1969 saw the first presentation of this relationship at an ASN meeting, in abstract form. Subsequently, intermittent attention surfaced, with presentations focused on the effects of phosphate depletion, parathyroid hormone (PTH), α-adrenergic catecholamines, renal nerve stimulation, and tubular lumen flow on the regulation of renal gluconogenesis. In the late 1980s, innovative molecular biology techniques were applied to the study of these phenomena, with two abstracts focusing on the regulation of phosphoenolpyruvate carboxy kinase (PEPCK) mRNA by acidosis.

In addition to the regulation of gluconeogenesis, there was also some interest in the impact of gluconeogenesis on other aspects of renal function. Studies in the perfused kidney initially in 1975 and isolated perfused proximal tubules subsequently in 1982 addressed the issue of whether under certain circumstances the energy demands for gluconeogenesis could affect the energy available for sodium transport. Dousa, Knox, and colleagues proposed that an increase in nicotine adenosine dinucleotide (NAD) produced by gluconeogenesis might account for the inhibition of phosphate transport produced by stimuli such as PTH and starvation, which are known to enhance gluconeogenesis.

In a symposium in 1979, Guder reviewed the studies performed with his colleagues that delineated the nephron localization of the enzymes critical for both gluconeogenesis and glycolysis. These data established definitively that gluconeogenesis is localized to the proximal tubules, whereas the more distal nephron segments are glycolytic. In that same year, Kurokawa and his colleagues described radioisotopic studies of glucose metabolism by selected nephron segments, confirming the absence of significant glycolysis in proximal tubules and suggesting the presence of the pentose phosphate pathway in cortical collecting duct. Thus, 1979 ushered in for the ASN the focus on metabolism by selected nephron segments. Interest in glucose-using pathways was relatively quiescent until the late 1980s, when Seifter and Schubert described the predominantly medullary localization of fructose 2,6 bisphosphate, a recently discovered potent regulator of glycolysis. At about the same time, altered glucose metabolism was demonstrated in the proximal tubule of the X-linked hypophosphatemia mouse, an influence of glucose metabolism mediated through the pentose cycle on the lipid composition of proximal tubule brush border membrane was suggested, and glycogen metabolism in papillary collecting duct cells was described.

Glucose metabolism by cultured renal epithelium was another broad area of interest that developed in the 1980s. Studies in this area paralleled the application of innovative cell culture techniques to nephrology. In 1982, the transport and metabolism of glucose by primary cultures of proximal tubular cells were reported by Sakranhi and Fine. This was followed by a detailed examination of the conversion of this gluconeogenic tissue to a glycolytic profile by Tannen and his coworkers and a 1989 abstract from Osaka delineating the induction of mRNA for glycolytic enzymes in the presumably regenerating epithelium of the ischemia-reperfused kidney. In 1985, Gasthranthaler and Handler reported development of a clone of LLC-PK_1 cells with gluconeogenic capability. A role for the hexosemonophosphate shunt in the protection of cultured proximal tubule cells from oxidant injury was described in 1987.

Coupling of Metabolism to Ion Transport

Renal blood flow through the kidneys accounts for approximately 25% of the cardiac output, and the amount of oxygen delivered to the kidney in blood exceeds the amount of oxygen consumed by this organ. The relation between renal blood flow to the kidney and oxygen consumption differs from that of other organs. In resting muscle, for example, oxygen consumption remains constant while blood flow may vary; in the kidney, oxygen consumption rises as renal blood flow increases. It has been suggested that the augmented oxygen consumption as blood flow increases is due to a rise in glomerular filtration rate and consequently in the amount of solute delivered to the tubules. Oxygen consumption is correlated with tubular reabsorption processes because a large fraction of the metabolism of the kidney is coupled to the reabsorption of sodium. Because a number of organic and inorganic solutes are coupled to sodium reabsorption and in turn hydrogen ion secretion is coupled to sodium reabsorption in the proximal tubule, the reabsorption of sodium at the basolateral border of tubular cells via the sodium potassium ATPase represents the major energy expenditure of the kidney.

In the 1960s, several studies were published in which different levels of sodium reabsorption by the kidneys were correlated with oxygen consumption. Sodium reabsorption was modified by changing glomerular filtration rate, by administration of hypertonic saline, by osmotic diuresis, by the administration of diuretics, by inhibition of the sodium pump, and by changes of ureteral or venous pressure. Most of the information that emerged from such studies suggested that the amount of oxygen used for sodium reabsorption remained constant and that for each mole of oxygen consumed, 28 to 33 moles of sodium were reabsorbed.

Most of the studies that correlated sodium reabsorption to oxygen consumption by the kidney appeared between 1961 and 1969 and were undertaken by research groups in Germany, in Scandinavia, and in this country. Starting in 1968, a series of abstracts was presented at the American Society of Nephrology, dealing with the coupling of energy to transport and with the segmental organization of metabolism within the nephron. These abstracts have provided a more comprehensive picture of the mechanisms coupling metabolic needs to sodium transport as well as to other processes of the kidney such as gluconeogenesis and hydrogen secretion.

At the second meeting of the ASN in 1968, George Porter, from the University of Oregon Medical School, reported an increase in Na transport as the temperature was raised from 18° to 30°C in the isolated toad bladder. There was a parallel increase in O_2 consumption. At temperatures higher than 30°C there was a fall in Na transport, which was attributed to diversion of energy into nontransport functions of the cell rather than to an overall reduction in the rate of cellular metabolism. At the same meeting, Dr. Franklin Epstein (Yale University) gave a state-of-the-art lecture, "Relation of Metabolism to Electrolyte Transport in the Kidney." In studies using the addition of metabolic substrates to the toad bladder to examine the coupling of sodium transport to metabolism, Maffly et al. (Stanford University) suggested that in this tissue, and probably in other epithelial tissues, the metabolism that supports transepithelial sodium transport is functionally separate from the metabolism that supports other processes.

Beauwens and Al-Awqati (University of Iowa) reported at the 7th Annual Meeting of the ASN on the constancy of energy cost of sodium transport in individual toad bladders. Changing sodium transport by altering either the activity of the Na "pump" or the passive entry step at the mucosal border of the epithelium did not affect the relation between sodium transport and CO_2 production in individual bladders. Dr. Robert Pitts et al. (Cornell University) reported at the same meeting on the effects of hypoperfusion (produced by partial aortic occlusion in anesthetized dogs) on the renal metabolism of glutamine and lactate. The authors concluded that (*1*) the observed stoichiometric relation between total renal CO_2 production and sodium reabsorption is consistent with the postulate that the major renal energy need is for sodium reabsorption; (*2*) there is a good correlation between renal energy needs and the use of glutamine and lactate; (*3*) energy for basal renal work derives from glutamine metabolism; and (*4*) energy from lactate metabolism is used predominantly for sodium reabsorption.

At the 8th Annual Meeting of the ASN (1975) two abstracts, one from the University of Iowa (Beauwens and Al-Awqati) and another from Walter Reed Hospital (Norby and Schwartz), examined the coupling of H^+ transport to metabolism in the turtle bladder. Beauwens and Al-Awqati reported on the relation of H^+ transport to oxidative metabolism, using the rate of glucose oxidation as an index of the metabolic activity of the epithelium. The results demonstrated that the hydrogen pump is tightly coupled to oxidative metabolism and that the shunt conductance for protons is normally negligible but can be markedly increased by dinitrophenol, an uncoupler of oxidative phosphorylation.

In 1976, Al-Awqati and Harten reported that aldosterone stimulates hydrogen secretion in the turtle bladder by an effect on the pump and that the stimulation was accompanied by a secondary increase in metabolism ($^{14}CO_2$ production from ^{14}C-glucose). In 1979, Dixon and Al-Awqati (Columbia University) reported at the 12th Annual Meeting of the ASN that the hydrogen pump in the turtle bladder regulates the rate of cellular metabolism by changing the free energy of ATP hydrolysis.

Norby and Schwartz explored the role of the pentose shunt and of glycolysis in hydrogen transport in the isolated turtle bladder. Inhibition of hydrogen transport with acetazolamide or by acidification of the mucosal solution resulted in a decrease in activity of the pentose shunt, whereas stimulation of H^+ transport by alkalinization of the mucosal fluid increased pentose shunt activity. The authors concluded that glucose metabolism via the pentose shunt is closely related to the rate of hydrogen transport. At the 9th meeting of the ASN in 1976, Norby, Lawson, and Schwartz reported on additional studies that supported the role of the pentose shunt in the process of urinary acidification.

In 1979, Dr. Leah M. Lowenstein moderated a symposium entitled, "Advances in Renal Metabolism." The topics on the program included "Is the Energy Cost of Sodium Transport Overestimated?", Julius Cohen (Rochester, NY); "Evaluation of Membrane Transport of Amino Acids," Stanton Segal (University of Pennsylvania); "Metabolic Steps in the Adaptation to Acute Nephron Loss," Leah M. Lowenstein (Boston University); and "Localization of Carbohydrate Metabolism Along the Nephron," Dr. Walter Gruder (University of Munich, Munich, Germany). At the same meeting, Professor Francois Morel (Paris, France) presented the Homer W. Smith Award lecture, entitled "Sites of Hormone Action in the Mammalian Nephron."

At the ASN meeting of 1975, Silva, Epstein, and their associates (Harvard Medical School, Beth Israel Hospital) reported on the relation between sodium transport and gluconeogenesis in the isolated perfused rat kidney. Kidneys obtained from fed rats required glucose for optimal Na transport when perfused in vitro. When fatty acids (butyrate) were the sole substrates, there was less sodium reabsorption, and the subsequent addition of glucose immediately increased tubular reabsorption. This relationship was reversed by maneuvers that greatly increased renal gluconeogenesis. Pretreatment of rats with methyl prednisolone or prolonged feeding of a noncarbohydrate diet yielded kidneys that reabsorbed sodium optimally with butyrate but not when glucose was the only exogenous substrate. Sodium reabsorption, however, was greatly increased in such kidneys when gluconeogenesis was blocked by mercaptopicolinate. This prevented the utilization of pyruvate for glucose synthesis and permitted its further oxidation. Simple addition of pyruvate had the same effect on sodium reabsorption. The authors concluded that pyruvate oxidation is critical for optimal reabsorption of sodium by the kidney and that under some circumstances renal gluconeogenesis may compete with metabolic needs for sodium transport.

At the 13th Annual Meeting of the ASN (1980), J. J. Cohen (University of Rochester) provided evidence that free fatty acids derived from renal tissue lipids can support a significant portion of the sodium reabsorption in the proximal tubule.

At the 1982 meeting, Lazaro Mandel (Duke University) discussed "Relations Between Renal Transport and Metabolism" at a symposium chaired by Dr. Stanley G. Schultz (University of Texas, Houston) and entitled "Advances in Epithelial Physiology." Mandel and his associates also presented an abstract describing the preparation of tubule suspensions from rabbit kidney enriched in thick ascending limbs.

At the 17th Annual Meeting of the ASN in 1984, Soltoff and Mandel reported that the proximal tubule uses mainly fatty acids as endogenous substrates to supply energy for the sodium pump during basal as well as pump-stimulated conditions. At the same meeting, Vandewalle et al. from Inserm and Hopital Tenon (France) described the isolation of distal cell populations from rabbit kidney by immunoadsorbent chromatography. This method has been useful in biochemical studies and in the production of monoclonal antibodies against distal cell subpopulations.

In 1985, Brezis, Spokes, Silva, and Epstein (Hadassah University and Harvard University) reported that L-lactate appears to increase potassium secretion by preferential metabolic stimulation of the distal tubule, a process that may help to prevent the development in vivo of hyperkalemia in the setting of lactic acidosis.

At the 19th Annual Meeting of the ASN in 1986, Lazaro J. Mandel gave an invited lecture, "Metabolic Regulation of Proximal Tubule Transport" in the portion of the meeting devoted to free communications on renal metabolism. Studies by Dillingham (University of Colorado) presented at the ASN meeting of 1987 demonstrated that basolateral glucose uptake and oxidation are required for arginine vasopressin (AVP) stimulated hydraulic conductivity in the rat cortical collecting tubule. This, to the best of our knowledge, represents the first attempt to characterize the metabolic requirements necessary to support AVP-stimulated hydrosmotic response in the mammalian cortical collecting tubule.

At the same meeting, the group of Vinay and Gougoux (University of Montreal) presented evidence that a large fraction of basolateral lactate entry in the thick ascending limb is coupled to the efflux of chloride by a 4-acetamide-4′-isothiocyanostilbene-2,2′-disulfonic acid (SITS)-sensitive anionic exchanger. The authors suggested that such a mechanism ensures a stoichiometry between the transepithelial flux of NaCl and the availability of substrates to support the energy requirements of cells of the thick ascending limb. The same investigators reported in 1988 on the effect of ATP and phosphorylation potential on the sodium pump of dog cortical tubules. Their findings suggested that (*1*) the Na-K ATPase is not regulated by ATP in intact tubules when the ATP is at or above the normal concentration, and (*2*) the stoichiometry of Na/ATP is probably constant when one or more of the following are altered: the ATP/ADP ratio, the phosphorylation potential, and the free energy released from ATP hydrolysis. At the same meeting (ASN, 1988), Dillingham (University of Colorado) reported on the regulation of ATP content in microdissected rat cortical collecting tubules (CCT). ATP was measured in individual CCT using a chemiluminescence technique. Studies using different inhibitors of oxidative phosphorylation or glycolysis revealed that both of these processes generate ATP in the CCT. However, oxidative phosphorylation is the major synthetic pathway for ATP, since oxidation of pyruvate without glycolysis maintained ATP levels whereas glycolysis without oxidative phosphorylation did not.

At the 22nd meeting of the ASN in 1989, Brain Ross et al. at the Huntington Medical Research Institute in Pasadena, California, reported, based on measurements of ATP gradients in intact porcine kidney using ^{31}P-NMR, a tight coupling between Na^+ transport and ATP levels. They found that reversible increases in renal ATP levels accompany reduction in total sodium reabsorption, indicating tight coupling of sodium transport and metabolism. At the meeting of the ASN in 1990, Vinay et al. reported on the metabolism of glycogen in canine papillary collecting ducts in vitro. They found synthesis of glycogen in collecting ducts, a synthesis significantly stimulated by the presence of ouabain. They concluded that small glycogen stores are present in dog papillary collecting ducts. The glycogen synthesis and/or breakdown in this area is regulated by the balance between production and use of ATP. They also found that glycolysis was required for optimal energy production in this nephron segment.

Hormone and Peptide Metabolism by the Kidney

The year 1960 was a milestone in the history of endocrinological research. The new technique of Rosalyn Yalow and S. A. Berson, "Immunoassay of Endogenous Plasma Insulin in Man," reported that year, ushered in a new era. The capability to measure peptide hormones in both plasma and urine by radioimmunoassay techniques and the ability to radiolabel peptides and hormones allowed a detailed examination of hormonal metabolism and of the role of the kidney in this process. It also permitted the measurement of hormonal levels in the blood of patients with end-stage renal disease prior to and during maintenance hemodialysis.

At the time of the IIIrd International Congress of Nephrology, held in Washington, D.C., in September of 1966, only one abstract dealt with the degradation of a peptide by the kidney (amylase, a protein with a molecular weight of 45,000 kDa). Two abstracts (by Donadio et al. from St. Louis University and Eschbach and his associates from the University of Washington) called attention to the role of erythropoietin deficiency in the anemia of renal disease. Interestingly, 20 years later, at the plenary session of the 19th Annual Meeting of the American Society of Nephrology, Eschbach presented the first report on the use of recombinant erythropoietin in the treatment of the anemia of patients on maintenance hemodialysis.

Parathyroid hormone (PTH) is a 9.5-kDa protein containing 84 amino acids. It is found in the circulation both as the intact hormone and as fragments of the amino- and carboxy-terminal portions of the molecule. Advancing renal failure is almost universally accompanied by a rise in circulating levels of parathyroid hormone. Although Yalow and Berson had developed the radioimmunoassay for PTH and made some initial measurements in uremic subjects, it was at the time of the second meeting of the ASN in 1968 that three groups (Eric Reiss and associates from Michael Reese Hospital in Chicago, John Potts et al. from the Massachusetts General Hospital, and Genuth and Sherwood from Mt. Sinai Hospital in Cleveland and Beth Israel Hospital, Boston) reported elevated levels of parathyroid hormone in the blood of uremic subjects and called attention to the development of hyperparathyroidism in patients with mild renal insufficiency. The elevated levels of immunoreactive PTH are the consequence of both increased secretion of the hormone by the parathyroid glands and decreased degradation of the hormone in the liver and kidney. As discussed by Hruska et al. at the Annual Meetings of the ASN in 1973 and 1975, the liver and kidney appear to be the principal sites of degradation of intact parathyroid hormone, accounting for 61% and 31%, respectively, of intact hormone removal. On the other hand, the kidney appears to be the only site for the degradation of carboxy-terminal fragments of the PTH molecule. This degradation seems to occur exclusively by glomerular filtration, since the carboxy-terminal fragments do not exhibit receptor binding to peritubular capillaries.

The major sites of insulin degradation are the kidney and the liver. Rabkin and his associates reported at the 8th Annual Meeting of the ASN in 1975 that the kidney removed proinsulin, insulin, and C-peptide at a rate inversely related to molecular size. Because the metabolic clearance rate of these three peptides exceeded GFR, it seemed likely that proinsulin, insulin, and C-peptide were cleared by extraction from peritubular capillaries as well as glomerular filtration. Thus it is that the kidney accounts for one-third of the metabolic clearance rate of insulin (extrarenal organs, muscle, and liver account for 67% of its disappearance rate). Five years later, at the 13th Annual Meeting of the ASN, Rabkin and his associates at Stanford University reported on the metabolic characteristics of renal insulin uptake. They concluded that tubular insulin reabsorption was independent of Na reabsorption and that insulin uptake, unlike contraluminal uptake, appears to have the metabolic features of a pinocytotic process followed by lysosomal degradation. At the same meeting, Katz and his associates (University of Chicago) reported on the degradation of insulin by luminal and basolateral renal tubular membranes.

The kidney is also an important site of degradation of glucagon, accounting for one-third of its metabolic clearance rate. At the ASN meeting of 1975, Felig and his associates from Yale University reported on the clearance of glucagon by the kidney and described a substantial uptake of glucagon across the peritubular capillary surface of renal tubular cells. They suggested that a reduction in the clearance of glucagon by the kidney accounted for the elevated basal levels and lower metabolic clearance rates of glucagon in patients with renal failure. At the same meeting (1975), Rubenstein, Katz and their associates at the University of Chicago reported that immunoreactive glucagon in plasma is heterogenous. Only about one-fifth of the total immunoreactive hormone present in the circulation is the biologically active 3.5-kDa species. About 60% of the immunoreactive hormone in plasma is a 9-kDa form with little or no biological activity. The remainder is a large molecular weight form in excess of 40 kDa. It should be remarked that the 9-kDa species is rarely seen in normal subjects. When present, it is found in the pancreas and very likely represents a glucagon precursor.

In 1974, at the 7th Annual Meeting of the ASN, Shalhoub et al. from George Washington and Georgetown Universities reported high levels of calcitonin in the peripheral blood of patients with chronic renal failure. Subsequent studies demonstrated that the kidney accounts for approximately two-thirds of the total metabolic clearance rate of calcitonin, a peptide with a molecular weight of 3.5 kDa. Calcitonin seems to be degraded both at the level of brush border membranes of tubular cells and intracellularly in lysosomes. In renal failure, the metabolic clearance rate of calcitonin and the plasma levels of the hormone are increased.

In 1973, at the 6th Annual Meeting of the ASN, Davidson et al. from UCLA reported elevated serum levels of gastrin in renal failure. Their experiments in rats suggested that the kidney was important in the metabolism of gastrin and that gastrin could be removed by the kidneys by a process other than glomerular filtration. Subsequent studies demonstrated hypergastrinemia in patients with renal failure most likely due to reduced degradation of this heptadecapeptide by the kidney.

At the ASN meeting of 1975, Johnson and Maack at Cornell University reported on the role of the kidney in the turnover and regulation of growth hormone in the rat. In experiments in the isolated perfused kidney, they calculated that in the intact rat the kidneys may account for 70% of the daily catabolism of growth hormone. At the same meeting, elevated levels of growth hormone in patients with uremia were described by Ramirez and Bloomer from Utah College of Medicine. Because growth hormone has a molecular weight of 21.5 kDa, its filtration is about 70% that of inulin. The hormone is reabsorbed extensively along the nephron, so that less than 1% of the filtered load is excreted in the urine.

The observations described above and subsequent studies have indicated that the kidney is an important site for the degradation of small and medium size proteins (<50 kDa). Because most peptide hormones fall in this category the kidney has an important role in their catabolism and thus participates in endocrine homeostasis. The peptide hormones metabolized by the kidney include insulin, proinsulin, C-peptide, parathyroid hormone and its fragments, glucagon, calcitonin, growth hormone, prolactin, gastrin, vasopressin, angiotensin II, and gastrin.

Two mechanisms are largely responsible for the degradation of peptide hormones in the kidney: (*1*) glomerular filtration leading to intraluminal (brush border) or intracellular (usually lysosomal) degradation, and (*2*) uptake at the contraluminal site of tubular cells. Degradation of a peptide hormone by glomerular filtration does not depend on biological activity of the peptide but is conditioned by the permeability of the glomerular capillary to the peptide. Tubular uptake at the basolateral membrane, on the other hand, appears to require, at least for some hormones, that the peptide be biologically active. Thus, studies of hormone metabolism using radiolabeled peptides, a process that in some instances causes loss of biological activity, may provide an inaccurate picture of the metabolism of that particular hormone.

Nuclear Magnetic Resonance (NMR)

Nuclear magnetic resonance is a form of spectroscopy in which a radio frequency pulse is used to radiate a sample located within a strong magnetic field. The radio frequency pulse is selected to match the resonance frequency of the nucleus of the elements of interest. In turn, this frequency depends on the strength of the magnetic field. For a given magnetic field strength, the frequency is unique for the particular isotope under scrutiny. The sample will absorb a small amount of radio frequency energy and produce a change in sample magnetization, inducing a current signal that can be detected. When the radio frequency pulse is turned off, the total magnetization returns to equilibrium with a characteristic time constant, T1, the longitudinal or spin-lattice relaxation time. When the magnetization returns to a steady state, the current detected by the receiver coil in the XY plane diminishes. This is measured as a signal that decays with time, the so-called free induction decay. The rate of loss of the XY magnetization or the duration of a detectable free induction decay is dominated by a second time constant, T2, the transverse or spin-spin relaxation time. Both T1 and T2 are independently influenced by the intrinsic properties of the sample and are measurable quantities. The free induction decay is mathematically transformed from the time to the frequency domain to produce the usual NMR spectrum.

The first application of NMR studies to renal tissue appear to be those of Sehr and his coworkers in 1977 (Biochem Biophys Res Commun 77:195–202). They studied the effects of renal ischemia on a kidney transport model in the rat. Since then, ^{31}phosphorus NMR and spectroscopy of other nuclei, particularly those of ^{23}sodium and ^{13}carbon, have been used to examine several aspects of renal physiology and metabolism. In addition, ^{1}H (proton) NMR imaging or magnetic resonance imaging (MRI) has progressed to the stage where it is a useful clinical tool in the evaluation of renal morphology, particularly renal tumors, cysts, and obstruction of the urinary tract.

As mentioned above, the radio frequency used is specific for the compound of interest. In the case of ^{31}P the emission signal generated is different for each phosphorus nucleus and therefore can distinguish among inorganic phosphorus (P_1), ATP (α, β or $\surd$ phosphate groups), phosphocreatine, and glycerophosphorylcholine.

In 1979, Shulman (Yale University) reviewed in Science (205: 160–166) the cellular applications of ^{31}P and ^{13}C NMR. In the same year, Sehr and Radda (University of Oxford) reported "Non-Destructive Measurements of Metabolites and Tissue pH in the Kidney by ^{31}P NMR" (Br J Exp Path 60:632–641, 1979).

Abstracts on the application of NMR to the study of renal physiology and metabolism began to appear in the early 1980s at the Annual Meeting of the ASN. The first abstract on the use of NMR was presented at the 13th Annual Meeting of the ASN in 1980. Weiner et al. (VA Medical Center, University of California, San Francisco) reported on the feasibility of using ^{31}P NMR to study kidney metabolism in vivo "in a continuous and non-destructive fashion."

The following year (1981) Balaban and Knepper from the National Institutes of Health reported on NMR studies using ^{14}N on the in vivo and in vitro mammalian kidney. One of the important findings reported was that the papillary cellular content of phosphocholine in the rabbit kidney is very high. The authors indicated that "the physiological significance of this previously unrecognized concentration of phosphocholine in the papilla remains to be established." Of course, subsequently the role of these compounds in the concentration process was uncovered. The role of organic osmolytes in the urine concentration process is discussed elsewhere in this chapter.

In 1982, two abstracts from the University of Oxford (by Radda, Ross, and their coworkers) were published in the Abstract book of the 15th Annual Meeting of the ASN. One of these abstracts was presented: combining classic DMO determinations with ^{31}P NMR techniques to measure pH in isolated rabbit cortical tubules, Adler, Shoebridge, and Radda reported that (*1*) both DMO and ^{31}P-NMR provide valid measurements of intracellular pH in renal tubular cells; (*2*) pH measured with NMR applies to the cytosol; and (*3*) the differences obtained by these two techniques allow for the measurement of cytosolic and intramitochondrial pH in the same cells over a wide range of extracellular pH.

One of the interesting uses of NMR is for the determination of metabolic events in an intact tissue. It is possible to label one reactant magnetically, then determine the rate at which this labeled reactant is converted into another by the altered magnetization of the subsequent metabolite. This method is usually referred to as "saturation transfer." The labeling process (saturation) can be accomplished by rapid or continuous pulsing with a second radio frequency source. Transfer is determined in a typical NMR experiment by quantitating the relevant peak in separate spectra obtained with or without labeling. When the saturated species is √ATP and the observed species is P_1, the rate measured is the metabolic rate of ATP synthesis. Using this technique of saturation transfer, Freeman and associates from Oxford University studied the regulation of sodium transport by ATP in the perfused rat kidney. The concentration of P_1 was found by NMR to be 0.6 mM or only 27% of that determined chemically; the concentration of ADP was 25% of that determined enzymatically. Chemical exchange between P_1 and √ phosphate of ATP was demonstrated. The oxidative phosphorylation rate was 16 μmol/min/g kidney, and O_2 consumption was 3.3 μmol O_2/min/g kidney. The P:O ratio was 2.4 ± 0.3. The amount of Na transported by ATP in these experiments was four times that attributable to the action of Na,K-ATPase (3 moles of Na per mole of ATP). However, the free energy yield of ATP calculated by NMR from the phosphorylation potential was 59.7 K^J/mole. The authors suggested that the free energy of ATP hydrolysis rather than a stoichiometric relationship between ATP and Na-K exchange may determine the rate of sodium transport.

The following year at the ASN meetings of 1983, Weiner and his associates from the Veterans Administration Hospital, University of California, San Francisco, using the saturation transfer technique, quantitated the rate of ATP synthesis in the rat kidney in vivo. They found a rate of 13 μmol/kidney/min when the renal inorganic phosphorus was assumed to be 1.7 mM. These experiments were apparently the first to quantitate ATP turnover in the kidney in vivo.

Also in 1983, Shulman, Siegel, Kashgarian, and their associates from Yale University reported on the measurement of cellular ATP in vivo by

NMR during the recovery phase of ischemic renal failure in rats. They found a rapid fall in ATP during the ischemic period. After the ischemic insult, ATP levels returned to 50% of control values within 10 minutes but rose no higher than 65% of normal after 2 hours. Rats given ATP-$MgCl_2$ had an accelerated recovery of cellular ATP. The authors concluded that infusion of ATP-$MgCl_2$ enhanced the recovery of ATP levels postischemia and that repair of metabolic disorders precedes the functional and morphological recovery in this model of acute renal failure.

At the same meeting, Ross, Radda, and their associates examined perfused human renal carcinoma samples obtained at nephrectomy. Spectra were obtained from the normal renal parenchyma and the tumor. The investigators found a predominant glycolytic metabolism in the tumor and suggested that such metabolic differences "could form the basis of future diagnostic or therapeutic tests for human tumors in vivo."

At the 1986 meeting of the ASN, Robert G. Shulman of Yale University chaired a symposium on nuclear magnetic resonance. This symposium was devoted to the application of NMR techniques to the study of kidney function and metabolism in health and disease. Participants included Robert Balaban (NIH), who spoke on "NMR Spectroscopic Studies of Kidney Biochemistry and Function"; Norman J. Siegel from Yale University, who discussed 31 NMR studies of renal metabolism; and Steven R. Gullans, now at the Brigham and Women's Hospital in Boston, who addressed the topic "Intracellular Na in the Proximal Tubule."

In 1987, the group at Yale (Shulman and Siegel et al.), using NMR techniques, reported that inhibition of ATP degradation during ischemia will ameliorate the metabolic and functional consequences of the renal insult in a manner similar to that seen with infusion of exogenous adenine nucleotides. In a separate communication, the same group reported that inhibition of 5′-nucleotidase enhances postischemic recovery of renal ATP levels. In additional studies, reported at the ASN meeting in 1988, they provided further evidence that restoration of high-energy metabolites is a fundamental determinant of recovery from renal ischemia. The following year, at the 22nd meeting of the ASN, Siegel and Shulman reported that adenosine transport contributes to the beneficial effect of injecting ATP-$MgCl_2$ after renal ischemia.

Heilig and Gullans reported in 1987 that hypernatremia in rats resulted in an increase in total trimethylamines in the brain, whereas in the inner medulla of the kidney trimethylamines remained nearly constant because of an increase in betaine and a slight decrease in glycerophosphorylcholine. Gullans also studied rats with diabetes insipidus (Brattleboro rats) to determine the independent effects of antidiuretic hormone (ADH) and dehydration on the levels of glycerophosphorylcholine in the inner medulla of the kidney. Marked dehydration, in the absence of ADH, did not increase the levels of glycerophosphorylcholine. In contrast, ADH replacement, without dehydration, resulted in a 4.5-fold increase in the concentration of glycerophosphorylcholine. These data suggested a role for ADH in the modulation of osmolytes in the inner medulla of rats with diabetes insipidus. Additional studies by Gullans, reported at the 1988 meeting of the ASN, identified the osmolytes that accumulated in rat brain during hypernatremia, and examined the regulation of organic osmolytes in Madin Darby Canine Kidney (MDCK) cells using nuclear magnetic resonance techniques. At the same meeting, Shulman and Siegel (Yale University) reported the demonstration of trimethylamine osmolytes in human kidney in vivo by ^{1}H NMR.

Nuclear magnetic resonance (NMR) has been and continues to be a useful tool to examine metabolic events in vitro, in the intact tissue, and in vivo. It was instrumental in the study of osmolytes in the inner medulla and has been used effectively to examine the metabolic consequences of renal ischemia. In addition, magnetic resonance imaging (MRI) is a rapidly evolving diagnostic tool. MRI of the kidney is an excellent complementary method when nuclear medicine, ultrasound, or computed tomography fails to provide the desired information. Magnetic resonance spectroscopy using ^{31}P promises to provide greater specificity in the study of various renal diseases and of metabolic events in the human kidney.

Cell Volume Regulation and Organic Osmolytes

During the 1940s and 1950s, it was established that maintenance of normal cell volume depends on a balance between passive salt entry and active extrusion. When the active transport is inhibited, the unopposed effect of electrically charged intracellular colloid causes progressive cell swelling. This relationship was formalized in pump-leak models proposed by Hoffman and Tosteson, Leaf, and Ussing in about 1960. Subsequent studies have shown that, when the volume of cells is perturbed, immediate recovery generally depends on changes in the permeability to Na, K, and Cl rather than on altered active transport.

In the usual experimental model of volume regulatory decrease (VRD), acute hypotonicity is used to swell cells. VRD then occurs through efflux of solutes and water, which shrinks the cells back toward their original volume. The usual model of volume regulatory increase (VRI) uses hypertonicity acutely to shrink the cells, which then recover by influx of solutes and water. The initial studies that established these principles used nucleated red blood cells and were reported in the early 1980s. Many other kinds of cells were subsequently examined, extending these results. The focus at the ASN has been on VRD and VRI in epithelial cells, especially those in the kidney tubules.

Between 1975 and 1978, Linshaw, Grantham, and their collaborators presented three reports at ASN on cell volume regulation in kidney tubules. They dissected individual proximal straight tubules and estimated total cell volume by measuring tubule diameter and length with a microscope ocular micrometer. Cell swelling was induced by inhibiting active electrolyte transport with ouabain. The swelling is restricted by the mechanical strength of the tubule basement membrane, as well as by addition of colloid to the medium.

In 1981, Spring gave a symposium talk on epithelial cell volume regulation, including a description of studies on Necturus gall bladder. He had developed a quantitative light microscopy method, involving computerized focusing, video imaging, and image reconstruction to measure continuously the volume of individual cells in living specimens. The method has proved generally useful and has been adapted for numerous tissues, including single kidney tubules. At the 1983 ASN meeting, there were three reports on cell volume regulation in different tubule segments, based on variations of Spring's method, and many more have followed.

The usual experimental model of volume regulation, consisting of a large step change in osmolality, is convenient but does not match any realistic physiological circumstance. In 1985, Lohr and Grantham reported at ASN that, if the change in osmolality is made gradually, the cells continuously accommodate, with the result that their volume remains constant despite eventual large alterations in tonicity. This probably is a more appropriate representation of the actual response of tissues in vivo.

Cell volume regulation became the subject of numerous reports starting with the 1987 ASN meeting, as investigators tried to understand what the signaling pathways are and what solutes are involved. Changes in intracellular calcium levels are implicated in the genesis of VRD. This was first reported by Chase for toad bladder in 1984 and was confirmed in other kinds of cells by presenters at subsequent meetings. It has not been clear, however, why the calcium level changes or what role this plays in the volume regulation. Another factor being examined is that cell swelling stretches the plasma membrane, which can directly increase ion permeability. At the 1988 and 1989 meetings, there were several reports of stretch-activated K currents in renal cells. With regard to the solutes involved, K and Cl currents have been reported in VRD and increased cell NaCl has been reported in VRI. Also, addition of short-chain fatty acids increases volume regulation, but it is not clear whether they act as osmolytes or regulators. Steven Hebert was active in presenting on this subject, giving an invited lecture in 1987 and a symposium presentation in 1989.

In 1956, Karl Ullrich measured high levels of glycerolphosphorylcholine (GPC) in the inner medullas of dogs. He and his collaborators recognized that the intracellular GPC helps balance the osmotic pressure of the high NaCl in the medullary interstitial fluid. They also incidentally noted high tissue inositol. Their discovery helps understand how medullary cells adapt to their hypertonic environment. Over the next 25 years, however, little additional research on renal medullary organic osmolytes was recorded.

At the ASN meeting in 1981, Balaban and Knepper reported on the first use of 14N-NMR in biological studies. An unintended result of their study was the rediscovery of renal medullary GPC, in this case in rabbits. They also noted that other trimethylamines were present in large quantities in the renal medulla. Like most nephrologists, they had been unaware of Ullrich's earlier work. In 1982, Yancey et al. reviewed in Science the widespread occurrence of intracellular organic osmolytes in water-stressed organisms and analyzed the protective roles of these compounds as "compatible" and "counteracting" solutes. This publication led Balaban and Knepper to the realization that GPC, and the other trimethylamines, are counteracting solutes that protect renal medullary cells from the perturbing effects of the high urea in the renal medulla, and they included this theory when they published their NMR results. In 1986, Bagnasco et al. discovered that in addition to GPC and inositol, there are also large amounts of sorbitol and betaine in rat and rabbit renal medullary cells, that these compounds vary with diuretic state, and that they presumably serve as compatible and counteracting osmolytes.

Since then there have been numerous studies of organic osmolytes in vivo and in vitro (where they are easier to study). The experiments aim at defining the changes in cell contents of these compounds under different conditions, the mechanisms by which the solutes are accumulated, how they are controlled, and how their presence affects the cells.

In 1985, Bagnasco et al. submitted an abstract to the ASN describing how the level of sorbitol in renal medullary cells in tissue culture increases with hypertonicity because the activity of aldose reductase, the enzyme that catalyzes its synthesis from glucose, rises. At the 1986 ASN meeting, Nakanishi et al. showed that MDCK cells accumulate betaine, inositol, and GPC in hyperosmotic medium. Since then, these cell lines have been used extensively for studying the organic osmolytes.

By 1987, the work on organic osmolytes had advanced far enough for Burg to give a state-of-the-art lecture on the subject, and five related papers were presented. Organic osmolytes were shown to vary with hypertonicity in both the kidney and the brain. Also, the osmoregulated accumulation of inositol was shown to depend on uptake from the extracellular fluid.

In 1988 there was a poster discussion group on cell volume regulation, featuring several presentations on organic osmolytes. The regulation of these compounds by brain and kidney cells was further characterized in vivo, in cell cultures, and in suspensions of medullary tubules. Several more presentations in 1989 followed along the same lines. In addition, the application of molecular techniques began providing evidence that osmoregulation of inositol and sorbitol involves changes in gene expression.

Renal Cell Culture

Culture of tissue explants began in the first decade of this century and expanded in the 1950s with the widespread use of dispersed primary cell cultures and continuous cell lines. Renal cell lines that were established early include LLC-PK_1 (started in 1958 from trypsin-dispersed porcine renal cells);

A6 (started in 1965 from *Xenopus laevis*); and OK (started in 1975 from opossum). Application of cell culture technology to studies of nephrology began with the discovery by Leighton et al. (1969) that renal cells form highly differentiated epithelia in culture. These investigators recognized that the blisters (often referred to as "domes" or "hemicysts") in monolayer cultures of MDCK cells represent pockets of fluid that are transported by the cells and accumulate between the cell layer and the support on which it is grown. Further, Leighton et al. observed that the epithelium formed by MDCK cells in culture is basically similar to renal tubular epithelium. The MDCK epithelium is morphologically polarized. There are numerous microvilli on the apical surface that faces the medium but very few on the basal surface that faces the support. Also, tight junctions join adjacent cells at their apical surface. Leighton et al. also recognized that the medium was analogous to a tubular lumen and that the domes were analogous to interstitial collections of resorbed components of the glomerular filtrate. Thus, the stage was set for using MDCK and other renal epithelial cell lines for nephrological studies.

Misfeldt et al. grew MDCK epithelia on filters, so that the solutions bathing both the apical and basolateral surfaces could be easily accessed. In 1976, they published on the electrical and transport properties of this system. Cereijido et al. developed a similar preparation independently. These results caught the attention of nephrologists, who began learning cell culture techniques. At the 1977 ASN meeting, Ausiello et al. showed that LLC-PK_1 cells increase their cyclic AMP content in response to vasopressin and calcitonin. At the same meeting, Mills, Ausiello, et al. presented a paper on interactions of ouabain with these same cells. At an ASN symposium in 1978, Karnovsky discussed glomerular cells in culture, and two studies were presented based on this preparation.

In 1981, Handler gave a state-of-the-art address entitled "Renal Cells in Culture: A Promising New Approach." In that year, enough abstracts of studies using cell culture were submitted to warrant a separate free communication session devoted to the subject. Since then, renal cell culture methodology has lived up to its promise. The technique has proved to be exceedingly useful. It is now widely used in nephrology, and at current ASN meetings there are numerous papers presented using cell culture as a general and widely applicable tool.

Renal Molecular Biology

The basic concepts of molecular biology were in place by 1967, when the ASN was founded. Watson and Crick has postulated the double-helix model of DNA in 1953, DNA and RNA polymerases had been discovered, DNA replication and RNA transcription were known, the genetic code was deciphered, and the function of messenger RNA had been discerned. Nevertheless, it took more than 15 years after the founding of ASN for studies using the powerful tools of molecular biology to appear regularly in its programs.

The striking exception was at the first ASN meeting in 1967, where in a prescient symposium, "Mechanism of Action of Aldosterone," Isidore Edelman proposed that aldosterone exerted its action by increasing gene expression. He had noted in the early 1960s that aldosterone binds to nuclear receptors and postulated that the steroid acts by increasing mRNA transcription and protein synthesis. He presented this theory in the symposium. At that time the supporting evidence included the blocking of the electrolyte transport effects of aldosterone by inhibitors of RNA and protein synthesis. Jack Orloff had organized the symposium and chaired it. He invited, as the second speaker, W. French Anderson, now a pioneer in gene therapy but at that time a beginning molecular biologist at NIH. Anderson's role was to instruct the nephrologists on gene transcription and mRNA translation. The third speaker was Alexander Leaf, who presented an alternative theory of aldosterone action. Anderson recalls that Orloff asked him to evaluate the merits of the competing theories, and, being in awe of Leaf and Edelman, who were already at that time distinguished professors, Anderson tried to be diplomatic by saying that both theories probably would turn out in the future to have merit. However, he remembers vividly that he was acutely embarrassed when Orloff later pointed out to him that he had misspoken and had inadvertently said that both professors probably were wrong!

Aside from only two abstracts in the 1970s relating aldosterone action to DNA and mRNA, the next recorded mention of molecular biology apparently was Edelman's in his Homer Smith Award address, "Receptors and Effectors in Hormone Action in the Kidney," in 1980.

At the 1984 ASN meeting, two papers described studies in which recombinant proteins were used as reagents, and another paper described a study in which angiotensin mRNA was localized in the kidney by RNA-DNA dot blot hybridization. By 1985 the number of studies using molecular biology was increasing rapidly. There were at least six at that meeting, including a study by Breuning et al. localizing the adult polycystic gene to chromosome 16, and a symposium talk, "Biology and Genetics of Complement Receptors," by Fearon.

Since that time there have been numerous presentations at the ASN meetings of original works using molecular biology techniques, as well as symposia and state-of-the-art addresses. The earlier state-of-the art addresses on molecular biology included those on anion and glucose transporters by Lodish in 1986, applications in clinical medicine by Baxter in 1987, and renin by Corvol in 1987. Also, in 1987 a symposium on membrane transport proteins included a talk by Lingrel on the molecular biology of the Na,K-ATPase and a talk by Pouyssegeur on the Na/H exchanger. The increasing frequency of presentations of work using molecular biology reflects the fact that, although most members of ASN have only recently begun using these tools, the approach is rapidly becoming routine in their laboratories.

9

Hormones and Hypertension

Thomas F. Ferris, Juha P. Kokko, and Michael J. Dunn

A Quarter Century

A review of the presentations on hypertension and hormones at the American Society of Nephrology (ASN) meetings over the past 25 years is a rewarding experience. It is a record of extraordinary accomplishments in understanding the physiology of hypertension and in the application of research to therapy. The development of immunoassays allowed for accurate measurements of the several hormones important in hypertension, and therapeutic advances were made with development of blockers of these hormones as well as drugs that interfere with contractility of vascular smooth muscle. The diagnosis of renal hypertension was a major clinical problem 25 years ago and is now a rather pedestrian clinical problem. Malignant hypertension, a major cause of mortality in the 1950s and 1960s, has virtually disappeared. How aldosterone causes sodium transport across epithelial cells has been elucidated, and natriuretic hormones, long the Holy Grail for renal investigators, have been isolated, although their physiological role remains unclarified.

We have arbitrarily divided this chapter into two sections, one dealing with reports on renal hypertension emphasizing advances in understanding the role substances of renin, angiotensin, prostaglandins and other vasoactive substances as well as natriuretic hormones, and a separate section on the mechanism of aldosterone action.

Renin-Angiotensin-Prostaglandins

At the time of the first ASN meeting in 1967, there was little understanding of the clinical significance of measurements of plasma renin. For instance, the low plasma renin activity (PRA) in diagnosing hyperaldosteronism was a major problem. Hyporeninemia was found in 15 of 35 black hypertensives, in whom only 2 had elevated aldosterone excretion. The fact that low plasma renin was present in a large number of patients with essential hypertension was not reported until the early 1970s. The role of renin in the hypertension of chronic renal disease was also unclear, since one found variable plasma renin and no correlation with systemic hypertension. Hypertension following acute experimental glomerulonephritis in the dog was not associated with an increase in plasma renin, yet hypertension in patients on chronic hemodialysis was reported to resolve following bilateral nephrectomy. The potential of renal renin concentration in predisposing to acute tubular necrosis was raised, since saline loading was noted to protect kidneys in glycerol-induced and other models of acute renal failure. Distal sodium delivery was found to be a factor in renin secretion, since the increase in renal venous renin in response to ethacrynic acid was prevented by ureteral occlusion. Renin was found in the plasma of four of six anephric women on chronic hemodialysis, and the site of renin production was presumed to be the uterus. Two lipids were isolated from the renal medulla, prostaglandin E_2 (PGE_2) and a second neutral lipid, which lowered the blood pressure of hypertensive dogs. The angiotensin infusion test, one measure of AII sensitivity, was reported to be of no value in the detection of surgically correctable renal hypertension, whereas high renal vein PRA from the kidney with an anatomical stenosis was reported to be predictive of a correctable lesion.

In 1968, the first of several symposiums held at ASN meetings on hypertension was presented. Over the 25 years, more symposia have focused on hypertension than any other topic. The first symposium was chaired by John Laragh with Louis Tobian, Merlin Bumpus, and Arthur Grollman panelists. Unfortunately, no record of these symposia exists, and at the first symposium the title was simply "Hypertension." A provocative report in 1968 was of six patients with malignant hypertension and renal failure who underwent bilateral nephrectomy; four received renal transplants and one was alive2 1/2 years later with only minimal hypertension. The potential role of renal prostaglandins in hypertension was emerging with PGE_2 reported to be higher in the renal vein of patients with renal artery stenosis. Reduction in the granularity of renal medullary interstitial cells, known to be the site of PGE_2 synthesis, was noted in rats following institution of desoxy corticosterone acetate (DOCA) and a high-salt diet, and transplantation of the renal medulla into the peritoneum of rats made hypertensive by renal artery clipping was reported to decrease blood pressure.

Two symposia on hypertension were held in 1969. One was on the regulation of renin secretion with Arthur Vander as Chairman and a panel consisting of Carlos Ayers, Andrew Michelakis, and William Ganong, and a second was on preeclampsia with E. A. H. Sims as Chairman and a panel of Leon Chesley, Robert McCluskey, Herbert Langford, Victor Pollak, and Marshall Lindheimer.

Patients with renal artery stenosis who had a ratio greater than 1.5 of renal vein renin from the involved kidney compared to the contralateral kidney were reported to have better results with surgical revascularization. In contrast to findings in anephric animals, four anephric patients were reported to be insensitive to angiotensin II, and anephric patients were noted to have higher plasma aldosterone concentration prior to dialysis with no change in PRA. Hyperplasia and hypergranularity of the juxtaglomerular cells were reported in biopsies of patients with Bartter's syndrome at this meeting.

In 1969, the distribution of renal cortical blood flow was thought to be a potential mechanism of controlling sodium excretion. Inner cortical nephrons were postulated to be less natriuretic than nephrons in the outer cortex because of their long loops of Henle. However, when xenon washout techniques and distribution of radioactive microspheres were used, infusions of PGE_1 were noted to increase urinary sodium excretion with a redistribution of blood flow to the inner cortex.

In 1970, another symposium on hypertension was held with John Laragh as Chairman and Louis Tobian, Arthur Guyton, James Davis, and Ed Biglieri as discussants. The topics covered included arteriolar changes in hypertension, the overriding dominance of the kidneys in the control of blood pressure, factors controlling renin secretion, and steroid-induced hypertension. In 1971, a symposium on hypertension featured James Melby speaking on mineralocorticoid hypertension. James Hunt reported on renal vascular hypertension, and Frank Finnerty discussed treatment of the hypertensive crisis. In 1971, stimulation of renin release by the β-adrenergic nervous system was first reported, and high renin concentration was reported in the uterine vein of nephrectomized rabbits. Angiotensin II was found to increase uterine blood flow by decreasing uterine vascular resistance thought to be caused by increased uterine prostaglandin synthesis. Production of PGE_2 by renal medullary interstitial cells grown in tissue culture was reported. Potassium was reported to decrease renin secretion, and the mechanism was thought to be increasing distal sodium delivery since potassium had no effect in the nonfiltering kidney.

The meeting in 1973 was opened with an address by John Laragh on "Renal and Endocrine Mechanisms in Hypertension." Several studies of the effect of the new competitive AII inhibitor, saralasin, were presented. Malignant hypertension in rats induced with DOCA was not prevented by saralasin nor was hypertension induced by renal artery clipping in the rabbit. The role of angiotensin II in causing renal hypertension remained perplexing because saralasin had an intrinsic AII-like effect. Several reports of the potentiating effect of prostaglandin inhibition in causing acute renal failure were presented, suggesting again a role for renal prostaglandin synthesis in controlling renal blood flow.

In 1974 the syndrome of low renin hypertension was discussed in a symposium by John Laragh, James Melby, and Gordon Williams. Two papers demonstrated that although renin secretion increased following uranyl nitrate, angiotensin given to animals receiving uranyl nitrate did not increase the severity of tubular necrosis. The complexity of factors controlling sodium excretion was evident in that although suppression of renin occurred in patients on propranolol, plasma aldosterone increased normally on a low sodium intake and pregnant women escaped from high sodium intakes in spite of persistent elevation of plasma renin and aldosterone. Plasma renin and aldosterone were noted to fall with aging, and at this meeting the success of an angiotensin I converting enzyme inhibitor in treating patients with malignant hypertension was reported. Measurement of plasma angiotensin converting enzyme demonstrated unexplained elevations in patients with carcinoma of the lung, pulmonary embolism, and acute viral hepatitis. (Sarcoid was not included in this study.) The increase in renal blood flow caused by furosemide and ethacrynic acid was found to be dependent on increased renal synthesis of PGE_2.

The 1974 meeting opened with a presentation by Stanley Peart on signals for renin release. AII blockade was reported to reduce blood pressure in pregnant women and in patients with cirrhosis, suggesting that the elevated AII maintained blood pressure in these conditions. Sodium bicarbonate was found not to inhibit renin secretion, in contrast to sodium chloride, suggesting a role for distal chloride absorption in inhibiting renin secretion.

In 1975, a patient with the syndrome of hyporeninemic hypoaldosteronism was reported to have low urinary PGE_2 excretion, suggesting that impaired prostaglandin synthesis might be a cause of the syndrome. Several interesting reports on PGE_2 were reported, including stimulation of synthesis by AII, bradykinin, and arginine vasopressin (AVP), and PGE_2 was found to inhibit sodium transport in the cortical collecting tubule.

Renal prostaglandins was the subject of a symposium for the first time with Joe Handler, Aubrey Morrison, and Myer Leifshitz participating. Topics covered were the role of prostaglandin synthesis on the renin-aldosterone axis and the antagonism of ADH by PGE_2. Inhibition of prostaglandin synthesis was noted to decrease single nephron glomerular filtration rate (SNGFR), with an increase in afferent and efferent resistance causing reduction in glomerular plasma flow. The efficacy of captopril on the treatment of renal vascular hypertension in humans was reported in 1976.

The first report of the efficacy of calcium channel blockers in preventing the vasoconstrictive effect of angiotensin, norepinephrine, and vasopressin was presented in 1977, and the application of transluminal angioplasty to correct renal artery stenosis was reported.

The first paper on the signal transduction pathways activated by prostaglandins was presented in 1977 with the report that PGE_2 stimulated adenylate cyclase and increased intracellular cyclic AMP in specific nephron segments. PGE_2 was found to reduce vasopressin-stimulated adenylate cyclase, thereby down-regulating water re-absorption in the rabbit medullary collecting tubule. PGE_2-stimulated adenylate cyclase was also documented at several sites along the rat nephron, including the medullary thick ascending limb of the loop of Henle and the cortical and medullary collecting tubules. PGE_2 was also found to antagonize vasopressin-stimulated sodium reabsorption in the thick ascending limb of the loop of Henle. Inhibition of active chloride transport by PGE_2 in the thick ascending limb of the rat was first reported in 1978. At this meeting, the term *type IV renal tubular acidosis* was used to describe the syndrome of hyperkalemia acidosis, with diminished renin and aldosterone secretion.

In 1979, the efficacy of captopril on the treatment of patients with scleroderma and malignant hypertension was reported. Captopril was noted to have had two unpredictable effects: (*1*) decreasing uterine prostaglandin synthesis with a reduction in uterine blood flow in pregnant rabbits and (*2*) a type IV renal tubular acidosis (RTA) in azotemic patients. AII receptors were reported in mesangial cell cultures of rat glomeruli, and increased PGE_2 and thromboxane synthesis in rat glomerular epithelial cells from spontaneously hypertensive rats (SHR) was reported.

Another symposium on the endocrine aspects of hypertension was presented in 1981 with John Laragh speaking on the renin-angiotensin-aldosterone system. Allen Cowley on vasopressin in experimental and human hypertension, Jean Sealey on inactive renin, and Michael Dunn on renal and vascular prostaglandins.

In 1982, prostaglandin synthesis in glomeruli was found to be important in modulating angiotensin II induced glomerular contractility. In rats with steptozotosin-induced diabetes mellitus, the diminished renal vasoconstrictor response to angiotensin II was found to be caused by increased prostaglandin synthesis. The correction of essential hypertension in blacks with malignant nephrosclerosis following renal transplantation pointed to the role of the kidney in causing the hypertension. Also, increased red blood cell (RBC) sodium-lithium countertransport, previously reported to be a marker of essential hypertension, was reported in women who developed hypertension during pregnancy.

At the 1982 meeting, there was general agreement that prostaglandins stimulated adenylate cyclase, thereby increasing cyclic AMP not only in glomeruli but also in various tubular epithelial segments. Although vasopressin also mediates its action through increases in intracellular cyclic AMP, paradoxically PGE_2 appears to down-regulate vasopressin-stimulated adenylate cyclase in selected nephron sites, thereby antagonizing the action of vasopressin, both in the loop of Henle and in the collecting tubule.

The postreceptor signal transduction pathways activated by angiotensin II did not receive attention at ASN meetings until 1983, when it was reported that angiotensin II activated phospholipase A_2 and phospholipase C in cultured glomerular mesangial cells. The activation of phospholipase A_2 seemed predominantly responsible for the deacylation of arachidonic acid and the subsequent synthesis of PGE_2, thereby activating a negative feedback loop to down-regulate the contractile and other actions of angiotensin on the cell. In 1984, Bonventre and his coworkers presented a series of reports assessing intracellular (cytosolic) calcium using calcium-sensitive fluorescent probes. Angiotensin II dramatically increased intracellular calcium, and this increase was primarily due to mobilization of calcium from intracellular stores.

Antihypertensive therapy was the subject of a symposium in 1983 with presentations by Emanull Bravo on converting enzyme inhibitors, Joseph Izzo on calcium channel blockers, and Richard Weinshilboum on sympathetic inhibitors. Cyclosporine was reported to inhibit the renin-angiotensin system with impairment of potassium excretion in 1984, and lowering arterial pressure was noted to diminish albuminuria in rats with diabetes mellitus by lowering glomerular capillary pressure. After years of reports of evanescent natriuretic hormones, the synthesis of the atrial natriuretic factor was reported in 1984. It reduced blood pressure and directly inhibited aldosterone secretion by an effect on the adrenal cortex. A high potassium intake was found to prevent strokes in stroke-prone rats independent of change in blood pressure.

In 1985, a symposium was held on the role of hypertension in the pathogenesis of renal disease with Helmut Rennke, John Curtis, and David Baldwin as speakers. Where the 1970s saw an emphasis on studies of renal vasoconstrictors, the 1980s were marked by an emphasis on vasodilators. Several studies of endothelial derived relaxing factor were reported. Hyperfiltration in the remnant kidney was found to be due to increased glomerular prostaglandin synthesis, and atrial natriuretic peptide was found to increase glomerular filtration rate in the rat with an overall decrease in renal resistance but an increase in efferent resistance. The increase in GFR with protein feeding also was found to be due to renal prostaglandin synthesis.

During the 1986 meeting, an additional prostaglandin-stimulated signal transduction pathway was described. The vasoconstrictor prostaglandins, $PGF_{2\alpha}$ and thromboxane A_2, increased intracellular (cytosolic) calcium through activation of phospholipase C in cultured rat glomerular mesangial cells. In 1987, thromboxane A_2 and $PGF_{2\alpha}$ were reported to alkalinize the cytosol of cultured glomerular mesangial cells, an effect consistent with activation of phospholipase C and subsequent activation of sodium-hydrogen antiport (i.e., hydrogen extrusion and sodium entry into the cell) with subsequent cytosolic alkalinization. At this same meeting, PGE_2 was described as a direct inhibitor of sodium-potassium ATPase in inner medullary collecting ducts. It is noteworthy that $PGF_{2\alpha}$ did not have this effect, nor did $PGF_{2\alpha}$ reduce sodium flux. These results were consistent with the conclusion that increases in intracellular cyclic AMP (PGE_2 effect) mediated the reduction of ATPase and of sodium transport. In subsequent meetings, these conclusions were reinforced to yield the prevalent belief that PGE_2 and PGI_2 were vasorelaxant and inhibited cellular proliferation, especially in glomerular mesangial cells and vascular smooth muscle, through activation of adenylate cyclase and increments of intracellular cyclic AMP. Vasoconstrictor prostanoids such as $PGF_{2\alpha}$ and thromboxane did not alter adenylate cyclase activity but did stimulate phospholipase C, thereby increasing cytosolic calcium and activating protein kinase C. These effects, in concert, not only stimulate cellular contraction but in cultured mesangial cells activate mitogenesis and cellular proliferation.

In 1986, the term *autocoids* was used at the meeting for the first time.

There were several papers on the atrial natriuretic peptide in congestive heart failure. ANP receptors were found in the inner medullary collecting duct, and medullary blood flow increased following an infusion of ANP. The use of molecular biology demonstrated that messenger RNA expression for renin was found in most organs, not simply in the kidney. Signal transduction in mesangial cells with emphasis on the pertussis toxin-inhibitable G protein linked angiotensin II receptors to phospholipase A_2. Inhibition of this G protein with pertussis toxin diminished PGE_2 synthesis in response to angiotensin. Release of arachidonic acid and increased synthesis of PGE_2 in angiotensin-stimulated mesangial cells may be secondary not only to phospholipase A_2 activation but also to stimulation of phospholipase C. Angiotensin II also was found to induce membrane depolarization in cultured cells, and the depolarization was secondary to an increased chloride conductance probably activated by the changes of cytosolic calcium. The increased chloride conductance caused intracellular chloride to decrease, which, in turn, activated, in an unknown fashion, PGE_2 synthesis. The increase in PGE_2 was interpreted as a negative feedback pathway triggered by angiotensin, whereas the membrane depolarization initiated cellular contraction.

Several papers in 1987 centered on the role of ANF. ANF levels were increased during water immersion and in response to volume expansion following cardiac transplantation, in spite of cardiac denervation. However, in spite of all the research effort, its physiological role remained unclear. The renal artery was noted to be a major source of endothelium-derived relaxation factor (EDRF). Whereas the effect of autocoids, vasopressin, and angiotensin on blood vessels had been emphasized at previous meeting, in 1987 they were reported to have effects on cell growth. Endothelin, a newly described vasoconstrictor synthesized by endothelial cells, elicited great interest, with papers directed at its effect on contraction of mesangial and smooth muscle cells and its effect on intracellular calcium and sodium transport. Whereas over 50 years were needed following their discovery to elucidate the chemistry of renin and angiotensin, endothelin was described and synthesized in 1 year.

An additional action of angiotensin was described, namely the capacity of angiotensin II to decrease adenylate cyclase activity and intracellular cyclic AMP through activation of an inhibitory G protein in proximal tubular epithelial cells. By 1989, research interest on angiotensin-activated signaling pathways was focused on angiotensin actions in proximal tubular cells. There were several reports that angiotensin activated the sodium-hydrogen antiport in cultured proximal tubular cells as well as in the isolated, perfused rabbit proximal tubule. Furthermore, angiotensin activated a sodium-bicarbonate exchange on the basolateral surface of the isolated, perfused proximal tubular cells in contrast to the luminal activation of sodium-hydrogen exchange. The more proximal steps linking the angiotensin receptor to these acid-base transporters, such as stimulation of protein kinase C or alterations of intracellular cyclic AMP, were not evaluated. There was also an interesting report in 1989 that angiotensin II stimulated hypertrophy but not hyperplasia in a cultured proximal tubular cell line. This hypertrophy, induced by angiotensin, was linked to increased oncogene expression as measured by increased transcription of the proto-oncogenes, c-*myc* and c-*fos*.

Hence, by the end of the 1980s, it was clear that angiotensin II triggered intracellular events not only in vascular smooth muscle and glomerular mesangial cells but also in tubular segments, particularly the proximal tubule. In smooth muscle and mesangial cells, angiotensin activates phospholipase C, thereby increasing intracellular calcium and also stimulating protein kinase C, leading to contraction, hypertrophy, or hyperplasia. The activation of phospholipase A_2 with subsequent synthesis of PGE_2 constitutes a negative feedback pathway that down-regulates angiotensin's actions, perhaps by reducing phospholipase C stimulability and also by altering calcium/calmodulin-triggered events. Angiotensin also depolarizes contractile cells, at least in part, through an increase in chloride conductance with decrements of intracellular chloride concentration. In proximal tubular cells, angiotensin is apparently linked through an inhibitory GTP-binding protein to adenylate cyclase, thereby decreasing intracellular cyclic AMP. It is unknown which signaling pathway links angiotensin to luminal stimulation of sodium-hydrogen exchange and basolateral stimulation of sodium-bicarbonate exchange in the proximal tubule.

In 1989, a symposium was held on vasoactive autocoids with platelet activating factor covered by R. Neal Pickard, endothelial derived relaxing factors covered by Salvador Moncada, and endothelin covered by Tadashe Inagami. Recombinant human erythropoietin was shown to induce hypertension in the rat without a rise in hematocrit, confirming the belief of many clinicians that its hypertensive effect was in part independent of erythropoiesis. The finding that erythropoietin increased endothelin synthesis in hemodialysis patients might be relevant in this regard. Binding sites for endothelin were found in rat mesangial cells and aortic smooth muscle, and cyclosporine was found to stimulate synthesis of endothelin, which might be a factor in the glomerular vasculopathy induced by cyclosporine. Urinary excretion of endothelin increased after radiocontrast agents and in patients with the hemolytic uremic syndrome.

In 1990, Salvatore Moncada gave a state-of-the-art lecture on the discovery and biological relevance of the arginine nitric oxide pathway. Blockers of EDRF caused vasoconstriction in the normal kidney. The association of obesity, insulin resistance, and hypertension was covered in several papers, and a symposium was held on genetic markers of hypertension and diabetes mellitus with emphasis on lithium-sodium counter transport.

Aldosterone

Prior to the first meeting of the American Society of Nephrology in 1967, it had been established that aldosterone had a pivotal role in the regulation of net sodium balance in various animals species and in human beings. It also was well appreciated that aldosterone's primary effect on sodium homeostasis is exerted through its effect on nephron segments. It, therefore, is not surprising that nephrologists have been intrigued with the mechanism and site of action of aldosterone, as well as factors that affect aldosterone secretion. Indeed, during the first annual meeting of the ASN that was held in Los Angeles, a main symposium was entitled, "Mechanism of Action of Aldosterone." The chairman of that symposium was Dr. Jack Orloff, and the three participants included Drs. Alexander Leaf, I. S. Edelman, and French Anderson. Although this symposium was one of the most important overview presentations at that meeting, it is somewhat surprising that such a small number of abstracts on aldosterone have been submitted to the annual meetings of the ASN. In perusing the annual ASN abstract books, there have been roughly two and a half articles per year for the past 25 years. Only during the past 3 years has the number of these abstracts increased to approximately six abstracts per year. Although the number of these abstracts has been relatively small, their quality and importance has been quite high. In contrast to many other fields, it appears that the subsequent models depicting the mechanism of action of aldosterone that have been developed have been logical extensions of the framework of understanding that existed in 1967.

In the early 1960s, the toad urinary bladder became the primary in vitro tissue used to examine the mechanism of action of mineralocorticoids. This was a convenient model, since technically it was easy to set up in the Ussing chamber and to measure the transepithelial short circuit current, which was an indicator of transepithelial sodium transport. Using this technology, it was determined that not all steroids exhibited the same effect on net Na transport, but rather, there existed relative differences in sodium transport activity with various steroids. It was then thought that the primary reason for the differences in mineralocorticoid activity was due to the varying affinities that these steroids had to specific mineralocorticoid receptors. Where these receptors existed was a hot topic of discussion in the early to mid 1960s. Earlier studies were complicated by the realization that both nonspecific and specific binding of aldosterone existed in various subcellular fractions. Initial studies involving subcellular fractions of the adrenalectomized rat kidneys demonstrated that there were saturable binding sites in the nucleus. It, however, was not clear then whether these were true "receptors" or whether these were some other type of binding proteins. It was thought that aldosterone gained access to these binding sites by passive diffusive mechanisms and that once bound specifically to these receptors, a series of biochemical mechanisms were initiated that involved DNA-dependent RNA protein synthesis. This conclusion was based on the observation that actinomycin and puromycin inhibited the aldosterone-stimulated sodium transport without affecting the baseline rate of sodium transport. Although it was not known what the proteins were at that time, they nevertheless were coined as aldosterone-induced proteins (AIP).

In 1967 it was not clear how aldosterone-induced proteins influenced sodium transport, and a number of possible mechanisms were considered. However, it was suggested that more than a single mechanism might be operative. The general model that was developed in the early to mid-1960s suggested that AIP somehow increased the sodium conductance of the apical cell membrane without affecting the back diffusion of sodium from the serosal solution. Once sodium gained access into the cell cytoplasm, it was hypothesized that sodium was extruded by an active mechanism on the basolateral membrane. Alternate suggestions were that AIPs were critical to cell energy metabolism or to the number of sodium pumps or linkage between these two suggestions. These hypotheses that were formulated 25 years ago have been the basis of the conceptual framework of the hypothetical model that has been examined and refined during the subsequent years. The current (1990) understanding of the model as to how mineralocorticoids affect sodium transport transepithelially is schematized in Figure 9.1.

Decade of the 1960s

It is convenient and maybe even instructive to consider the advances made in our understanding of various aspects of aldosterone in specific decades of ASN existence. After the initial meeting of the ASN in 1967, the remainder of the 1960s was concerned primarily with further definition of the specificity of steroid receptors and their localization, as well as confirmation of the role that aldosterone-induced proteins had in sodium transport. These studies suggested that aldosterone receptors existed in both the nuclear and cytoplasmic fractions obtained from adrenalectomized rat kidney homogenates. Some evidence was put forth that there was more than a single corticosteroid receptor, at least in the isolated toad bladder. It was also shown in the toad bladder that after receptor activation, the physiological consequences of the aldosterone-induced protein were dependent on the presence of substrates such as glucose. Further, these stimulated proteins had a relatively long half-life.

Decade of the 1970s

The studies concerning aldosterone in the 1970s were directed primarily toward identifying the target tissues for aldosterone and the factors that regulated aldosterone secretion. Initial clearance studies on dogs showed that administration of aldosterone to bilaterally adrenalectomized animals had no effect on free water clearance or free water generation, and therefore it was concluded that aldosterone had no significant mineralocorticoid effect in the ascending limb of Henle. Subsequent in vitro microperfusion studies localized the primary mineralocorticoid effect to the cortical collecting tubule in contrast to the distal convoluted tubule. This view now is generally held, but later

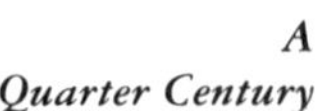

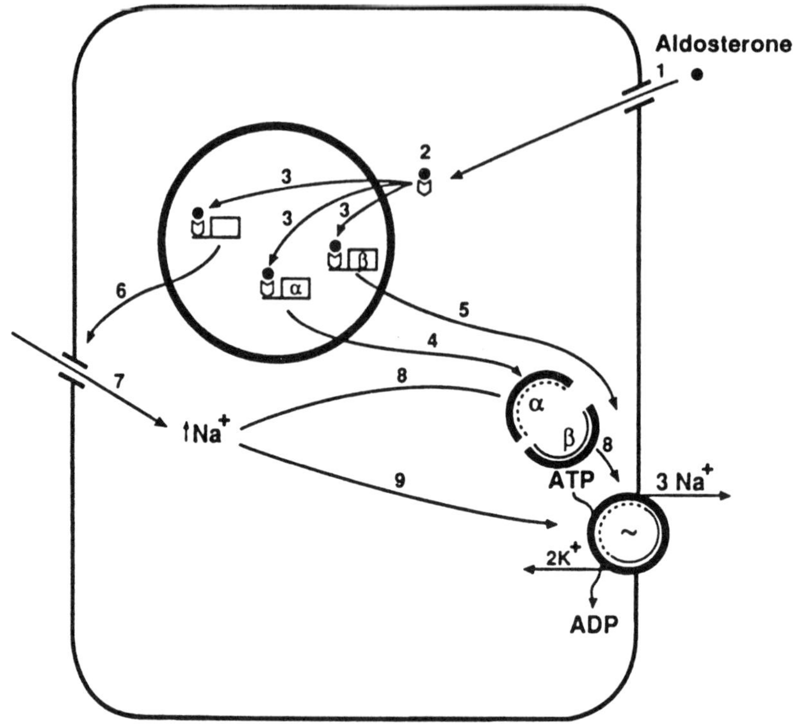

Figure 9.1. Schematics to depict the mechanism by which aldosterone increases sodium transport across the principal cell of the collecting duct: **1**, passive diffusion of aldosterone (*) into cytoplasm; **2**, specific binding of aldosterone to receptors (☐); **3**, binding of aldosterone to promoter regions of specific genes (☐); **4–5**, increased transcription of alpha (a) and beta (β) subunits of pump; **6**, transmission of information to increase Na channel activity; **7**, passive influx of Na; **8**, Na-dependent posttranslational processing of subunits into active pump; **9**, Na-dependent activation of NaK ATPase.

studies have indicated that mineralocorticoids in addition also modulate acidification processes in the medullary collecting duct segments. In agreement with these physiological studies were the autoradiographic observations that noted specific binding of tritiated aldosterone to receptors of high affinity only within the collecting tubule. In addition it was shown that physiological concentrations of mineralocorticoids stimulated sodium potassium ATPase activity only in connecting and cortical collecting tubules in contrast to all other nephron segments that were studied. Thus, based on physiological measurements, as well as binding and biochemical studies, it was concluded that the cortical collecting tubule is the primary mineralocorticoid target site of aldosterone.

Studies on factors that regulate aldosterone secretion are quite interesting. Studies have shown that there is a circadian variation in plasma aldosterone. In normal individuals, there is a gradual rise of plasma aldosterone in the morning that peaks at approximately 12 noon and then reaches the lowest concentration between 9 P.M. and 3 A.M. This normal diurnal variation is lost in anephric patients, and therefore it was suggested that diurnal variation in plasma aldosterone requires an intact renin angiotensin system. Although the renin angiotensin system is an important modulator of aldosterone secretion, it was noted that plasma aldosterone concentration can increase in salt depletion even though the renin angiotensin system was suppressed by propanolol. In agreement with this conclusion was the observation that serum aldosterone concentrations were suppressed normally in response to water immersion in chronic renal failure patients without presumed resources of renal renin-angiotensin. It was also demonstrated that increases in ambient potassium concentration stimulate aldosterone secretion from the adrenal gland, but the possibility exists that various other factors might also influence aldosterone secretion in a significant manner. It is noteworthy that approximately half of the patients with chronic renal failure who have hyperkalemia are aldosterone deficient, while about half of the patients apparently have a defect for potassium secretion in response to aldosterone. Why this difference occurs is not clear.

Decade of the 1980s

In the early 1980s, it became clear that aldosterone had varying effects on different target tissues. In vitro microperfusion studies demonstrated that aldosterone stimulates hydrogen secretion across medullary collecting ducts. This was an important observation in two regards. First, this process occurred independent of sodium, and the process was clearly distinct from the effect aldosterone had on sodium transport across the cortical collecting duct. Also of interest was the abstract that demonstrated that aldosterone stimulates sodium resorption in both the distal and proximal rat colon. In the distal component, however, the stimulation of sodium absorption is by electrogenic mechanisms, whereas in the proximal segment aldosterone primarily stimulates electroneutral sodium transport. The sodium transport in the colon is also mediated by receptors, and it is of interest that these receptors increase in number quite rapidly following bilateral nephrectomy. It further was shown that the increase in potassium secretion in the colon can be dissociated from the effect on sodium absorption, as is the case in the medullary collecting tubule where aldosterone stimulates hydrogen secretion independent of sodium. Thus it can be concluded that the mechanism of aldosterone is not identical in all target tissues, and indeed aldosterone has more than pure mineralocorticoid effects since it affects hydrogen secretory processes.

The last decade has also seen a significant increase in the number of studies that have attempted to determine the exact cell type that responds to aldosterone, as well as examining the nature of biochemical coupling to sodium transport. It is now well accepted that chronic increases in plasma aldosterone increase basolateral membrane surface density of principal cells in rat collecting duct in contrast to lack of morphological effects in the mitochondrial rich cells. These types of studies as well as others have led to the conclusion that it is the principal cell that is a primary mineralocorticoid target cell for aldosterone. Both indirect and direct microelectrode studies have also demonstrated that chronic mineralocorticoid treatment increases both sodium and potassium conductance on the apical membrane of these cells. These observations have led to a series of sophisticated studies that have examined the mechanism of aldosterone-stimulated increase in sodium conductance across the apical membrane.

During the last decade, physiologists introduced the amphibian epithelial cell line A6 as a model of the principal cell and began to use it to explore further the mechanism of aldosterone action. It was demonstrated that these cells have an amiloride sensitive sodium channel that is functionally restricted to the apical plasma membrane with a resulting increase in apical conductance in response to aldosterone. Several questions of interest have been directed to these cells. First, there is the question of whether there is an increase in the numbers of these channels or whether there is an increase in open probability of existing channels. Second, what are the second messengers that cause an increase in apical conductance? With the development of antisodium channel antibodies, it was shown that the total pool of sodium channels was not increased but rather there must exist some posttranslational modification of the 70 kD subunits of the channel that may provide a mechanism by which aldosterone regulates net sodium channel conductance. It has been suggested that the GP70 is a component of the amiloride sensitive conductive sodium channel and that the GP70 is the only polypeptide that is induced by aldosterone. How this GP70 glycoprotein is involved with increased sodium channel activity is conjectural, but it could be dependent on a methylation reaction. It is quite possible that the probability of opening of these channels is regulated in part by methyl donor S-adenosyl-methionine and that its activity is partially regulated by a decarboxylase enzyme in A6 cells that in turn is regulated by aldosterone. Studies also on A6 cells suggest that a modest increase in intracellular calcium in response to aldosterone may be the second messenger that links the activated aldosterone receptor to an incompletely defined protein that ultimately increases apical conductance for sodium. The time delays in intracellular calcium transits in response to aldosterone are consistent with the view that calcium is a second messenger for aldosterone-induced electrogenic sodium absorption.

The time course of action of aldosterone has also been of interest. It is well recognized that there is some delay before the antinatriuretic and kaliuretic effects of aldosterone are seen in vivo. Studies on A6 cells or from cell lines that originate from toad urinary bladder have shown that the early effects of aldosterone can be attributed to both an increase in apical membrane sodium conductance as noted by induction of the glycoprotein 70 complex within 30 minutes that continues to rise until 120 minutes.

The last 2 years have seen aldosterone research enter a new era where the tools of molecular biology are used. This was well demonstrated in 1988 in a state-of-the-art lecture that was given by Bernard Rossier entitled "The Effect of Aldosterone on Renal Tubule Cells." While this presentation was not summarized, he did review much of the data in this chapter and as well presented cutting edge research results from his own laboratory. Some of his suggestions are incorporated in part in Figure 9.1 where he and his colleagues studied gene transcription in A6 cells in response to aldosterone. These studies demonstrated that there was a relatively fast increase within 15 minutes in the rate of transcription of the α and β subunits of NaK ATPase. These observations of NaK ATPase, when interpreted with previous studies that have demonstrated a delayed Na-dependent increase in NaK ATPase activity, suggest that there exists further Na-dependent posttranslational processing of these subunits into active pumps.

In a 1990 meeting, it was reported that the human mineralocorticoid receptor could be synthesized in vitro in rabbit reticulocyte lysate using human mineralocorticoid receptor mRNA. Competitive binding analysis indicated high mineralocorticoid specificity of the product. It was of interest that 60% of the human mineralocorticoid receptor synthesized in vitro assembles into an unactivated oligomeric steroid binding form, while 40% of the receptor synthesized does not bind aldosterone, suggesting that additional processing is required for binding. Further, in 1990 it was reported that the rat mineralocorticoid receptor was characterized to have 981 amino acids, and that the deletion mutants were being used to examine various domains with respect to function. It is this type of research that will usher a new era into our understanding of the mechanism of aldosterone action.

Conclusion

Figure 9.1 is a schematic representation of our current understanding of the mechanism of action of aldosterone at the cellular level. Step 1 involves the diffusion of aldosterone into the cytoplasm. Here it specifically binds to a cytoplasmic receptor (step 2) that has been synthesized directly by an identified messenger RNA or by an indirect route that requires additional unidentified processing at present. The aldosterone binds to form an active receptor aldosterone complex. There then exists intranuclear translocation of the aldosterone receptor complex to a promoter area of nuclear genes (step 3) that results in increased α_1 (step 4) and β_1 (step 5) subunit transcription in addition to transmission of information to increase sodium channel activity (step 6). This transcription of information may in part be mediated by a second messenger that involves intracellular calcium. There then appears to be induction of polymorphic glycoprotein complex GP67,70 that is a component of sodium channel derived from either preexisting proto channels or insertion of preexisting conducting sodium channels. Nevertheless, whatever the mechanism, there is an increase in passive intracellular entry of sodium (step 7). The increase in intracellular sodium and the response to aldosterone increases sodium-dependent posttranslational processing of these subunits into active pumps (step 8) and increases sodium-dependent activation of NaK ATPase (step 9), which results in increased efflux of sodium from the cell.

In summary, the general features of the mechanism of action of aldosterone were formulated as early as the first meeting of the American Society of Nephrology in 1967; however, numerous exciting advances have been made during the past 25 years. The annual meetings of the American Society of Nephrology have participated in transmission of this new information in a major way. It is now agreed on that aldosterone is the main hormone that regulates net sodium balance. While aldosterone has many target sites, the principal target for aldosterone with respect to sodium homeostasis is the kidney. Here, aldosterone regulates sodium, potassium, and hydrogen balance. The sodium and potassium balances are mainly regulated through aldosterone's effect, depicted in Figure 9.1, across the principal cells of the cortical collecting tubule. The effects of aldosterone on hydrogen balance are primarily mediated across the cells in the medullary collecting duct system. It is to be expected that the theoretical model depicted in Figure 9.1 will undergo revisions and modifications in the future with the development of new technical approaches to physiological studies and with the use of ever-expanding molecular biological techniques.

10

Transplantation

Charles B. Carpenter, Ronald D. Guttmann, and Lawrence G. Hunsicker

Where We Were in 1967

The first scientific meeting of the American Society of Nephrology was held just 5 years after the introduction of azathioprine, the first truly effective immunosuppressive drug. Because by 1967 several groups of investigators had acquired some experience with clinical kidney transplantation, the following subjects were presented as papers: lymphocyte depletion by way of thoracic duct drainage or irradiation as pretransplant therapy, methods of kidney preservation, application of immunofluorescence to the study of graft biopsies, and physiology of the transplanted kidney. Also presented was a report of 34 consecutive cases of cadaveric transplantation. In addition, a symposium on the science and philosophy of kidney transplantation was conducted, with participation by John Merrill, David Hume, Thomas Starzl, and Paul Terasaki. At that time transplantation was not considered a proper branch of immunology by many; nor was it yet certain that transplantation would turn into a major branch of the emerging discipline of nephrology. The nature of the rejection response was obscure and initially regarded by some as a perversion of the normal immune response or even as a surgical artifact unrelated to normal biology. Since understanding of the immune system was itself quite primitive by today's standards, these earlier controversies now mean very little. The formation of national and international scientific societies in the fields of clinical transplantation, transplantation biology, and immunogenetics did much to promote investigation and provided important stimuli and cross-fertilization of transplantation with both immunology and nephrology. At the same time, the ASN annual meetings provided an important forum for symposia and for plenary speakers to present timely updates on scientific and clinical progress. In addition, over the years, papers from member and associated laboratories also reflected many of the major new developments in transplantation research. We have assembled this review in a topical fashion, emphasizing the development of new knowledge rather than the contributions of particular laboratories.

Role of Histocompatibility

The first international histocompatibility workshop, held in 1964, attempted to compare techniques for identification of leucocyte antigens and to establish the genetics and functional significance of this newly appreciated genetic system. Many thought this genetic system might function as the major transplantation barrier analogous to H-2 in the mouse which turned out to be true; but it was not at all obvious at the beginning. In 1969 the first ASN paper on the subject dealt with strong and weak antigens of the "HL-A sublocus." In the following year a symposium on selection of donors by histocompatibility testing was held, as well as a symposium on the hazards and expense of transplanting incompatible kidneys. Part of the incompatibility problem had already been recognized as the development of antidonor antibodies, detected by a crossmatch test. In 1971, papers were delivered on the development of antibodies before and after transplantation, and animal models of "hyperacute" rejection mediated by such antibodies were described. By 1975 a symposium, "Is tissue typing worthwhile in transplantation?" was already necessary. During the same meeting it was reported that kidney graft recipients could develop antibodies that were directed to B lymphocytes but not to T lymphocytes. It had been known for 2 to 3 years that the human mixed lymphocyte culture phenomenon was not stimulated by the "HL-A antigens" being typed for on lymphocytes. These anti-B cell-specific antibodies were soon found to identify the class II HLA antigens responsible for MLC proliferation, and the new antigen system was subsequently found to be a very strong barrier to acceptance of transplants.

In 1977, reports of living related donor transplants and cadaveric donor transplants were presented. HLA identical sib donations yielded an 85% graft survival rate 4 years after transplantation; cadaveric grafts matched for HLA class I antigens yielded a 4-year graft survival rate of 80% if 2 or more of a possible 4 antigens were matched and 56% if less than 2 antigens were matched. In haplotype mismatched, living related transplants, outcome was negatively influenced by sensitization as evidenced by panel reactive antibodies and by a highly reactive mixed lymphocyte culture. In the following year, additional data on the effects of histocompatibility in living related donation reported that 1-year graft survival rates were 95% for HLA identicals, 91% for 1 haplotype matched with low mixed lymphocyte culture reactivity, and 47% for 1 haplotype matched with high mixed lymphocyte culture reactivity. When retrospective haplotyping of cadaveric donors was possible from family

HLA typings, transplant results were comparable to those with haplotype matched living related donors.

With evidence that tissue typing was relevant even before the definition of HLA-DR class II antigens, attempts were made to begin organ-sharing systems, and this development was marked in 1979 by a symposium on this subject. A rapid readout mixed lymphocyte response (MLR) was proposed, based on evidence that early activation events in the mixed lymphocyte culture could be detected within 18 to 20 hours of tissue culture. The first such report in 1979 involved the insulin receptor. Evidence was also presented that deliberate transfusion of high-risk (high mixed lymphocyte culture) 1 haplotype matched cases with donor blood, a procedure known as donor specific transfusion (DST), improved survival of subsequent transplants if anti-HLA antibodies did not result from the transfusions. In 1980 the results of a local area organ-sharing program using HLA matching reported improved graft survival rates.

Two new developments marked the decade of the 1980s: the emergence of cyclosporine and the ability to define the HLA-DR class II system serologically. Both have had a demonstrable impact on graft survival, and because of this they became competitors in the eyes of many clinicians. Before reviewing the chronology of developments in HLA, it is important to point out that serial studies throughout the 1970s and into the 1980s had already demonstrated a steady progressive improvement in patient and cadaveric graft survival without significant application of HLA matching or use of cyclosporine. This changing baseline made it difficult to assess the true significance of any new element, especially as the 1-year cadaveric graft survival rate approached 85% overall.

With definition of the class II DR system the relative contributions of class I and II antigens as targets for rejection became an important theme. In 1981 it was reported that HLA-DR was a target for cytotoxic T cells. In addition, evidence was presented that a non-HLA antigen system expressed on monocytes and endothelium could elicit an antibody response of importance in graft injury. With the growing backlog of HLA-sensitized patients awaiting transplantation and the demonstration that many patients fluctuated from month to month in their antibody reactivity to particular HLA antigens, a study addressing the question of whether one could ignore positive crossmatches from previous months concluded that only the sera from the past 6 months was needed for the final crossmatch. In 1982 the increased sensitivity of the flow cytometric crossmatch was first evaluated. In subsequent trials this technique appeared to be most useful when dealing with repeat transplants, although others using augmented cytotoxicity assays, such as with antiglobulin reagents, have claimed similar sensitivity. In 1983 another single center study demonstrated the value of organ sharing based on HLA-DR matching, and another rapid mixed lymphocyte culture assay based on de novo expression of interleukin-2 (IL-2) receptors seemed promising. However, application of class II typing by serology subsequently supplanted the need for the more cumbersome culture technique. Plenary sessions during this period dealt with blood transfusions, HLA matching, cyclosporine, and therapeutic monoclonal antibodies. In 1984 a paper describing the additive beneficial effects of blood transfusion and HLA-DR matching in cadaveric transplantation was presented. By 1984 the debate between cyclosporine and HLA typing was in full swing and included such "sound bites" as "an ounce of histocompatibility is worth a pound of cyclosporine." In fact, representatives from both sides of the debate made valid points, the problem being that not everyone awaiting transplantation had a reasonable expectation of obtaining a well-matched graft.

By 1985 the relative scarcity of donors had raised the question of whether or not to use living nonrelated volunteers, featuring a debate on the subject. In 1986, the HLA-versus-cyclosporine debate was taken up again; by 1988 it was becoming apparent that the long-term rate of graft loss was lower in well-matched cadaveric cases, with half-lives of 12 years compared with 7 to 8 years for poorly matched cases. In fact, cyclosporine, though improving the survival rate at 1 year, was yielding the same half-life of graft loss after 1 year as azathioprine had yielded. At a plenary session in 1989 participants were updated on the rapid strides being made in defining the structure and function of HLA molecules as peptide-binding antigen-presenting molecules. A plenary session in 1990 included a report on HLA matching.

Therapeutics

The ASN began its relationship with renal transplantation very much in medias res. By 1967, both related and cadaveric renal transplantations were being performed with reasonable success at several institutions. In the United States as transplantation spread out from the Peter Bent Brigham Hospital, it was becoming largely a surgical undertaking, and surgeons to a large extent determined immunosuppressive management (Fig. 10.1). Perhaps for this reason there were few free communications at the ASN about immunosuppressive therapy. The invited presentations and symposia on transplantation were mostly delivered by surgeons—in 1967, Hume and Starzl with Merrill and Terasaki; in 1968, Hume; in 1969, Starzl; and in 1970, Paul Russell and Olga Jonasson with immunologists Felix Milgrom and Henry Winn.

Azathioprine and Steroids. During the first 4 years of the ASN we counted only 3 abstracts discussing immunosuppression or immunosuppressive agents. In fact, azathioprine and prednisone had been established as the cornerstones of immunosuppressive therapy about a decade previously with Joseph Murray's classic studies in dogs. Although earlier in the 1960s several immunosuppressive agents had been tried as alternatives to azathioprine and although an occasional patient was still treated with thioguanine or cyclophosphamide because of hepatotoxicity, by 1967 no immunosuppressive

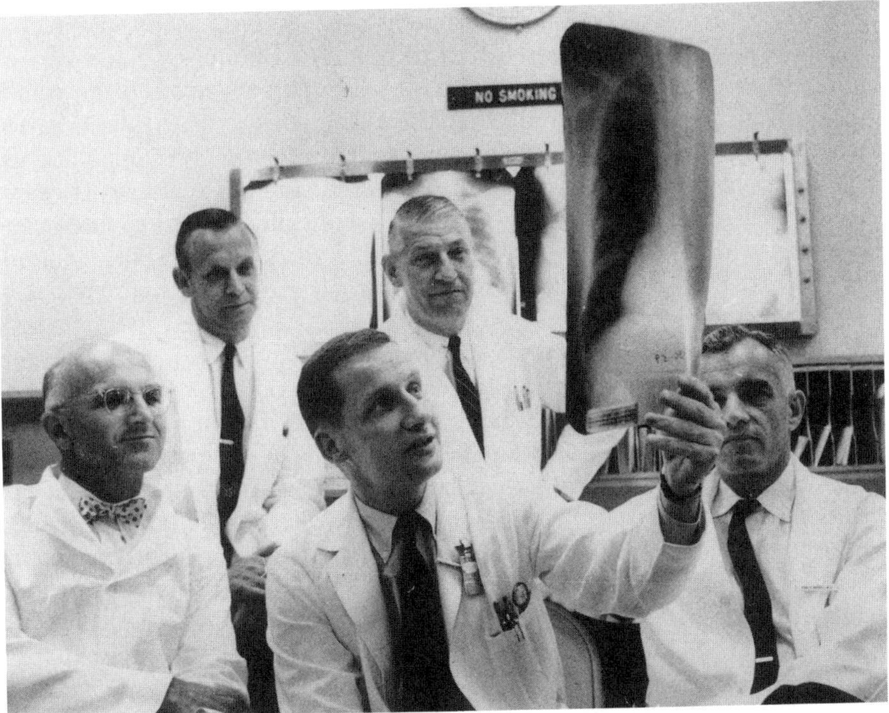

Figure 10.1. Members of the transplant team involved with the first identical-twin renal transplants at the Peter Bent Brigham Hospital in 1954. From left to right: Joseph Murray, plastic surgeon and innovator of the surgical procedure (1990 Nobel Laureate); J. Hartwell Harrison, urologist; James Dealey, radiologist and radiotherapist; Gustave Dammin, pathologist; and John Merrill, nephrologist and innovator of both dialysis and transplantation.

agents were in serious competition with azathioprine. In our review of the history of transplantation as it was reflected in the presentations at the ASN annual meetings, it was quite striking that no papers or symposiums have focused principally on azathioprine. Azathioprine was a surgeon's drug. Its dosing was straightforward and largely unchanged by changes in renal function. Although it produced some significant side effects—principally, leukopenia and, occasionally, hepatotoxicity—these seemed managed easily enough by dose reduction. It had no toxicity for the kidneys. Its mode of action was well-known; it was one of the first "designer" drugs, designed to slow the proliferation of rapidly dividing cells. Though its mode of action was known, the target cells for this action were unknown; as a result there was no sensible way to monitor the dose. Because patients were still rejecting their kidneys while on azathioprine therapy, our treatment was simply to administer as much of the drug as patients could tolerate, checking periodically that we hadn't lowered patients' white-cell blood count too much.

On the other hand, ASN members have had a good bit to say about the use of glucocorticoids in renal transplantation. The first mention, in 1974, was a report on the successful use of methylprednisolone, administered as a large intravenous bolus, to reverse acute rejection. But mostly, and this is significant, the ASN reports focused on the side effects of steroid therapy and ways to minimize them. After all, steroids were internists' (and pediatricians') drugs; we had acquired experience with steroids through treating patients suffering from lupus and nephrotic syndrome. In 1975 2 papers were presented suggesting that steroids could be successfully tapered to alternate-day dosing with no adverse effect on renal allograft survival. It was reported that only 20% of patients converted to alternate-day steroids suffered any deterioration of their renal function. Most of the 20% with "escape" regained stable therapy when daily steroids were reinitiated. In 1978 it was reported that transplanted patients placed on alternate-day steroids experienced reversal of their hyperlipidemia. Another paper reported that T-lymphocyte numbers and function were more nearly normal in the patients on alternate-day steroids, while delayed hypersensitivity was equally suppressed. In 1981, it was again reported that 75% to 85% of transplant recipients could be successfully converted to alternate-day therapy, that the graft survival of patients converted was equal to those on daily steroids, and that the patient survival of those converted to alternate-day steroids was superior. A controlled trial confirmed the benefits of alternate-day steroids in lowering lipid levels. A third paper reported that lower doses of pulse methylprednisolone (250 mg daily for 4 days) was as effective in reversing rejection as the traditional course of 4 1-gram boluses, with equal 1-year graft survival. Virtually each year since 1981 one or more papers have reported the advantages of alternate-day steroid therapy for renal transplant recipients. We have found only one ASN report suggesting a significant risk of conversion to alternate-day steroids; in 1987 it was reported that children with cadaveric grafts, treated only with azathioprine and prednisone, suffered a 50% failure rate requiring reinstitution of daily steroids. Based on reading only the ASN abstracts over these years, a reasonable person would conclude that alternate-day steroid dosing had become standard in transplantation. This is, of course, not the case. Most transplant centers still administer steroids on a daily basis to most of their patients. One must assume that the papers supporting daily steroid dosing were presented at other meetings.

If steroids can be reduced to alternate-day dosing in many patients, are there some patients in whom steroids can be completely discontinued? This was first suggested at the ASN in 1982, during the azathioprine-prednisone era. In a report, of 83 kidney recipients—51 receiving cadaver kidneys and 32 receiving kidneys from living donors—all reporting stable and normal renal function more than 1 year following transplant, all but 7 were initially successfully tapered off steroids and only 5 had to be readministered steroids within a few weeks. The thirty patients successfully withdrawn permanently from steroids lost excess weight, required less antihypertensive therapy, and developed lower plasma lipids. Few others were willing to risk steroid withdrawal in the precyclosporine era; more recently, however, a greater number of centers have tried steroid withdrawal in patients receiving cyclosporine, often together with azathioprine. In 1989 one of these centers reported some preliminary success in total steroid withdrawal.

In addition to therapeutic aspects of immunosuppressive medicines, ASN members have been concerned with the mechanisms of actions. Because glucocorticoid use has been part of transplantation longer than any other immunosuppressive agent, it is perhaps fitting that glucocorticoids were among the first whose mechanism was understood at a genetic level. In 1985 a solution to the longstanding riddle of antiinflammatory glucocorticoid action was presented. The data showed that dexamethasone, presumably bound to its cytosolic receptor, completely inhibited the transcription of IL-1 messenger RNA in human monocytes.

Blood Transfusions. The effects of blood transfusions have been a major concern over the years. No area of transplantation has been more controversial. Many of the important trends and issues in this area have been reflected during ASN meetings. As already noted in the histocompatibility section, sensitization to histocompatibility antigens is a major hazard after blood transfusions. In the early 1970s, however, it was also noted that untransfused graft recipients as a group experienced the worst graft survival rate. Although this effect might be explained by a process of negative selection in which patients are provoked by transfusions into developing antibodies to HLA antigens to which they are inherently most reactive, and thereby spared from receiving kidneys they will vigorously reject, the beneficial transfusion effect was also found in patients who did not produce anti-HLA antibodies after transfusion. By the time that cyclosporine was being introduced into the clinic in 1979, the beneficial effect of transfusion in cadaveric transplantation was in decline, principally because nontransfused patients were doing better. After the addition of cyclosporine to the armamentarium, the benefit all but disappeared, with the following exceptions: (*1*) if a patient suffered a rejection episode, recovery was more likely if pretransplant transfusions were administered, and (*2*) if the blood donor shared 1 HLA-DR antigen with the recipient, the recipient was less likely to lose the graft from rejection, as well as less likely to manufacture anti-HLA antibodies, in comparison with recipients of mismatched blood. At the ASN in 1981 1 study reported that sharing of HLA-A,B antigens between the blood donor and the graft donor was beneficial; recent Dutch data, not presented at ASN, indicate benefit only if the blood donor and recipient share one HLA-DR or one HLA-DR plus one HLA-B antigen.

The degree of HLA matching for unrelated blood donors described above, occurs in most cases of living related donor transplants who are pretreated with donor-specific transfusion (DST), since most such cases are selected as having a 1 HLA haplotype match. As mentioned in the histocompatibility section, evidence revealed that HLA haplotype mismatched family donor grafts from donor-recipient combinations that were highly reactive in mixed lymphocyte cultures were at higher risk for rejection unless the recipient underwent such a DST. Even when early accelerated type rejections occurred in such patients, they were readily responsive to treatment. Criticisms of these protocols were directed at the lack of randomized controls, and it was pointed out that random blood donors were also beneficial. Before these matters could be sorted out, cyclosporine entered the scene; the hype and excitement of acquiring a new drug after 20 years convinced many that all rejection problems were overcome and that questions about the role of transfusions and HLA matching were no longer relevant. Since these early hopes for cyclosporine were only partially realized, the true immunological meaning of the blood transfusion effect has been recently reconsidered; this area is the subject of renewed research in pursuit of the elusive goal of true tolerance.

Antilymphocyte globulins. Destruction of lymphocytes or inhibition of their function by antibodies was an early experimental tool in animal experiments. During the mid-to-late 1960s, horses and rabbits were immunized with human cells (thymus, thoracic duct cells, or B lymphoblastoid cell lines), the sera absorbed with human serum proteins and red cells, and gamma globulin fractions prepared. These were first administered intramuscularly, and later intravenously, in efforts to prevent or reverse rejection episodes. Over a period of several years, effectiveness was revealed, but with considerable uncertainty of how to standardize and predict the immunosuppressive potency of a given product or lot thereof. The treatment was not without side effects, including thrombocytopenia, fevers, and aches and pains suggestive of serum sickness. In 1968 the first ASN abstract on this topic was a report of adverse reactions. In 1970 it was reported that these products needed testing for the presence of cross-reacting anti-basement membrane antibodies that could induce an anti-GBM (glomerular basement membrane) disease. By the 1980s controlled trials were being reported, and some of these reports appeared at the ASN. In 1980 a horse anti-human ATG (antithymocyte globulin) administered prophylactically was revealed to delay onset of rejection but not reduce overall morbidity and mortality. In 1982 another study revealed that the addition of ATG to steroid pulse therapy for rejection did improve both the graft survival rate and creatinine clearances in the ATG group. In 1986 a follow-up of a similar group of patients, in which rejection reversal was improved with addition of ATG, disclosed that the benefits were maintained over a 4-year period. Another trial reported in 1986 compared the same horse ATG with a rabbit antithymocyte serum (ATS) and found similar beneficial and adverse effects.

Monoclonal antibodies. The development of the procedure for making monoclonal antibodies was one of the landmark scientific contributions to immunology. The immediate prospect of producing well-characterized and standardized antibodies in unlimited quantities and of having these precisely targeted to a selected cell surface molecule was first exploited in 1980 in Boston where a pan T-cell antibody, first termed *anti-T3*, from the Dana Farber Cancer Institute, was administered to renal transplant recipients at Massachusetts General Hospital. At the time there was no definition of the

T cell receptor complex. The antibody, later known as OKT3, was selected simply because it reacted with all T cells. The famous "first dose reaction," a continuing problem with the use of this antibody, was later found to be a direct consequence of initial T-cell activation because the target molecule is a component of the T-cell receptor activating system. In 1982, a study on the immunological effects of OKT3 in vivo disclosed that the treatment reduced responsiveness to lectin stimulation of lymphocytes, an effect that was reversible when therapy was stopped. As multicenter trials progressed, annual updates on the results revealed substantial benefit in reversal of acute rejections. In 1988 the prophylactic use of OKT3 in patients with delayed graft function was reported to be beneficial in terms of length of dialysis and in graft survival. In the following year, evidence was presented that the "first dose reaction" was caused by cytokine release and principally attributable to tumor necrosis factor (TNF). In 1990 3 papers were presented on the prophylactic use of OKT3, 2 of them randomizing with ALG. The studies all indicated benefits in terms of delay in time of first rejection and better initial graft function, particularly when cyclosporine was not given during the first few days. However, in subsequent follow-up studies of such sequential therapy protocols using antibodies, there is no clear evidence that initial prevention of rejection by this means improves long-term graft success rate. Several other monoclonal antibodies have been used in clinical trials and are under active development. Many of these antibodies have been demonstrations in animal models, and those used in humans so far have not been as effective as OKT3. New generations of "designer" monoclonal molecules, based on gene constructs and fusion proteins, were reviewed in a 1990 symposium. These promise to be more selective to the effector pathways in the rejection process and more effective in preventing specific lymphocyte functions for longer periods of time.

Cyclosporine. The introduction of this immunosuppressive drug was marked in 1980 by a presentation at the ASN of the first 9 patients treated at the Brigham Hospital in Boston. The presentation demonstrated both the immunosuppressive and nephrotoxic potential of the drug and presaged a decade of reports on its benefits and difficulties. This was not a "designer" drug. It was serendipitously salvaged from a collection of many fungal products being screened for new antifungal antibiotics. The subsequent partial elucidation of cyclosporine's effects on cell biology has opened new areas in immunosuppression, in addition to stimulating much study by nephrologists on its renal toxicity. Papers or symposia were presented in subsequent years documenting the potential benefits of the drug. In 1983, the development of renal failure in cardiac transplant recipients was reported, clearly demonstrating the direct clinical nephrotoxic effect on normal kidneys when high doses were used. In 1984 its use as a rescue drug for acute rejections was reported, and, at the same meeting, the production of intraglomerular microthrombi, in the absence of hemolytic uremic syndrome, was established to be a distinct complication of cyclosporine. The complication of hyperkalemia was attributed to the drug's inhibition of the renin-angiotensin system in a 1983 paper. In 1984 acute administration of the drug in rats was revealed as producing renal vasoconstriction and reduced renal blood flow; at the next meeting 3 papers were delivered on the same subject: one paper indicated that renal vasoconstriction in rats could be blocked with an ACE inhibitor; the others reported on 2 studies in patients indicating that the drug decreased blood flow and glomerular filtration rate (GFR). In 1985 and 1986 several studies on the conversion of cyclosporine to azathioprine demonstrated improved short-term renal function, although some patients subsequently developed rising creatinines from poorly controlled rejection activity. Other reports noted favorable experience with continued maintenance on low-dose cyclosporine. In subsequent years, many centers have preferred the latter approach, although the financial costs of long-term cyclosporine use still provide a formidable burden for some patients.

At present we are entering another period of clinical trials with new drugs. A 1990 symposium reviewed the structural and mechanistic relationships of cyclosporine, FK-506, and rapamycin. FK-506 is very similar in action and in nephrotoxicity to cyclosporine, and its relative clinical value is yet to be established. Rapamycin has the effect of blocking response to cytokines such as IL-2 rather than inhibiting cytokine production, the main action of the other 2 agents. Other drugs that are azathioprine-like also show some promise. The question of whether any of these will substantially improve the odds of inducing stable states of tolerance will be a central theme for the future. At present, the ability of the drugs to sustain survival without the continuous use of suppressive drugs is lacking, with exception of a small number of cases reported anecdotally.

Mechanisms of Rejection and Graft Prolongation

The significant progress made in understanding the pathogenesis of rejection by using a variety of experimental models of renal transplantation was presented as early as 1968 to the ASN at annual meetings. In that year, studies on hemodynamic changes in renal allograft rejection were presented, in addition to a study of weak histocompatibility differences leading to a chronic glomerulopathy in the inbred rat model of renal transplantation. In 1969 work on the pathogenesis of rejection using the rat model of renal transplantation revealed that an antitubular cytotoxic response was generated by effector lymphocytes. Another report disclosed a possible role for platelets in the vascular injury of rejection. In 1970 the inbred rat renal transplant model and bone-marrow chimeras were used to demonstrate that "passenger leukocytes" functioned as specific targets of enhancement as well as rejection.

In 1971, 3 papers focused on sensitization and rejection. Two focused on studies of patients, relating transfusions as a source of alloimmunization, and 1 on the allograft rejection response with production of antibody. In 1973, more data were presented about donor pretreatment as a mechanism to reduce allograft immunogenicity by reducing "passenger leukocytes." In 1975, the capillary necrotic lesions of machine perfusion injury during renal preservation were reported. These lesions were associated with poor allograft function but no etiologic factor could be determined. Researchers believed these were non-HLA related. Another study described the lesions of chronic rejection and speculated about their association with the phenomenon of antibody dependant cellular toxicity.

In 1977 a clinical study on measures of rejection activity revealed that antibody-dependent cellular cytotoxicity (ADCC) or complement dependent cytotoxicity (CDC) antibody assays were associated with rejection episodes while lymphocyte mediated cytotoxicity (LMC) was not. The failure of steroids to convert ADCC reactivity to negative was associated with graft loss.

In 1978, a study of suppressor cells and their relationship to long-term survival in rat renal allografts was reported. During the next decade the detailed dissection of alloimmunity was illustrated by the 1987 presentation demonstrating how peptides of as few as 8 amino acids can induce or suppress immune recognition and as little as a 1 amino acid change in the HLA-A2 sequence can alter immune recognition. The structure-function relationships could be detailed now that the crystal structure of A2 was known.

Other important papers on rejection mechanisms discussing specific issues such as lymphokines began to appear in 1981 when the significance of IL-2 as a mediator in rat allograft rejection was demonstrated. This was followed in 1982 by further study on lymphocyte activation, proliferation, and the relationship to IL-2 production using an in vitro system. After recognizing the significance of IL-2 and IL-2 receptor interactions in immune responses in 1984, researchers reported that prolonged graft survival in the mouse was produced by administering an anti-IL-2 receptor monoclonal antibody; in 1989 a report was presented on the use of anti-IL-2-diphtheria-toxin conjugate in vivo to suppress delayed-type hypersensitivity (DTH) in mice.

In the area of the nature, phenotype, and function of graft infiltrating cells, a 1978 report disclosed that gamma globulin secreting cells were concentrated in lesions of rejecting renal allografts and that this finding was associated with humoral rejection. With the availability of highly specific monoclonal antibodies that can be used histochemically, it was shown in 1981 that monoclonal antibodies could elucidate the phenotypes of cell infiltrates. An increased ratio of T8/T4 lymphocytes in interstitial infiltrates by using similar techniques was also reported. Subsequent work by other laboratories found the reverse ratio in a different set of biopsies, and the field went through a period of fine tuning discrepancies based on technique. In 1983 2 papers reported on modulation of class II antigens on renal tubular cells stimulated by lymphocytes. These papers represent the new era of molecular dissection of interactive rejection events.

Long-Term Outcomes

Beginning at the 1974 ASN meeting, a series of significant papers were delivered about long-term outcomes of renal transplantation. The field was only 10 years old and already a focus on many important medical complications was being established. In 1974 a report on hyperlipidemia posttransplant in children appeared; in 1976 hypertension became a focus for study, with the appreciation that successful renal transplantation could relieve the hypertension of chronic renal failure and that a causal relation existed between renal artery stenosis and increased renin secretion posttransplant. Case studies described that in more than 10% of recipients nephrotic syndrome posttransplant developed in association with the lesions of chronic rejection. Additionally, a report on serum factors associated with accelerated vascular disease posttransplantation appeared. A symposium in 1976 focused on these and other long-term complications and outcomes of both renal transplantation and chronic renal failure.

In 1977, studying the pathophysiology of increased serum lipids posttransplantation was again emphasized. Studies of outcomes of second renal transplants were featured on the program as well.

In 1978 information about the long-term outcome and survival of large numbers of patients from Massachusetts, Michigan, and Minnesota was reported. Improvement in the management of immunosuppressive drugs leading to decreased mortality was emphasized. Dialysis and transplantation were identified as complementary rather than competing treatment modalities. Further studies detailed the role of infection and malignancy in long-term morbidity.

In 1979 a study reported on the relationship of chronic chemical immunosuppression to delayed-type cutaneous anergy and the subsequent association with risk for hepatitis, sepsis, and the development of cancer in a significant number of these patients.

In 1982, a paper on rehabilitation of long-term patients postrenal transplant found that while patients experienced significant incidence of complications, most considered their rehabilitation and quality of life improved or the same following renal transplantation.

From Montreal and Boston from 1982 to 1984, further observations of long-term results in renal transplantation were presented with respect to patients who were hepatitis B carriers. The presentations documented the progression of histological changes in the liver in carriers of hepatitis B virus and noted the high mortality rate in these patients from sepsis. That patients of non-B hepatitis experienced relatively better outcomes was reported as well.

Pediatric Transplantation

Renal insufficiency presents special problems in children: in addition to all the difficulties faced by adult patients, children suffer from arrested growth, development, and maturation. Although it was clear from the beginning that dialysis would not correct these problems, it seemed possible that renal transplantation might. The history of pediatric transplantation over the past 25 years reflects more than anything the concern of the pediatric community about these issues of growth and development. In 1969 and 1971 papers presented at the ASN annual meetings revealed that children and young adults who underwent transplantations could grow, mature sexually, and become parents. But by the end of the 1970s the picture seemed less optimistic. In 1977 it was reported that while most children less than 12-years-old began growing again following transplantation, only 13% experienced normal growth. Short stature was the rule and led to low self-esteem, poor social adaptation, and serious problems with noncompliance with the immunosuppressive regimen. Transplantation affected not only physical stature. In 1984 the Minnesota group reported that the adverse effects of uremia on psychomotor development of infants was largely reversed by early transplantation, establishing the importance that infants undergo transplantation at as young an age as possible.

In the late 1970s and early 1980s, factors predicting good growth in the pediatric renal transplant recipient were identified: age less than 7 years, well-preserved renal function, and use of alternate-day rather than daily steroids. With the introduction of cyclosporine in the early 1980s, one group reported that cyclosporine monotherapy, omitting steroids altogether, was feasible in many children and was associated with normal growth hormone levels. But by and large, little could be done to improve the growth of children with transplants. Two papers presented in 1989 summarized the experience up to that time of long-term growth following renal transplantation. The first documented that, though catch-up growth often occurred early after transplantation, subsequent growth failure occurred in the majority of children even if they continued to experience good renal function. In addition, few continued to experience catch-up growth. The second paper, from the North American Pediatric Renal Transplant Cooperative Study (NAPRTCS), confirmed that catch-up growth was found only in younger patients and, then, only during the first year following transplantation. But also in 1989 we saw the first reports of the use of recombinant growth hormone in these children, demonstrating its effectiveness in inducing catch-up growth. Another paper in 1990 reported that many children with transplants experienced abnormal nocturnal endogenous growth hormone release, confirming the effectiveness of exogenous growth hormone in inducing catch-up growth. So, as the ASN approaches its 25th anniversary, perhaps this problem which has occupied ASN's attention since its founding may be nearing a solution.

Public Policy Issues

As early as 1970, important public policy issues were being presented at the ASN annual meetings. The meeting in 1970 reported on the hazards and expenses incurred for transplanting incompatible kidneys. In 1979 a special symposium was held to focus on many issues surrounding organ sharing. In 1986 the unfair distribution of kidneys was noted, emphasizing gender and racial inequities. In 1988 the use of elderly donors as a mechanism for increasing the supply of kidneys was detailed, representing the increase in effort toward fulfilling the expanding demand for renal allografts. In 1989 the effect of decreasing or ending cyclosporine therapy because of financial reasons was reported. The economic effects of renal transplants on health-care financing and insurability were now being considered.

Considerable concern was directed toward the issue of the impact of live donor nephrectomy on long-term donor outcome. In 1982, a hypothesis based on rat research suggested that unilateral nephrectomy in man may be related to long-term complications of proteinuria, hypertension, and focal sclerosis. In 1983 4 papers on the long-term outcome of living donors presented no support for this hypothesis. In 1984, using correct family and sibling controls, more studies presented evidence against this hypothesis. At least for the 10–20 year period of observation after unilateral nephrectomy, there was no general increased risk of development of renal failure or hypertension. In 1985 a symposium debating the use of living donors presented no clear evidence that the practice should be abandoned.

Expanding indications for transplantation were first heralded in 1970 in a report on the transplantation in high-risk recipients. In 1971 there was a report on successful transplantation in patients with diabetic nephropathy. In 1973, levels of preformed reactive alloantibody (PRA) were found to be uncorrelated with outcome, thus expanding the population that could benefit from transplantation.

In 1974 success of transplantation in patients with previous cancers were reported. In 1977 more reports indicated the effectiveness of second transplants, and in 1981 the first study was issued signifying that a current negative crossmatch in the face of a positive historic crossmatch could be correlated with a favorable outcome. In 1982 transplants in reformed heroin addicts were described, and in 1986 2 reports disclosed favorable outcomes in patients 50 years of age and older.

Four papers between 1985 and 1988 focused on the subject of race and outcome in renal transplantation. These papers illustrated some new issues regarding differences in particular medical problems associated with racial minorities, such as incidence of end-stage renal disease, severity of hypertension, and priorities in organ distribution.

Thus, over a 20-year period, studies on biological factors, original disease, previous allograft, age, and race factors have both expanded and restricted prognostic factors for therapy of patients, and at the same time raised many new public issues.

Contributions of Transplantation to Nephrology and Immunology

Several areas of nephrologic research have been directly influenced or even created by the existence of successful renal transplant programs. Earlier in the ASN's history a focus was placed on distinguishing the consequences of renal versus systemic disorders in various forms of renal disease. Physiologists were given the opportunity to study the effects of the uremic milieu on a normal rather than a damaged kidney. The ability to correct the uremic state more completely than possible with dialysis provided subjects for study of metabolic bone disease, especially in relation to parathyroid function. The hemodynamic alterations in the uninephrectomized living donor with increasing flow and GFR provided fundamental knowledge on functional compensation to reduction in renal mass. The role of the kidney in the genesis of hypertension has been studied both in animal models and in the clinic by observing recipients of kidneys from hypertensive versus normotensive donors. Immunologists and clinical nephrologists, similarly, were able to identify which diseases were of local and which of systemic origin. The recurrence of various glomerulonephritides in transplants provided evidence that such diseases were systemic diseases of the host, with secondary effects on the kidney. The report of the recurrence of anti-GBM disease in a transplanted kidney, delivered in 1967 at the first meeting of the ASN, offered the first clear proof of antibody as a causative agent in an autoimmune disease. Equally important was the evidence, reported in 1975, that diabetic lesions developed in the transplanted kidneys of diabetic recipients; this evidence offered strong proof that the lesions resulted from abnormal glucose or insulin metabolism rather than from an independent abnormality of basement membrane structure, as some had hypothesized. Renal transplantation also offered the first opportunity for testing the effectiveness of "gene therapy." The transplantation of individuals with cystinosis was first reported at the ASN in 1969. By 1975 it had been shown that, while renal transplants into children with cystinosis did not cure the systemic enzyme deficiency, the renal tubular cells of the transplants did not develop the cystine deposits characteristic of the native kidneys, nor did Fanconi's syndrome reappear.

In later years the major contribution of renal transplantation to other aspects of nephrology and medicine has occurred in the area of viral infection in the immunosuppressed patient. As early as 1974 cytomegalovirus (CMV) infection was recognized as a problem in recipients of renal transplants, and the incidence of CMV disease and seroconversion was found to be correlated with long-term graft function. Over the years debate has continued to focus on which is the chicken and which the egg in the relationship between CMV infection and allograft rejection. The introduction of antilymphocyte antibodies led to the recognition that their use likely led to symptomatic CMV disease; this, in turn, led to the recognition of the role of T-lymphocytes in protecting against reactivation of the CMV virus. More recent papers have focused on the prevention and treatment of CMV disease with anti-CMV antibody and ganciclovir, paralleling studies in neonates and patients with AIDS. Other ASN papers have discussed the transmission of hepatitis C by transplantation and the course of hepatitis B and C in the immunocompromised host. Since the level of immunosuppression can be adjusted in the transplant recipient, unlike in the patient with AIDS or malignancy, study of the transplant recipient may permit better dissection of the role of immunosuppression in the pathogenesis of many of these opportunistic viral diseases.

With regards to transplantation's impact on immunology, it can be said that the empiric success in renal transplantation provided the major stimulus for the study and definition of the major histocompatibility (MHC) system. As it turned out, the major transplantation antigens did not evolve simply to frustrate attempts at transplantation, but are the central controlling molecules in the initiation and development of any full-blown immune response. These antigens also are likely to make crucial contributions to the autoimmune processes that underlie many of the primary renal diseases resulting in renal failure. Research in the MHC has progressed since the 1960s. In the 1980s some of the complexities of events subsequent to the MHC + antigen interaction were unraveled, and it appears that cytokine growth and differentiation factors are central to molding the nature of inflammatory or healing events. In this regard, work in transplantation immunology parallels work in other areas of immunobiology. One can anticipate that immunobiological topics common to transplantation and other areas of nephrology will be an important part of future ASN meetings.

11

Physiology of Salt and Water Transport

James A. Schafer, John W. Boylan, and Thomas E. Andreoli

Introduction

At the time of the first ASN meeting in 1967, the contemporary understanding of salt and water transport processes in the nephron had just been elegantly summarized in the second edition of Robert Pitts' (Fig. 11.1) classic textbook on renal physiology, *Physiology of the Kidney and Body Fluids* (Yearbook Medical Publishers, Inc., Chicago, IL, 1968). The extensive application of micropuncture and clearance technology during the preceding decade had provided a wealth of new information concerning the localization of the most important solute and water transport processes in the proximal and distal convoluted tubules of the mammalian nephron. Physiologists in 4 major centers were responsible for developing most of this information and for training other renal physiologists who extended it: the laboratories of Erich Windhager, Gerhard Giebisch (Fig. 11.2), and Gerhard Malnic at Cornell University; the Laboratory of Kidney and Electrolyte Metabolism at the NIH under the direction of Robert Berliner (Fig. 11.3); the laboratory of Carl Gottschalk (Fig. 11.4) at the University of North Carolina; and the laboratory of Karl Ullrich at the Free University of Berlin. As reflected in Pitts' book, micropuncture technology had proven its utility in demonstrating the fundamental transport requirements of the countercurrent hypothesis, and the focus of investigation was shifting to characterization of the individual membrane transport mechanisms in the various nephron segments. Electrophysiological techniques, including intracellular microelectrodes, were just emerging as powerful tools for identifying the contributions of the individual cell membranes to transepithelial transport and for determining the kinetic characteristics of the transporters involved.

At this important juncture in the history of renal and epithelial physiology, 5 important concepts, originating largely in the domain of general physiology, had recently evolved to dominate the future course of investigation. These were: the Ussing frog skin model for vectorial sodium transport in

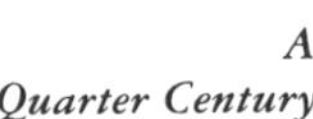

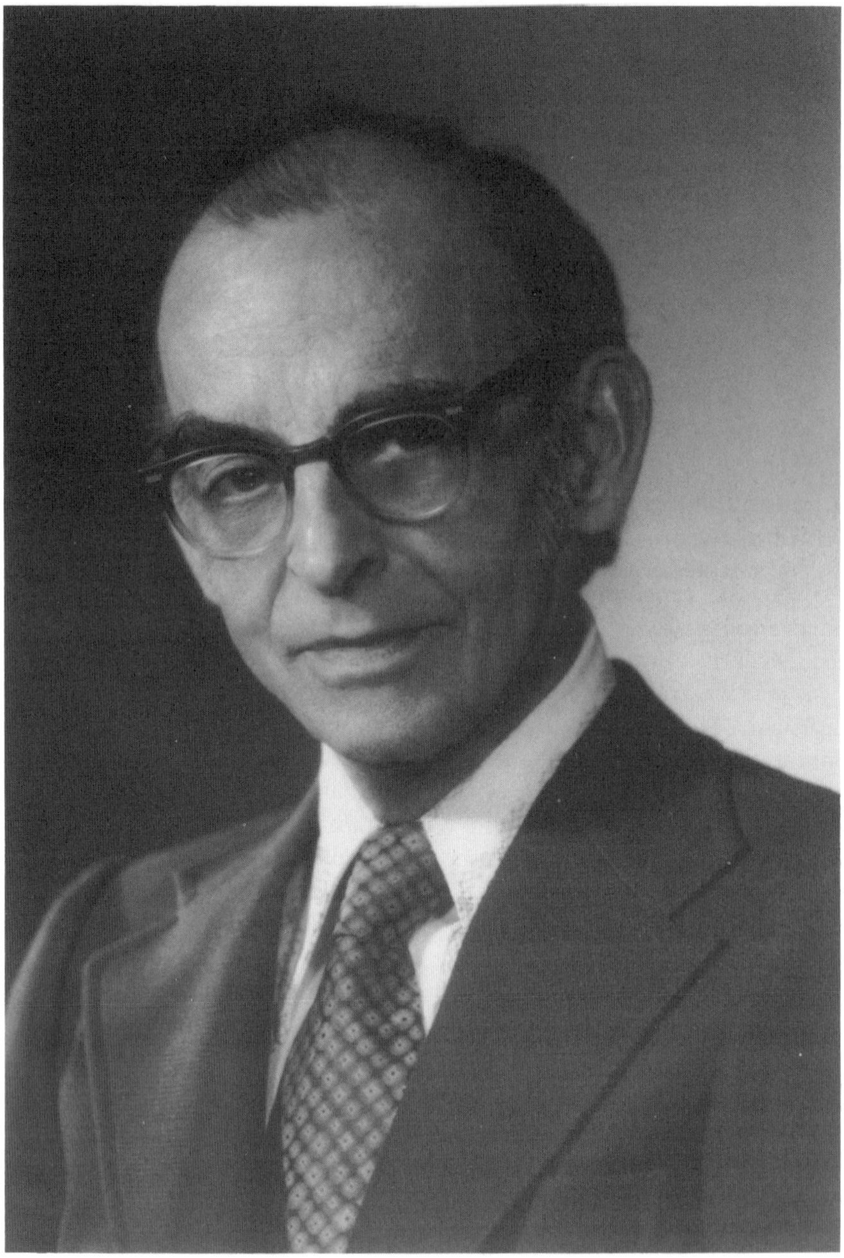

Figure 11.1. Robert F. Pitts (photo courtesy of Erich E. Windhager).

epithelia, the concept of the coupling of solute flows by way of membrane transporters, the development of models by which water flow could be coupled to transepithelial solute transport, an appreciation of the functional significance of the structural complexity of an epithelium, and an understanding of how the functions of discrete nephron segments could be integrated in a system such as countercurrent multiplication.

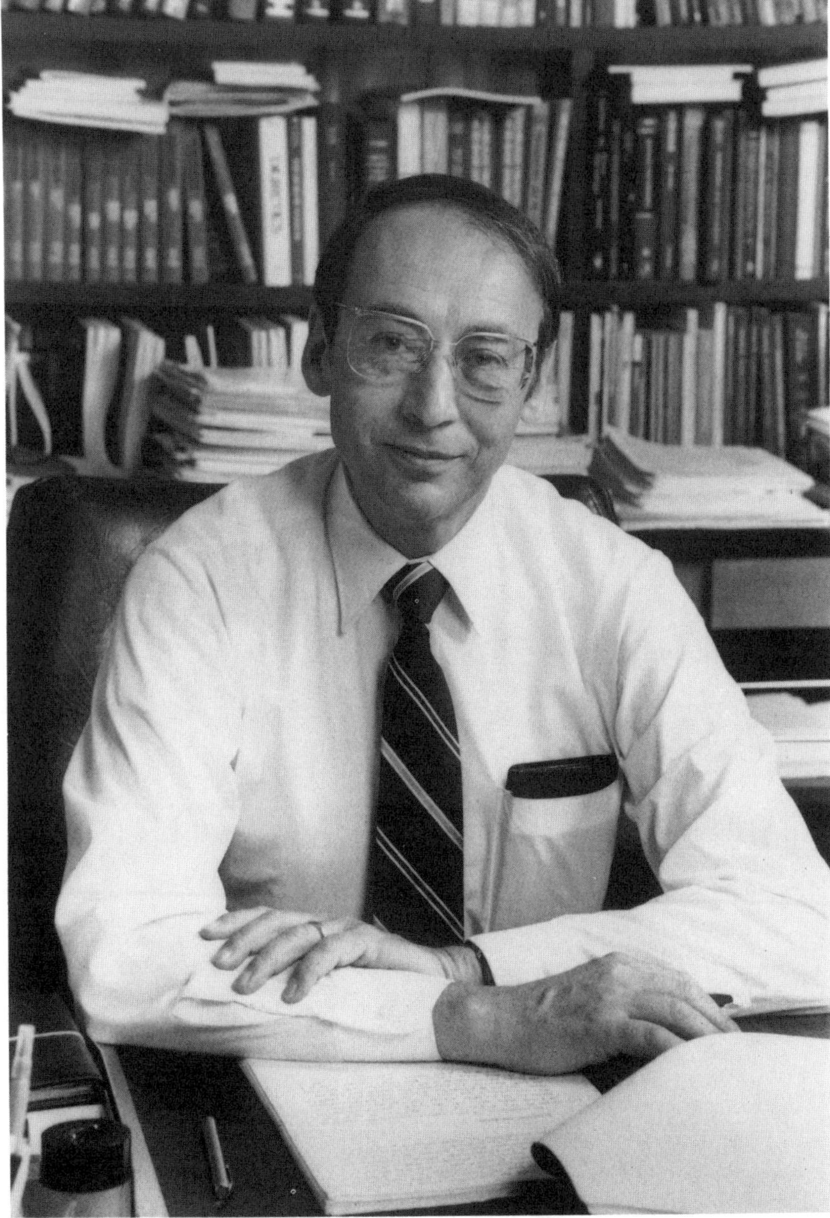

Figure 11.2. Gerhard H. Giebisch (photo by David Ottenstein).

The Ussing Frog Skin Model. Perhaps the single most important contribution to the biology of epithelial transport processes was the model of Na^+ transport in the frog skin advanced by Hans Ussing (Fig. 11.5) in the 1950s. As Figure 11.6 reveals, this model explained the vectorial reabsorption of Na^+ as a consequence of the asymmetrical distribution of transport mechanisms between the apical and basolateral membranes. Na^+ entered the

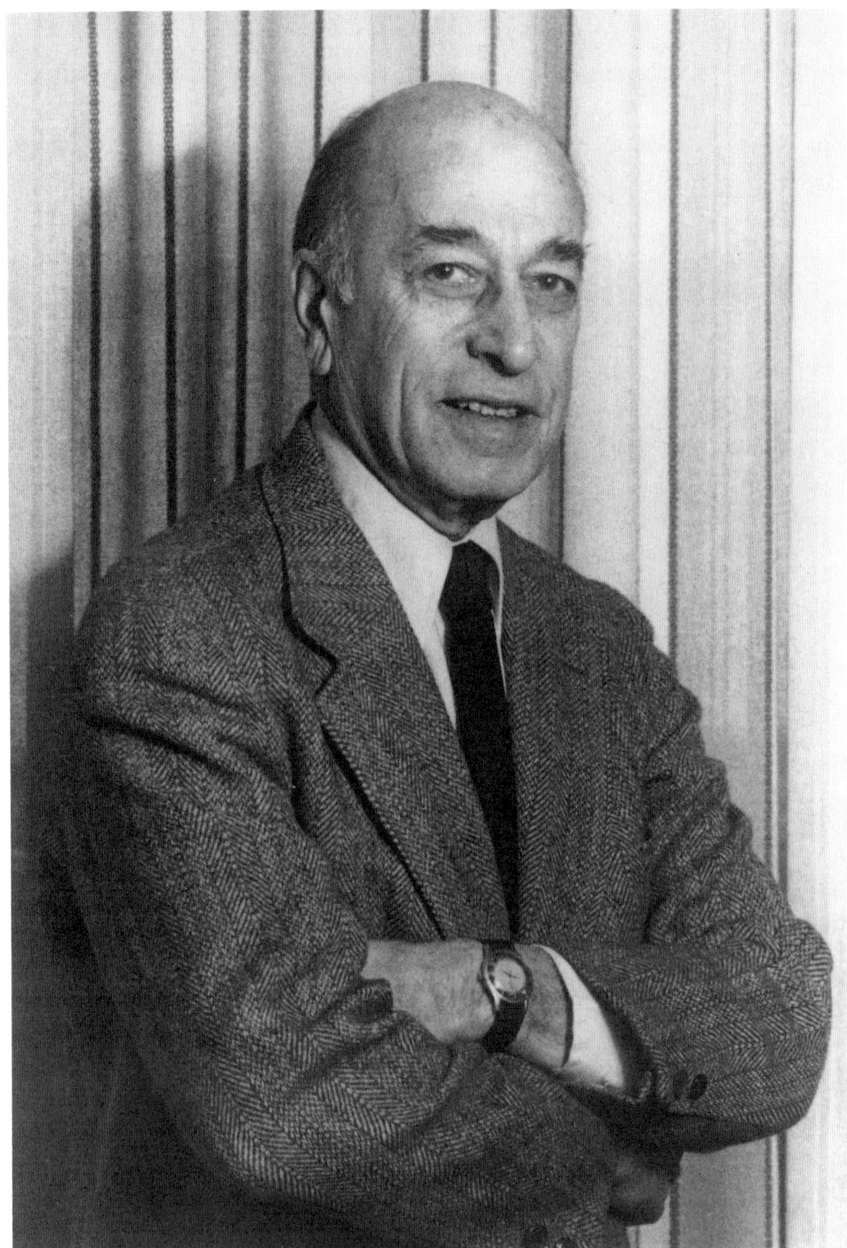

Figure 11.3. Robert W. Berliner (photo by T. Charles Erickson).

cell across the luminal membrane and down its electrochemical potential gradient, by a process left unspecified in the model. Nevertheless, the passive entry of Na^+ across the apical membrane coupled with (adenosine-triphosphate-dependent) extrusion across the basolateral membrane explained the vectorial transepithelial Na^+ transport from apical to basolateral side against

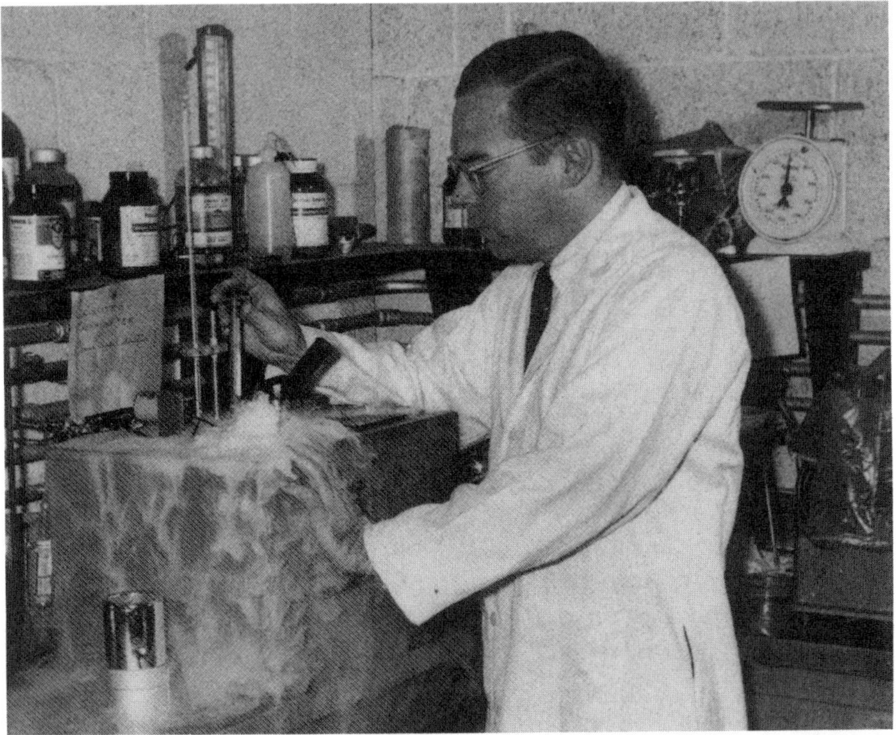

Figure 11.4. Carl W. Gottschalk.

a large electrochemical potential gradient. Thus the (Na^+ + K^+)-ATPase, which had only recently been described by Jens Skou at the University of Aarhus, served as the generator that maintained the extracellular to intracellular ionic concentration gradients.

Coupling of Solute Flows. A second conceptual breakthrough was the recognition that the movement of a solute down its electrochemical potential gradient could be coupled to the movement of a second solute, even against the second solutes electrochemical potential gradient, if the solutes shared a common membrane transporter. In the late 1950s the description of exchange diffusion, which Ussing and Erich Heinz in Germany independently referred to as counterflow or antiport, provided the first experimental demonstration of solute flux-coupling.

But the most intriguing aspect of coupled flows was the demonstration of secondary active transport driven by cotransport of solutes with Na^+. In the early 1960s Robert Crane at Rutgers demonstrated that active glucose absorption in the small intestine was driven by a specialized transporter in the luminal membrane which mediated the simultaneous transport of glucose and Na^+ as Figure 11.7 reveals. This work was followed by similar demonstrations of Na^+ and amino acid cotransport in the small intestine by Stanley Schultz and Peter Curran at Harvard. Using electrophysiological techniques, these investigators also found that Na^+-coupled sugar and amino acid processes

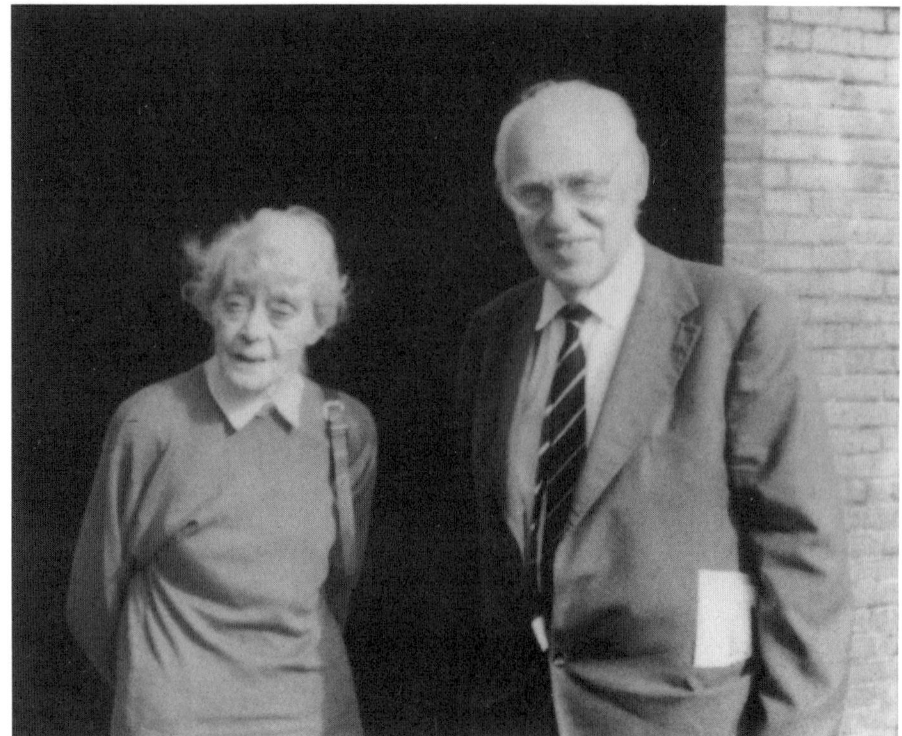

Figure 11.5. Hans H. Ussing and Mrs. Ussing (photo courtesy of Stanley G. Schultz).

were electrogenic, that is, they involved net change transfer across the luminal membrane, as Figure 11.8 indicates. The theoretical foundations for energy transfer in coupled transport systems had also been established through the formalism of irreversible thermodynamics in the early 1960s by Ora Kedem and Aaron Katchalsky in Israel, Eric Heinz in West Germany, and Peter Curran and Clifford Patlak in the United States. The coupling of Na^+ entry to the secondary active transport of glucose or amino acids required only the presence of an as yet unidentified transporter that mediated cotransport of Na^+ and sugar or amino acid, resulting in net charge transfer.

Coupling of Water Flow to Solute Flow. The production of a highly concentrated urine and the absorption of water in the gastrointestinal tract provided examples of movement of water against an apparent transepithelial osmolality difference. In the 1940s and early 1950s it was proposed that the reabsorption of water in such systems might be an active transport process, coupled directly to metabolic energy. However, the thermodynamic analysis of active water transport by William Brodsky and his coworkers in 1954 found that the direct absorption of water would require far more energy than was available from oxidative metabolism. These investigators reasoned that in some manner the reabsorption of water would have to be coupled to the reabsorption of solutes.

There was no ready explanation for such coupling until it was recognized than anisotonic compartments might exist within the epithelial cell layer itself.

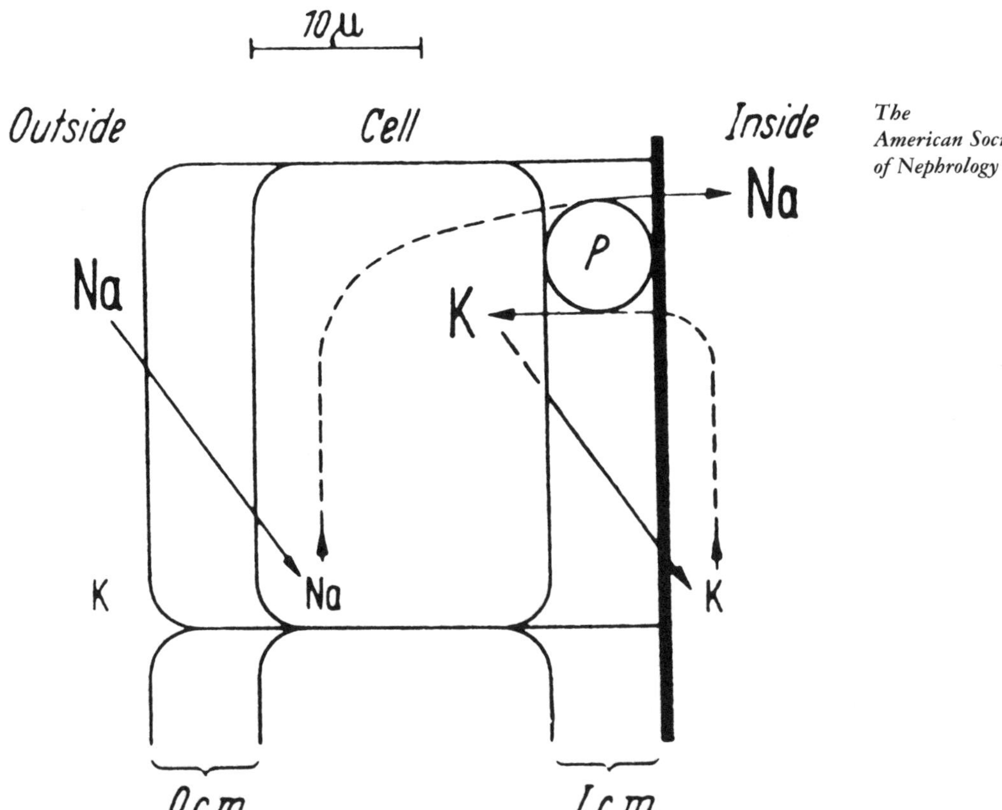

Figure 11.6. The Ussing model for active Na^+ absorption across the frog skin. Na^+ was proposed to enter the epithelial cell by an unspecified mechanism across the outer membrane, and was transported out of the cell across the inner membrane by the (Na^+ + K^+)-ATPase (P). (V. Koefoed-Johnsen and H. H. Ussing. Acta Physiol. Scand. 42:298–308, 1958.)

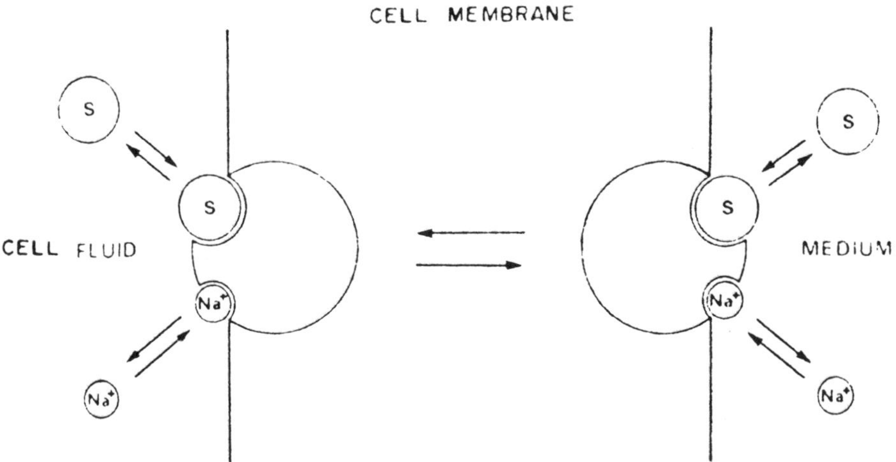

Figure 11.7. The intestinal Na^+-glucose cotransporter. This cotransporter was envisioned to contain sites for both Na^+ and the sugar, thus coupling the downhill movement of Na^+ and the uphill movement of sugar into the cell. (R. K. Crane. Gastroenterology. 24:1000–1006, 1965.)

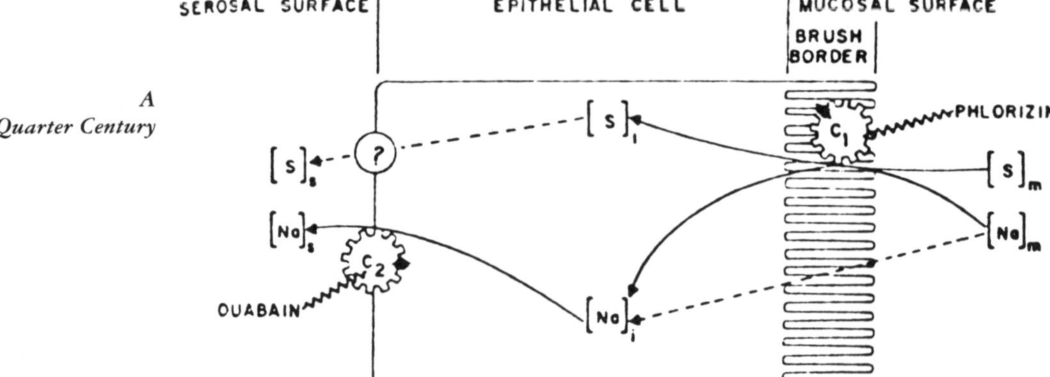

Figure 11.8. Model for electrogenic cotransport of Na^+ and sugar (S) across the microvillus membrane of the small intestine. The coupled phlorizin-sensitive, cotransporter (C_1) was located in the brush border of the microvillus, and an unidentified and unspecified facilitated diffusion mechanism for the exit of sugar in the serosal membrane. Energy for the entire process was provided by the ouabain-sensitive Na,K-ATPase (C_2). (S. G. Schultz and R. Zalusky, J. Gen. Physiol. 47:1043–1049, 1964.)

A model to explain water transport against an osmotic gradient was developed at the Biophysics Laboratory of Harvard Medical School in the late 1950s, initially through informal discussions among investigators including Richard Durbin, Erich Heinz, Jared Diamond, and Peter Curran. The model proposed the existence of 3 compartments composed of the 2 solution compartments on either side of an epithelium and an intermediate compartment within the epithelium. The model first published by Heinz in 1960 and, subsequently, in more detail by Curran and MacIntosh in 1962 as Figure 11.9 demonstrates.

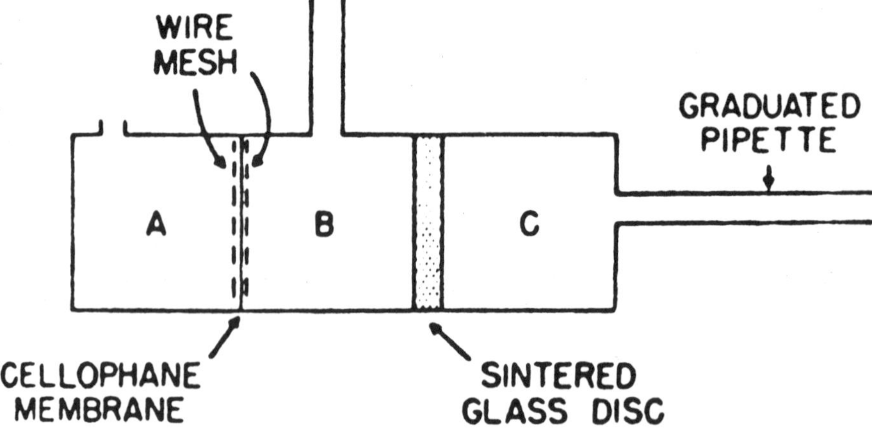

Figure 11.9. The 3-compartment model for explaining water transport against an apparent trans-epithelial osmolality difference. The model proposed that net water transport could proceed from a more concentrated compartment A to compartment C if the middle compartment B were hyperosmotic to both. Pressure developed in compartment B, produced by the osmotic pressure developed across the semipermeable cellophane membrane, would force water flow across solute permeable sintered glass disk, which could develop no osmotic pressure. (P. F. Curran and J. R. MacIntosh. Nature. 193:347–348, 1962.)

Theoretical support for the model based on irreversible thermodynamics was developed by Clifford Patlak and his coworkers in 1963, and the model has come to be referred to as the "3-compartment model." The model revealed that, as long as the middle compartment was maintained hypertonic by active solute transport and a slow rate of diffusional solid exit, net transepithelial water flow against an osmotic gradient could occur if the middle compartment was bounded by membranes of differing solute and water permeability characteristics.

Although the original Curran-Patlak model did not postulate the location of the middle compartment, in 1964 Richard Whitlock and Henry Wheeler at Columbia proposed that it might be the lateral intercellular spaces between adjacent epithelial cells. This suggestion was amplified in the work of Jared Diamond who expressed that if active sodium transport were directed primarily into the long, tortuous lateral intercellular spaces, these spaces would become hypertonic and drive transcellular water flow, resulting in the formation of a standing osmotic gradient along the lateral intracellular spaces, as demonstrated in Figure 11.10.

The development of a hyperosmotic intraepithelial compartment could also be invoked to explain water reabsorption in the proximal tubule, which occurred in the apparent absence of any strikingly significant transepithelial osmolality differences. However, in his book, The Kidney, Structure and Function in Health and Disease, Homer Smith stated simply that in the proximal nephron, water absorption "followed" Na^+ absorption. Implicit in Smith's statement was the notion that if the water permeability of the

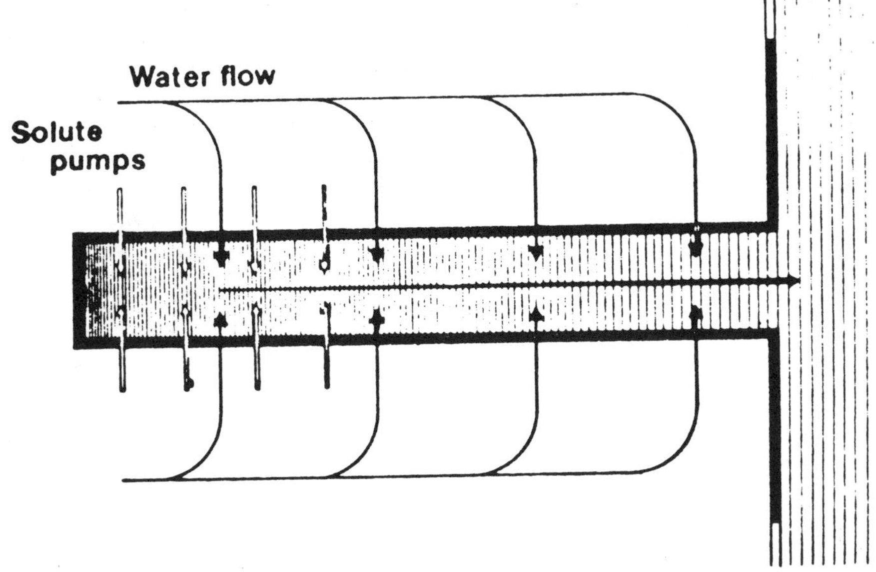

Figure 11.10. The Diamond and Bossert model for a standing osmotic gradient in lateral intracellular spaces. Active pumping of solute such as Na^+ into the closed end of the lateral intracellular space would raise its osmolality, thus driving transcellular water flow into the space. J. M. Diamond and W. M. Bossert. J. Gen. Physiol. 50:2061–2083, 1967.)

proximal tubule were sufficiently high, water reabsorption might require only very small transepithelial osmolality differences. Further examination of the process of isosmotic volume reabsorption in the proximal tubule depended upon the appropriate analysis of the osmotic water permeability and osmolality differences in this segment.

Structural Complexities of Epithelia. The Curran-Patlak model incorporated 1 aspect of the complexity of epithelial structure to explain the coupling of solute and water transport. In the mid-to-late 1960s, it became increasingly evident that solutes and water might also cross the epithelium by way of a paracellular route, proceeding through the junctional complexes and lateral intercellular spaces. Although the Diamond and Bossert model (Fig. 11.10) had assumed that the junctional complexes were impermeable to salt and water, electrophysiologic experiments by Erich Windhager, Emile Boulpaep, Gerhard Giebisch, and others indicated that the low transepithelial resistance observed in the proximal tubule might reflect a high permeability of the junctional complexes to ions. Direct experimental support for this hypothesis was obtained by Eberhard Frömter and Jared Diamond in the Necturus gallbladder in 1972. As shown in Figure 11.11, they proposed that there were 2 routes of transepithelial transport, the first route involving movement through apical and basolateral membranes and the cytoplasm, and the second route proceeding through the junctional complexes and lateral intracellular spaces. Frömter and Diamond proposed that in "leaky epithelia" such as the proximal tubule and the gallbladder, most passive ion movement might occur paracellularly; whereas, in other epithelia such as the frog skin, toad bladder, and distal tubule, transepithelial movement would be predominantly transcellular because of a low permeability of the junctional complexes.

Alexander Leaf had also raised the possibility that the individual plasma membranes of the apical and basolateral surface might be more complex than a simple homogeneous barrier. In the early 1960s Leaf and his coworkers had explained the effect of vasopressin to increase water permeability on the basis

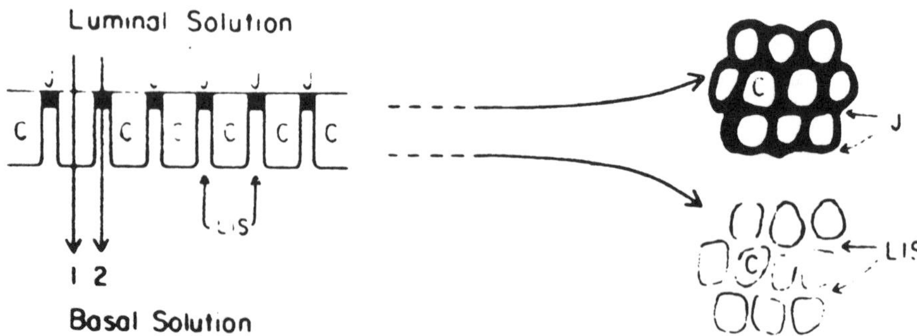

Figure 11.11. Paracellular and transcellular routes of solute and water flow in epithelia. It was recognized that solute and water transport across an epithelium could proceed not only by the transcellular route (1), but also paracellularly (2) through the junctional complexes (J) surrounding the individual cells of the epithelium, and then proceed into the lateral intracellular spaces. (Nature New Biol. 235:9–13, 1972.)

of an enlargement of aqueous pores in the luminal membrane of the toad bladder. However, the low solute permeability of the toad bladder was inconsistent with the presence of aqueous pores of sufficiently large diameter to explain the water flow. In answer to this dilemma, Hans Ussing and, later, Alexander Leaf and his associates at the Massachusetts General Hospital proposed that the apical membrane might consist of 2 barriers in series as Figure 11.12 indicates. Whereas the outer layer would provide a diffusional restriction to the movement of solutes, the underlying porous barrier would be regulated by vasopressin.

Thus the recognition of the complexity of epithelial structure set the stage for a more detailed examination of epithelial transport processes and their localization to apical and basolateral membranes, and to the paracellular pathway.

The Countercurrent Hypothesis. In the early 1960s there was considerable excitement in the field of renal physiology because the basic tenets of the countercurrent hypothesis had been validated by micropuncture. As Wirz, Hargitay, and Kuhn proposed in 1951, countercurrent multiplication in the loop of Henle combined with active sodium chloride transport out of the thick ascending limb could result in the hypertonicity of the medullary

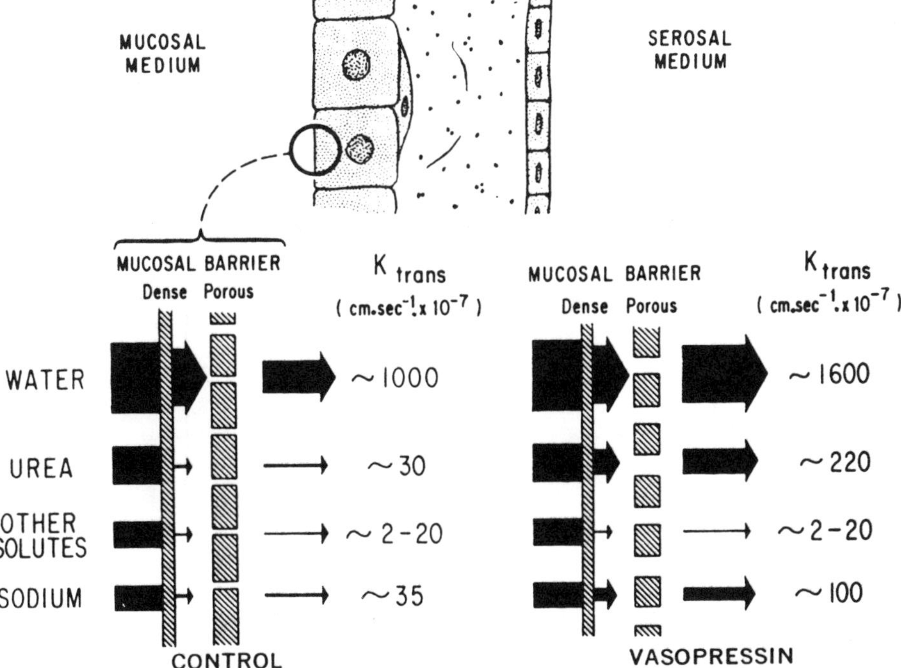

Figure 11.12. The double barrier model. In order to explain water permeabilities characteristic of a pore in combination with low solute permeabilities, it was proposed that the luminal membrane of vasopressin-responsive epithelia might consist of an outer dense diffusion barrier limiting the access of solutes to an underlying porous barrier. Vasopressin would act to increase the pore size of the second barrier and the permeability of the dense outer barrier. (A. Leaf, Am. J. Med. 42:745–756, 1967.)

interstitium and the delivery of a dilute urine to the early distal tubule. As Figure 11.13 reveals, the classical micropuncture experiments of Carl Gottschalk and Margaret Mylle at the University of North Carolina confirmed that the tubular fluid entering the distal tubule always remained dilute, irrespective of the final osmolality of the urine. These observations set the stage for later studies examining the transport properties of those nephron segments that comprised the loop of Henle and the collecting duct system.

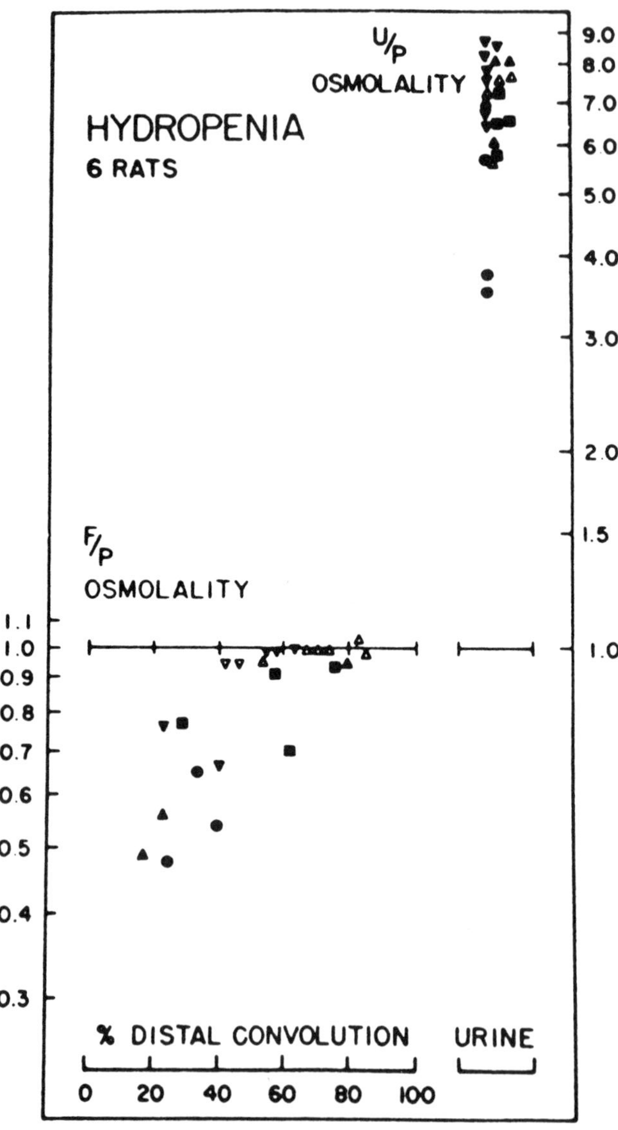

Figure 11.13. Demonstration of hypotonicity of early distal tubule fluid samples. The osmolality of micropuncture samples of tubular fluid from the early distal tubule were consistently less than the plasma osmolality, in spite of a high urine to plasma osmolality ratio in hydropenic rats. (C. W. Gottschalk and M. Mylle, Am. J. Physiol. 196:927–936, 1959.)

It was in the context of these 5 contemporary conceptual advances, documented in part in Pitts' book, that renal physiologists began to examine the details of salt and water transport in different segments of the nephron in the late 1960s. Research in this area was considerably advanced by several important methodological advances that occurred in the early years of the ASN.

Advances in Methodology

Methodologic advances have assumed special importance in the study of salt and water transport processes in individual nephron segments. These studies focused on several technical hurdles that related to the microscopic size of the nephron and the diversity of epithelial types along its length. The resulting heterogeneity in transport processes necessitated the development of ultramicro techniques for studying individual nephron segments and in analyzing nanoliter volumes of fluid collected from them. The technological advances that resulted from necessity provided methods of studying not only individual nephron segments, but also subcellular systems ranging from individual plasma membranes to transport proteins themselves. The increased sophistication and diversity of methodologies were widely reflected in the programs of annual ASN meetings. In order to provide as wide a dissemination of newer technologies as possible, workshops were introduced in association with the ASN meeting, beginning in 1986. These workshops provided a forum for disseminating information regarding a number of new techniques including patch-clamping, the use of intracellular fluorescent dyes, antibody techniques, nuclear magnetic resonance (NMR), membrane vesicles, renal cell culture, and molecular biology.

In the early years of the ASN, the most dramatic methodologic advances occurred in new techniques for the isolation and study of individual nephron segments that were not accessible by in vivo techniques. These approaches were augmented by the use of electrophysiology to study the conductive properties of the epithelium and its individual membranes. The introduction of isolated membrane techniques, including transport studies in isolated membrane vesicles, allowed the characterization of transporters associated with luminal or basolateral membranes of different segments of the nephron. This technology was later extended by procedures to isolate, purify, and reconstitute many transport proteins. The development of new optical techniques permitted important correlations between structural and functional changes and in discrete types of renal cells, and the development of fluorescent dyes provided convenient ways of monitoring changes in intracellular ion concentrations in vitro. In the late 1970s the application of cell culture and the methods of cell biology and molecular biology opened important new avenues of investigation that have allowed the pursuit of the physiology of the nephron from the cellular to the molecular level.

In Vitro Perfusion of Isolated Nephron Segments

In the 1960s the widespread use of in vivo micropuncture provided extensive information about the localization of transport processes to the proximal tubule, loop of Henle, and distal tubule. However, this technique was constrained by the inability to study nephron segments that did not reach the cortical surface. Thus, most of the information derived from the proximal convoluted tubule and distal convoluted tubule of superficial nephrons and the functional properties of the other nephron segments had to be inferred from changes in solute and water flow between the proximal and distal convoluted tubules and between the distal convoluted tubule and the urine. A limited number of micropuncture studies had been conducted in the thin segments of the loop of Henle by exposing the renal papilla in vitro. A few studies had also been conducted by in vitro microperfusion of inner medullary collecting ducts in situ.

In the mid-to-late 1960s a dramatic advance occurred with the development of the methodology for complete isolation and perfusion of all nephron segments. This important methodologic advance was made in the Laboratory of Kidney and Electrolyte Metabolism at the NIH by a group under the direction of Maurice Burg (Fig. 11.14) which included: Maurice Abramow, Jean Cardinal, Gustavo Frindt, Jared Grantham, Sandy Helman,

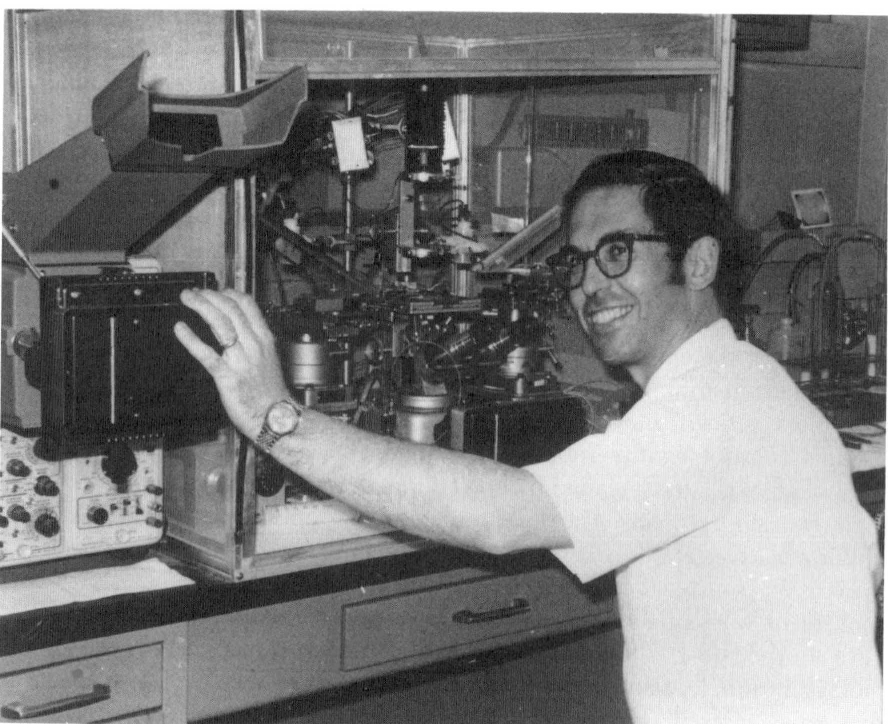

Figure 11.14. Maurice B. Burg.

L. C. Isaacson, Juha Kokko, and Bruce Tune. As these postdoctoral fellows and research associates left the NIH to establish their own laboratories during the late 1960s and early 1970s, the technique spread throughout the world. During these early years the technique was also adopted and modified in other laboratories, including those of William Dantzler at the University of Arizona; Thomas Andreoli and James Schafer at Duke University and, later, at the University of Alabama at Birmingham; and Gerhard Giebisch and Emile Boulpaep at Yale University.

The development of the technique of in vitro perfusion coincided almost exactly with the first meetings of the ASN. At these early meetings during the late 1960s and early 1970s, the results of numerous studies with previously inaccessible nephron segments were presented. Studies from the cortical collecting duct provided information about the basic transport characteristics of this segment, the hormonal regulation of ion and water transport, and allowed the characterization of pathways for water flow and the nature of the vasopressin-induced permeability change at the luminal membrane. Studies were also presented concerning the mechanism of salt and water reabsorption by the proximal tubule, including the previously inaccessible proximal straight segment.

Perhaps the most significant advance made from such information was the further substantiation of the countercurrent model for urinary concentration and dilution. A rapid succession of studies conducted from 1969 to 1972 in the laboratories of Maurice Burg and Juha Kokko in collaboration with Masashi Imai and Antonino Rocha established the basic transport characteristics of the 3 components of the loop of Henle. The thick ascending limb was found to have a very low, vasopressin-insensitive water permeability and active NaCl reabsorption; thus, this segment possessed the necessary "single effect" required by the countercurrent model of Wirz, Hargitay, and Kuhn. The descending thin limb of the loop of Henle was found to have a high water permeability and lower permeabilities for urea and NaCl, while the thin ascending limb had an essentially zero water permeability and no evidence of active solute reabsorption. It was also demonstrated that the urea permeability of all nephron segments from the tip of the loop of Henle to the outer medullary collecting duct was extremely low; whereas, the inner medullary collecting duct had a higher urea permeability which could be augmented by vasopressin. These observations led directly to an extension of the countercurrent model to explain urea concentration in the inner medulla without the necessity of active transport in the thin segments, as Juha Kokko and Floyd Rector published in 1972.

Studies in isolated perfused nephron segments also provided the basic parameter values required for the development of a more comprehensive mathematical model of the countercurrent system by John Stephenson, the so-called *central core model*. Although the question of whether there is any active transepithelial transport in the thin ascending and descending limbs is still open, the basic transport properties of the model had been demonstrated.

The further study of individual nephron segments by in vitro perfusion from the mid-1970s until the present also revealed what was at first a bewildering heterogeneity in the transport properties of nephron segments previously assumed to be homogeneous. Abstracts presented at ASN meetings during this period showed differences in the ionic permeability properties of proximal tubule segments deriving from superficial and juxtamedullary nephrons. Functional differences were revealed among the early and late distal convoluted tubule, the connecting segment, and the cortical collecting duct; between the medullary and cortical regions of the thick ascending limb; and even among different regions of the collecting duct, including the outer and inner medullary collecting duct. At the 1984 ASN meeting, the first functional studies of the isolated perfused macula densa region of the thick ascending limb were presented, and symposia at the 1987 and 1990 meetings provided new information about the special properties and hormonal regulation of urea and ion transport in the inner medullary collecting duct.

The earliest studies with in vitro tubule perfusion were conducted exclusively with rabbit nephron segments. Throughout the 1970s and 1980s these studies were extended to nephron segments from the mouse, rat, psammomys and hamster; and to reptilian, amphibian, and avian species including the snake, Amphiuma, Abystoma, and Necturus. These studies demonstrated some interesting functional differences in the transport properties and their hormonal regulation among species. The utility of the technique was also expanded by combining it with other methodologies including electrophysiology with intracellular microelectrodes, the measurement of intracellular solute concentrations, direct collection of absorbate from the proximal tubule, and optical techniques.

Electrophysiology

Until the end of the 1960s there existed only a limited number of electrophysiologic measurements in individual nephron segments, and these were limited primarily to determinations of transepithelial voltage and resistance and some intracellular voltages of surface nephron segments. In the late 1960s and early 1970s Eberhard Frömter, Gerhard Giebisch, Emile Boulpaep, Takeshi Hoshi, and others used electrophysiologic techniques, including intracellular microelectrodes, to characterize ion conductance and coupled ion and electrolyte flows in proximal and distal convoluted tubules in vivo. Isolated perfused tubules extended these electrophysiologic techniques for use in the thick ascending limb and regions of the collecting duct. At the 1970 ASN meeting, Giebisch received the Homer Smith Award for his contributions; in 1983 and 1986 Frömter and Boulpaep, respectively, were similarly awarded.

As several abstracts presented at the ASN meetings in the early 1970s reported, electrophysiologic studies established the electrical leakiness of the proximal tubule segments and the thick ascending limb. They also confirmed the low transepithelial voltage previously measured in vivo in the proximal tubule and explained that it could be determined to a large extent by diffusion potentials established by transepithelial ion concentration differences. The demonstration of a lumen-positive transepithelial voltage in the thick ascending limb led ultimately to the identification of the electroneutral Na^+:K^+:$2Cl^-$ cotransporter in this nephron segment. From the mid-1970s to the present, there were numerous reports at ASN meetings using the techniques of intracellular microelectrodes to determine luminal and basolateral membrane conductances of discrete nephron segments. These studies provided important information on the distribution of ion transporters between luminal and basolateral membranes.

Many of these studies also made good use of amphibian nephron segments for intracellular microelectrode measurements because of the advantages that their large cell sizes provided. The Necturus proximal tubule and the Amphiuma distal tubule or diluting segments provided good models for their corresponding mammalian nephron segments. Intracellular microelectrodes, first applied to the rabbit proximal straight tubule and cortical collecting duct, were extended in the late 1970s and early 1980s to the thick ascending limb. The development of liquid ion exchange resins permitted the development of ion-specific microelectrodes to replace the older, less sensitive, glass microelectrodes in the early 1980s. This technology was particularly helpful in establishing the fact that the intracellular chloride activity in nephron segments such as the thick ascending limb was higher than predicted from electrochemical equilibrium, thus providing support for the presence of secondary, active chloride transport coupled to that of sodium.

The development of the patch clamp technique and its application to epithelia in the 1970s was a major advance. The first ASN abstract to report single channel activity in a cultured renal epithelium was presented by Erich Hunter from Gerhard Giebisch's laboratory in 1983. This technology was also the subject of an invited lecture by Larry Palmer at the 1984 meeting, and numerous studies employing this technology appeared in subsequent years. These studies have provided important information about the kinetics of ion channels, particularly in the thick ascending limb, cortical collecting duct, and inner medullary collecting duct. In combination with noise or fluctuation analysis in toad bladder and frog skin, patch-clamp technology was instrumental in demonstrating that the ion permeability conferred by channels was regulated primarily by the number of channels and the probability of their being open rather than by changes in their intrinsic conductances.

Isolated Membrane Techniques

At the 1974 ASN meeting, Irving Schwartz, Rolf Kinne, and their associates presented a new technology for separating luminal and basolateral membranes of discrete nephron segments. Starting with renal cortical or medullary homogenates, the methodology combined differential centrifugation techniques with a new technique of free-flow electrophoresis to separate membrane fractions from the cortex and medulla, based on differences in their density and charge characteristics. In their initial presentation, Schwartz et al. demonstrated that PTH-sensitive and vasopressin-sensitive adenylate cyclase activity were associated with basolateral membrane fractions from proximal tubules and cortical collecting ducts, respectively. On the other hand, phosphorylation of membrane proteins by cAMP-dependent kinases was associated with the luminal membranes.

Throughout the mid-to-late 1970s, an explosion of abstracts was submitted to the ASN using this methodology to localize and examine the characteristics of transport processes in renal membrane vesicles and later to reconstitute transport activity in artificial membrane systems. The methodology was already widely used in 1978, when Rolf Kinne presented a state-of-the-art lecture at the ASN meeting on "Isolated Membranes as Tools to Elucidate Epithelial Cell Function." In 1989, Kinne's pioneering work was recognized by the Homer Smith Award; Kinne presented the award lecture, "Selectivity and Direction: Plasma Membranes in Renal Transport."

The use of isolated membrane vesicles was particularly instrumental in establishing the characteristics of electrogenic Na^+ cotransporters in brush border membrane vesicles from the proximal tubule. Work appearing from the mid-1970s onward established the existence of cotransport mechanisms that actively accumulated various organic solutes and phosphate in proximal tubular cells as the consequence of cotransport with Na^+ across the luminal membrane. Later studies demonstrated antiport mechanisms, including sodium-proton exchange in proximal tubule brush border membranes and anion exchangers in basolateral membrane fractions. Kinetic studies of the sodium-phosphate cotransporter and sodium-proton exchanger also established that the number of transporters, or their maximal rate of action, were altered by hormones such as PTH and changes in vivo of the acid-base status.

The further development of isolated membrane technology in the 1980s led to the isolation and purification of many transport proteins and their functional reconstitution in artificial membrane systems. During this period, abstracts were presented at each ASN meeting discussing sugar, amino acid, and anion cotransporters; the sodium-proton exchanger; the amiloride-sensitive Na^+ channel; the Na^+:K^+:$2Cl^-$ cotransporter; and proteins associated with vasopressin-dependent water permeability in the cortical collecting duct.

Optical Techniques

In the early years of the ASN, new information about the functional characteristics of some nephron segments was obtained by the use of conventional light and electron microscopy. Abstracts were presented that examined the structural evidence for the pathways for water flow in the cortical collecting duct and in the proximal tubule. At the 1975 ASN meeting the first studies were presented in which freeze-fracture methodology demonstrated the presence of intramembrane particles related to transport. This methodology was used to particular advantage in subsequent years to correlate changes in intramembrane particle density with water permeability in the toad bladder and with changes in water and K^+ transport in the cortical collecting duct. Studies in the 1980s employed both high-resolution electron microscopy and colloidal gold-labelled antibodies to localize membrane transporters to different plasma membrane surfaces and intracellular organelles. Results of these studies have provided important, new information regarding the trafficking of transport proteins between cytoplasmic reservoirs and the plasma membrane.

Computer-assisted morphometric techniques were also used in association with isolated perfused renal tubules. Because the isolated nephron segment is composed of a single-cell layer and underlying basement membrane, it provided an ideal subject for examination by light microscopy using contrast enhancement procedures such as Nomarski microscopy. The combination of these technologies allowed contemporaneous correlation of structural and functional changes in the same nephron segments. These techniques were advanced, particularly by Ken Spring in the Laboratory of Kidney and Electrolyte Metabolism at the NIH and by Larry and Dan Welling at the University of Kansas Medical Center. Also, using morphometric techniques on electron microscopic sections, the latter investigators provided the first detailed information about luminal and basolateral membrane surface areas and cell shape in the proximal tubule, thick ascending limb, and cortical collecting duct. In the late 1970s and early 1980s, several abstracts examined changes in morphometrically measured cell volume associated with changes in transport and examined their role in the regulation of cell volume. Much of this work was summarized at the 1976 and 1985 meetings of the ASN in symposia discussing the use of morphological techniques and other optical techniques in renal physiology.

In the early 1980s several laboratories began to use ion-sensitive fluorescent dyes to measure intracellular concentrations of H^+, Ca^{++}, and Cl^-. With these dyes it was possible to obtain excellent temporal resolution of rapid changes in intracellular or intravesicular H^+ or Ca^{++} concentrations in isolated perfused nephron segments, isolated membrane vesicles, cell suspensions, and cell cultures. The application of fluorescent extracellular fluid-phase markers was also important in demonstrating membrane cycling as a mechanism for regulating the density of membrane transporters. This mechanism of transport regulation by shuttling transporters into and out of the plasma membrane was an important focus of research presented at the ASN meetings in the 1980s.

Cell Culture

The application of cell culture techniques to renal epithelia in the late 1970s offered the prospect of obtaining larger quantities of pure cell types for biochemical studies. Also, the development of techniques to grow these cells on permeable membrane supports provided a new experimental system for studying transepithelial transport that possessed all of the convenience of the frog skin or toad bladder models.

The earliest cell culture work in the laboratories of Dennis Ausiello at Massachusetts General Hospital and Joseph Handler and Maurice Burg in the Laboratory of Kidney and Electrolyte Metabolism at NIH used established epithelial cell lines derived from pig, dog, or toad kidney. The methodology was widely adopted; numerous abstracts based on cell culture have been presented at the ASN since the early 1980s, including work with primary cultures of mammalian proximal tubule cells, thick ascending limb cells, and cortical and inner medullary collecting duct cells. The rapid growth of the field was reflected in Handler's lecture, "Renal Cells in Culture," delivered at the 1980 ASN meeting and at a symposium held at the 1983 meeting. By 1986 free communication sessions at the meeting were devoted entirely to studies in cultured cell systems. The technique continues to present important, new opportunities for the study of membrane transporters and the regulation of their expression.

Biochemistry, Cell, and Molecular Biology

Throughout the last 25 years, the study of renal function at the subcellular level has been enhanced considerably by the development of new receptor ligands and specific inhibitors and promoters of intracellular regulatory processes. More recently, this area has exploded with the application of the techniques of cell and molecular biology to the study of membrane transporters and their regulation.

From the time of the first ASN meeting to the present, numerous abstracts relating to the regulation of nephron transport by aldosterone and vasopressin have been presented. As summarized at the 1980 ASN meeting, Isidore Edelman's Homer Smith Award lecture, "Receptors and Effectors in Hormone Action on the Kidney", a considerable body of knowledge had accumulated regarding the localization of aldosterone receptors in the cytoplasm and nucleus and the action of aldosterone inducing new protein synthesis. During the early 1970s numerous abstracts also demonstrated the involvement of cAMP as a second messenger in mediating the effects of parathyroid hormone (PTH) and vasopressin.

In the mid-1970s micromethodology was developed to measure cAMP production in single isolated nephron segments, and it became evident that several peptide hormones and β-adrenergic agonists augmented cAMP production in various nephron segments. Furthermore, some nephron segments, such as the thick ascending limb, responded to more than 1 hormone by increasing intracellular cAMP. These observations, as well as differences among species with regard to the hormone responsiveness of different nephron segments, were the subjects of Morel's Homer Smith Award lecture, "Sites of Hormone Action in the Mammalian Nephron," at the 1979 ASN meeting.

In the mid-1980s the availability of different promoters and inhibitors of cAMP production, including pertussis toxin, cholera toxin, and forskolin, demonstrated the involvement of GTP-binding proteins (G-proteins) in the regulation of adenylate cyclase activity. In the last 5 years, it has become abundantly evident that G-proteins are involved in numerous cellular regulatory processes in the kidney and may be directly associated with membrane transporters themselves. These exciting new findings were summarized at the 1987 ASN meeting in a symposium on G-proteins and at the 1990 meeting by Henry Bourne's lecture, "G-Proteins and Transmembrane Signals."

In the last 5 years, it has been recognized that many nephron segments possess an alternative signaling system—the phosphoinositide system—to regulate membrane transporters and other cellular processes. The activation of phospholipase C by a G–protein-linked receptor results in breakdown of phosphoinositides and the subsequent elevation of intracellular calcium and activation of protein kinase C. The involvement of this phosphoinositide system in transport regulatory mechanisms, the subject of numerous recent abstracts at the ASN meetings, was summarized at the 1988 meeting in Michael Berridge's state-of-the-art lecture on "Inositol Lipids and Cell Signaling" and a symposium on intracellular calcium as a second messenger. At the 1989 ASN meeting, Yasutomi Nishizuka presented a lecture, "The Role of the Protein Kinase C Family in Intracellular Regulation."

The developing importance of the disciplines of cell and molecular biology to renal physiology was recognized at the 1986 ASN meeting by a separate *abstract* category bearing this title. Over the past 4 years, abstracts have presented the primary amino acid structure of different membrane transporters, as determined from analysis of their corresponding cDNA. A symposium at the 1986 ASN meetings summarized progress on understanding transport function and its regulation by molecular cloning approaches, using the Na^+-glucose cotransporter, $(Na^+ + K^+)$-ATPase, and anion exchangers as examples. In 1987, a symposium presented recent advances in understanding the structure and function of transporters, and examined the different $(Na^+ + K^+)$-ATPase isoforms and the Na^+/H^+ antiporter as examples. Abstracts and invited lectures at the 1989 and 1990 meetings extended molecular biology approaches to the single nephron segment level by applying the polymerase chain reaction. These new techniques provide exciting new possibilities for examining the molecular details of transporter function and its regulation in discreet nephron segments.

Other Methodologies

The above sections have discussed only those new and emerging technologies that served most extensively in work presented at the ASN meetings over the past 25 years. However, other important new methodologies have also played a major role in advancing our knowledge. Among these were mathematical modeling methods that examined more complex systems. For example, the application of mathematical modeling to the countercurrent multiplication system provided important new insights about the integration of the functions of different nephron segments into the regulation of urinary concentration and dilution. Mathematical models of the proximal tubular epithelium and its transport processes also furnished new insights about the process of volume reabsorption and the coupling of solute and solvent flows.

In the mid-1970s, abstract presentations at the ASN were evidence of the addition of electronprobe methodology as an important new tool for analyzing nanoliter volumes of fluid and as measuring intracellular solute composition. Nuclear magnetic resonance (NMR) technology also introduced a potentially important new technology for in vitro and in vivo studies of metabolic and transport processes as a 1986 ASN Symposium chaired by Robert Shulman summarized.

Solute and Water Transport in the Proximal Tubule

At the time of the first ASN meeting, the present understanding of ion transport in the proximal tubule had been simply but elegantly summarized in a diagram from Pitts' Physiology of the Kidney and Body Fluids (Fig. 11.15). This model was not remarkably different from the Ussing frog skin model displayed in Figure 11.6; with the exception of the (Na^+ + K^+)-ATPase located on the basolateral membrane, the model left unspecified the mechanisms by which the major ions crossed both the luminal and basolateral membranes. From the time of the earliest ASN meetings, it was already clear that new strategies were being developed to open this black box and determine the transport mechanisms involved in the individual membranes. In his lecture, "Models for Proximal and Distal Tubule Electrolyte Transport," delivered at the second ASN meeting, Gerhard Giebisch laid out the current knowledge concerning these transport mechanisms in the proximal and distal tubule and the strategies by which electrophysiologic flux experiments could examine ion transporters in the individual membranes.

During the late 60's and early 70's, it was well recognized that the junctional complexes in the proximal tubule possessed a high electrical conductance and that the paracellular pathway was a potential route for large ion fluxes driven by transepithelial electrochemical potential differences. It was shown that changes in the permselectivity properties of the junctional complexes could alter ion flows in various segments and regulate transepithelial salt and water transport. These changes in the general view of the proximal tubule were reflected by the schematic representation of the proximal tubule in Pitts third edition of Physiology of the Kidney and Body Fluids, published in 1974, in which prominent lateral intercellular spaces and transjunctional ion movement were evident. At the 1978 ASN meeting, Erich Windhager's Homer Smith Award lecture summarized the important new membrane transporters and the significance of their regulation in the control of Na^+

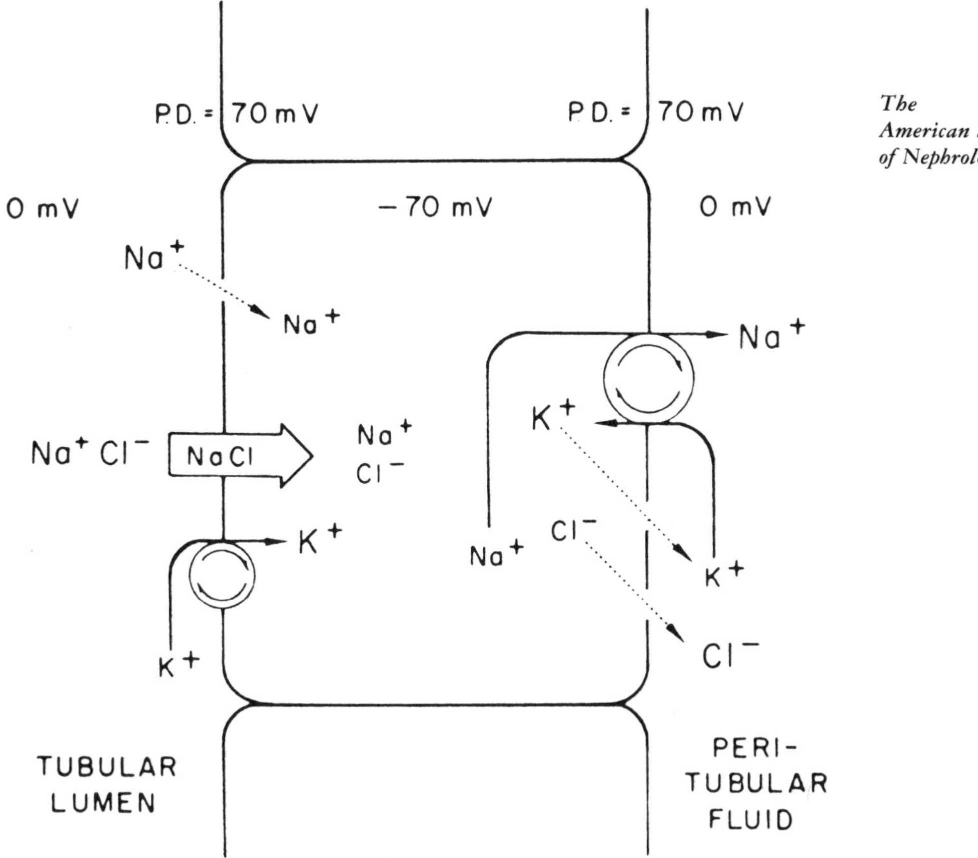

Figure 11.15. Model of ion transport processes in the proximal tubule in use at the time of the first ASN meeting. Copied from (R. F. Pitts, Physiology of the Kidney and Body Fluids. 2nd Edition, Yearbook Medical Publishers, Inc., Chicago, 1968, p. 102.)

transport along the nephron. These advances were particularly evident in 4 areas: the identification of symport and antiport mechanisms for coupled solute flows in the luminal and basolateral membranes, the use of intracellular microelectrodes to define individual membrane conductance properties and individual membrane electrochemical potential differences, the demonstration of high hydraulic conductivity and low reflection coefficients for some solutes in the proximal tubule, and the characterization of solute secretory processes.

Coupled Solute Transport Pathways

Since Crane's formulation of the Na^+-glucose symport mechanism in the early 1960's the presence of similar Na^+-coupled transporters in the luminal membrane of the proximal tubule had been regarded as likely. However, it was also recognized that similar coupling could occur among ion flows, given appropriate transporters. These concepts were summarized in a symposium at the 1970 meeting which focused on coupled ion transport pathways and included presentations on: K^+ and Na^+ exchange processes, reabsorption of Na^+ in exchange for H^+ secretion, and basolateral anion exchange mechanisms.

Work involving micropuncture and in vitro perfusion techniques in the early-to-mid 1970s demonstrated the existence of Na^+-dependent glucose, amino acid, and phosphate reabsorption in the proximal convoluted and proximal straight tubule. These studies in isolated tubules also demonstrated that the active transport mechanism was present in the luminal membrane, because of the higher concentration of the solutes in the cytoplasm. As discussed above, the application of the technique of isolated membrane vesicles allowed the complete characterization of the kinetics of Na^+-dependent cotransport processes for glucose; amino acids; phosphate; sulphate; and organic anions such as lactate, citrate, urate, and di- and tricarboxylic acids. All of these studies demonstrated quite clearly that a large fraction of Na^+ entry into the proximal tubule across the luminal membrane occurred in association with cotransport of all these various preferentially reabsorbed solutes.

In the late 1970s studies with isolated brush border membrane vesicles demonstrated that Na^+ entry across the luminal membrane also occurred in exchange for H^+ secretion. Thus, this antiporter appeared to be the connection between Na^+ reabsorption and H^+ secretion that had been postulated in both the proximal and distal tubule in Pitts' Physiology of the Kidney and Body Fluids. Subsequent studies indicated that the activity of this transporter could be regulated by in vivo acid-base conditions and by the actions of hormones such as adrenergic agonists and angiotensin.

In the late 70s and early 80s it was also recognized that chloride transport across the proximal tubule could occur both transcellularly and paracellularly. Furthermore, the transcellular pathway appeared to involve coupled transport systems in both the luminal and basolateral membranes. Experiments presented at ASN meetings during this period using membrane vesicle preparations, micropuncture, and in vitro perfusion methods demonstrated Cl^- transport across the luminal membrane in the form of symport with Na^+ or in exchange for hydroxyl or bicarbonate ions. Anion exchange mechanisms in the basolateral membranes were also demonstrated. The current concepts of transepithelial chloride transport in the proximal tubule were summarized in Rector's 1982 Homer Smith award lecture, "Sodium, Bicarbonate, and Chloride Reabsorption by the Proximal Tubule." In the 1980s, mechanisms of bicarbonate movement across the proximal tubule basolateral membrane were further characterized by many investigators.

Throughout the late 70s and 80s considerable work was accomplished on the reconstitution of Na^+-dependent symporters and antiporters isolated from membrane vesicles into artificial lipid vesicles. Presentations at various ASN meetings demonstrated solubilization and purification of the glucose transporter: similar advances with many of the symporters and antiporters led to their further biochemical and kinetic characterization. The late 1980s saw the application of the techniques of molecular biology to the cloning, sequencing, and expression of many of these transport proteins. For example, at a symposium in 1987 Jacques Pouyssegur presented the primary structure of an Na^+/H^+ antiporter analogous to that located in the luminal membrane of the mammalian proximal tubule. At a symposium the following year, Ernest Wright presented the structure of the Na^+/glucose cotransporter isolated from the small intestine, which now appears to be quite similar to that in the proximal tubule. During 1989 and 1990 papers appeared demonstrating expression cloning of the Na^+/myoinositol cotransporter and glucose and amino acid cotransporters. The increasingly intense focus on the molecular details of transporter regulation was exemplified by a free communication session during the 1989 meeting devoted to the physiology and molecular biology of the Na^+/H^+ exchanger, including its genetic linkage, specific monoclonal antibodies against the antiporter, and its regulation by atrial natriuretic peptide and dopamine.

Electrophysiology

Beginning with the earliest ASN meetings, quite sophisticated electrophysiologic techniques had characterized individual nephron segments and their component membranes. Intracellular microelectrodes allowed investigators to define the electrical driving forces for ion movements across the proximal tubule, beginning first with experiments in the larger amphibian proximal tubule segments and, later, applied to mammalian proximal tubules.

These approaches were particularly useful in defining the conductance properties of the individual membrane of the proximal tubule and demonstrating functionally the existence of electrogenic cotransport and antiport processes, including Na^+ cotransport processes in the luminal membrane and coupled Na^+-bicarbonate transport in the basolateral membrane. The tremendous advances these electrophysiologic techniques achieved were presented during the Homer Smith award lecture Eberhard Frömter delivered at the 1983 ASN meeting, entitled "Viewing the Kidney through Microelectrodes."

Further application of ion-specific microelectrodes from the late 1970s onward allowed the measurement of intracellular ion activities and established the presence of some cotransporters such as secondary active Cl^- transport into proximal tubular cells. The latter application of patch-clamp technology yielded the identification of different types of channels, including those responsible for K^+ and Cl^- transport across the basolateral membrane. It also identified some channels that appeared to be activated only for the purposes of volume regulation, including the stretch-activated K^+ channel of the basolateral membrane.

Coupling of Water and Solute Absorption in the Proximal Tubule

Through the 70s and early 80s considerable advances were made in understanding the driving force for volume absorption in the proximal tubule and the coupling between water and solute flows. These advances depend upon the development of two primary concepts. First, Schafer and Andreoli reported that the water permeability of the proximal tubular epithelium was remarkably high in comparison to most other epithelia. Second, the demonstrated leakiness of junctional complexes in the proximal tubule permitted the coupling of water and solute flows by solvent drag. The significance of these observations was that quite small transepithelial osmolality gradients would be sufficient to drive the rates of volume absorption observed in the proximal tubule. Furthermore, because of differences in the reflection coefficients among solutes, the cryoscopically measured transepithelial osmolality difference was not necessarily equal to the effective osmolality difference that would drive volume flow across the proximal tubular epithelium, an argument Rector and his associates had set forth some years previously.

More specifically, as ASN meetings in the early 1980s reported, solute absorption in the proximal tubule could result in the dilution of tubular fluid in comparison to the epithelium. Although the resulting transepithelial osmolality differences were small, the high hydraulic conductivity of the proximal tubule indicated that these differences could produce high rates of water reabsorption. It was further demonstrated that reflection coefficients for preferentially reabsorbed solutes such as bicarbonate and the organic solutes exceeded that of NaCl. Consequently, the rising concentration of NaCl in the lumen and the falling concentrations of the preferentially absorbed solutes enabled the development of an effective transepithelial osmolality difference that further augmented volume reabsorption. The existence of such an effective osmolality difference caused by reflection coefficient differences came to be referred to as the "passive" component of volume reabsorption. The demonstration of reflection coefficients lower than 1.0 for several solutes in the proximal tubule led to later evidence that the reabsorption of some ions was enhanced by solvent drag with reabsorbed water.

In spite of the demonstration of sufficient transepithelial osmolality driving forces for volume absorption, the route of water transport across the proximal tubule remained the subject of vigorous investigation during the mid-1980s. Rapid computer-assisted video techniques, which were developed to measure the water permeability properties of luminal and basolateral membranes in isolated perfused proximal segments, indicated that substantial water absorption could occur transcellularly, but did not rule out potential additive contribution from paracellular water flow.

During the late 1980s additional methodology, including NMR, was developed for measuring the diffusional water permeability properties of the proximal tubular basolateral membrane; at several meetings evidence was presented suggesting the existence of water channels that mediated water flow across proximal tubular membranes. Evidence also suggested that the interstitium could serve as a hyperosmotic compartment in vivo to augment the transepithelial osmolality difference.

Mechanisms of Solute Secretion in the Proximal Tubule

During the early-to-mid 1970s both micropuncture techniques and isolated renal tubule perfusion demonstrated active secretion of solutes such as para-aminohippurate (PAH) and uric acid in the proximal tubule. The technique of isolated renal tubule perfusion also indicated that the proximal straight portion of the proximal tubule was the primary site of active solute secretion. Beginning in the mid-1970s, vesicle studies demonstrated numerous symport and antiport mechanisms for PAH, nicotinamide, uric acid, oxalate, and other organic acids and bases, in both luminal and basolateral membranes. These studies defined the basic transport mechanisms involved in both luminal and basolateral membranes responsible for secondary active transport and facilitated diffusion resulting in the secretion of these various solutes.

It was also recognized during the early 1970s that the active secretion of solutes in the proximal tubule could, under certain circumstances, result in net fluid secretion or a diminution of fluid reabsorption. In 1973 J. J. Grantham and his associates demonstrated fluid secretion in the proximal straight tubule in the presence of uremic serum; evidence that metabolites accumulating in uremia could contribute to diminished proximal tubular volume absorption by virtue of their active secretion in the proximal straight tubule was also presented.

Mechanism of Sodium Chloride Absorption in the Thick Ascending Limb of the Loop of Henle

As preceding sections have noted, the technique of perfusing isolated nephron segments supplied the most direct access to the study of different segments of the loop of Henle. The most striking advance from the application of this technology, perhaps, was the localization and characterization of the "single effect" mechanism for salt reabsorption in the thick ascending limb of the loop of Henle. In 72 and 73, Rocha and Kokko at Dallas Southwestern and Maurice Burg at NIH's Laboratory of Kidney and Electrolyte Metabolism determined that the water permeability of the thick ascending limb of the loop of Henle was extremely low and that both Na^+ and Cl^- were actively reabsorbed. Because Cl^- was reabsorbed against a positive luminal voltage, chloride initially appeared to be the actively absorbed anion with Na^+ following passively. However, subsequent studies demonstrated the ultimate dependence of NaCl absorption on basolateral ($Na^+ + K^+$)-ATPase. Studies throughout the remainder of the 1970s established the full characteristics of the transport mechanisms in the thick ascending limb of the loop of Henle, as discussed below.

During the early-to-mid 1970s the focus of many presentations at ASN meetings was the question of whether or not active salt reabsorption occurred in the thin ascending limb of the loop of Henle as well as the thick segment. Although this question is still not fully resolved, the passive model of urea recycling proposed by Kokko and Rector and by Stephenson (see above) indicates that active NaCl reabsorption is not necessary in this segment. Nevertheless, this issue has remained a matter of controversy and was the subject of a 1975 symposium, "Active Versus Passive Movement in the Loop of Henle—Implications for the Countercurrent Mechanism."

During the late 70s and 80s, 2 additional models of coupled transepithelial Na^+ and Cl^- movement, examining the regulation of this important transporter, were developed: the shark rectal gland, which was found to actively secrete NaCl, and the Amphiuma diluting segment, which actively reabsorbed NaCl. Presentations at the ASN throughout this period produced evidence that these 2 structures, just like the thick ascending limb of the loop of Henle, contained a cotransporter for Na^+, K^+, and Cl^- in a stoichiometry of Na^+:K^+:$2Cl^-$. Work with intracellular microelectrodes in the Amphiuma diluting segment, and later in the mouse and rat thick ascending limb, further established that a conductive K^+ channel existed in the luminal membrane and that a conductive Cl^- channel as well as a KCl cotransporter existed in the basolateral membrane.

During the late 1970s, vasopressin was also found to stimulate sodium chloride reabsorption in the mouse thick ascending limb, and increased osmolality and prostaglandins were found to inhibit this process. This was the first indication that vasopressin regulated not only the water permeability of the cortical collecting duct but also medullary osmolality, with further negative feedback regulation exerted by rising medullary osmolality and prostaglandins.

During the 1980s subsequent work using plasma membrane vesicles from the shark rectal gland and from the mouse and rat thick ascending limb provided further kinetic characterization of the Na^+:K^+:$2Cl^-$ cotransporter and the regulation of individual ion conductances in these membranes. Subsequent studies also indicated that the activity of these transporters was regulated not only by vasopressin and the requirements of the countercurrent multiplication mechanism but in response to changes in cell volume. Work has continued in attempts to characterize the molecular nature of the Na^+:K^+:$2Cl^-$ cotransporter; the late 1980s saw studies on the functional molecular size of the cotransporter as well as studies on isolation and reconstitution. Work is progressing in several laboratories to clone and sequence this important protein.

Sodium Chloride Transport in the Distal Convoluted Tubule and Collecting Duct

At the time of the first ASN meeting, Na^+, K^+, Cl^-, and H^+ transport in the distal tubule was basically understood as shown in Figure 11.16, from

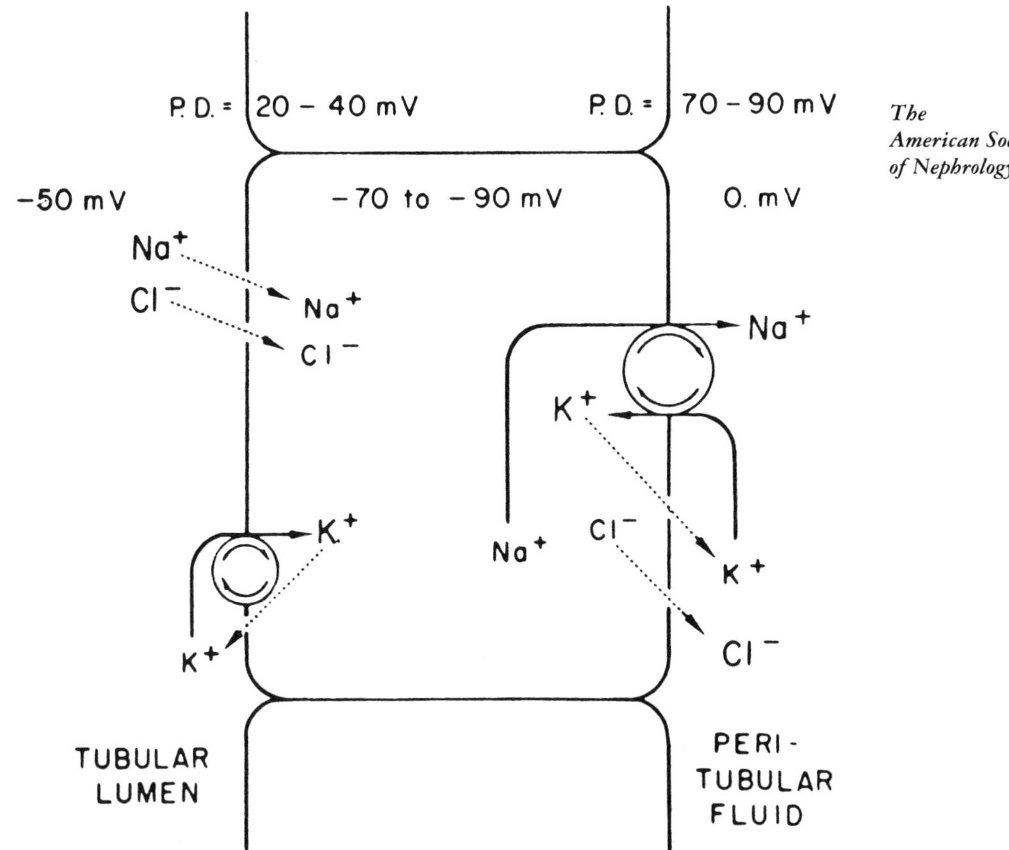

Figure 11.16. Model of ion transport processes in the distal tubule, as understood at the time of the first ASN meeting. (R. F. Pitts, Physiology of the Kidney and Body Fluids. 2nd Edition, Yearbook Medical Publishers, Inc., Chicago, 1968, p. 114.)

Pitts' Physiology of the Kidney and Body Fluids, second edition. Although free-flow micropuncture experiments, conducted during the mid-to-late 1960s by Gerhard Malnic, Gerhard Giebisch, and Erich Windhager, had demonstrated that Na^+ was actively reabsorbed and K^+ and H^+ were actively secreted in the distal convoluted tubule, the mechanisms and transporters involved were not identified. (Fig. 11.17 describes one such experiment.) Nevertheless, the transport of all 3 ions were correlated in a way that suggested Na^+ reabsorption might occur in exchange for K^+ and/or H^+ secretion. Similar research, later conducted on the isolated perfused cortical collecting duct, revealed the same relationships.

In 1975, it was demonstrated that Na^+ movement across the luminal membrane of the cortical collecting duct involved a conductive channel that could be blocked by amiloride. Based on assessments of transepithelial electrophysiological experiments, subsequent reports at ASN meetings indicated that in vitro dietary restriction or mineralocorticoid administration led to an increase in this membrane conductance. The effects of mineralocorticoids on the transport of Na^+ and K^+ were summarized in a symposium at the

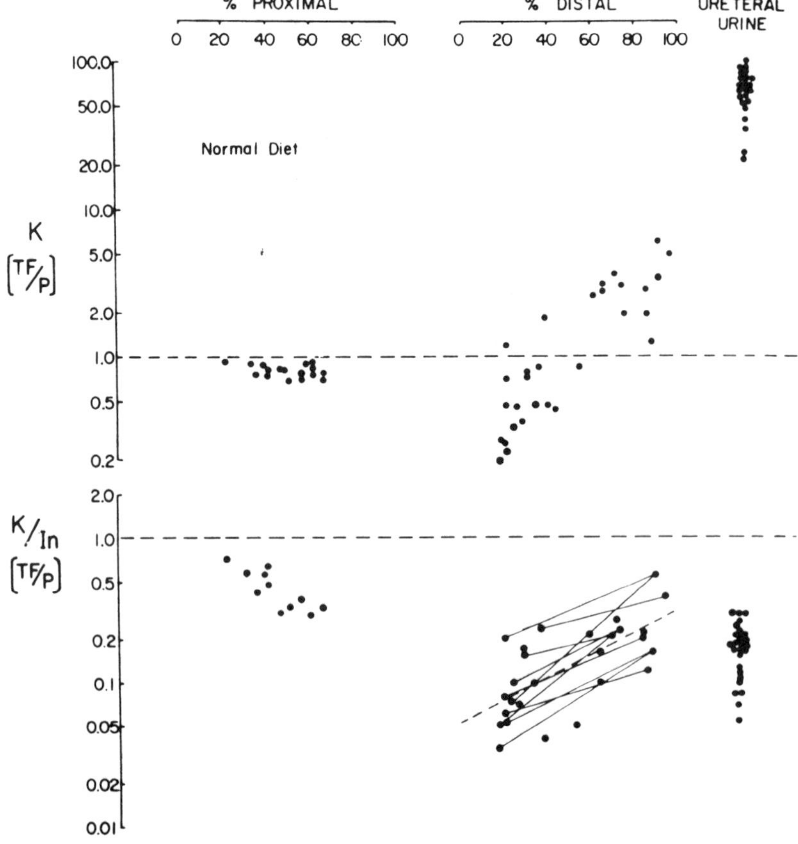

Figure 11.17. Sites of K^+ reabsorption in the proximal tubule and secretion in the distal tubule from the free-flow micropuncture data of G. Malnic, R. Klose, and G. Giebisch. Am. J. Physiol. 206:674–686, 1964.

1979 ASN meeting entitled "Regulation of Na^+ and K^+ Transport by the Cortical Collecting Duct." During the late 1970s, evidence also indicated that the Na^+ channel was regulated by the relative concentrations of Na^+ in the lumen and in the cell, as well as by the intracellular calcium concentration. Interest in the role of Na^+ entry and intracellular Na^+ concentration on the activation or increased synthesis of $(Na^+ + K^+)$-ATPase in the cortical collecting duct also continued. Mineralocorticoids were further found to increase the expression of specific mRNA related to the $(Na^+ + K^+)$-ATPase and the luminal membrane and Na^+ channel. Numerous studies also examined the functional relationship between Na^+ and K^+ transport in the cortical collecting duct; the changes in electrochemical potential driving forces for K^+ secretion were identified and were demonstrated to be correlated with changes in Na^+ delivery and flow rate in the distal nephron.

During the early 1980s, the first intracellular microelectrode studies in the isolated perfused rabbit cortical collecting duct established relative ionic conductances of the luminal and basolateral membranes as well as establishing the relative ionic conductances of the junctional complexes and identified changes induced by in vivo mineralocorticoid treatment. At the same time, it was also recognized that different segments of the collecting duct exhibited varied electrophysiologic properties. Differences in transport among segments of the outer medullary collecting duct (inner and outer stripe regions) and segments of the inner medullary collecting duct were presented at various ASN meetings. In 1987, a symposium was held focusing specifically on the varied functions of segments of the inner medullary collecting duct.

In 1985, patch-clamp results presented at the ASN meeting revealed the kinetics of individual Na^+ channels in the luminal membrane of the rat cortical collecting duct and the effects of mineralocorticoids on the Na^+ and K^+ transport properties of this segment. Throughout the mid-to-late 1980s numerous presentations addressed attempts to isolate, purify, and reconstitute amiloride-sensitive Na^+ channel components. The development of photoactive amiloride analogs and other amiloride-like ligands were critical to the isolation and purification of the channel. At a symposium in 1987, Dale Benos presented the first evidence indicating the size and subunit composition of the purified Na^+ channel protein, whose activity could be reconstituted in planar lipid bylayers or membrane vesicles.

In the 1980s evidence of the thiazide-sensitive NaCl cotransporter, a second mechanism of Na^+ movement across the distal tubule and the cortical collecting duct, was also presented. Later studies on thiazide-binding sites and their isolation attempted to purify this separate cotransport mechanism.

Throughout the 1980s growing data also revealed that numerous autacoids were capable of regulating the activity of the luminal membrane Na^+ channel and the NaCl cotransporter. Early reports during the late 70s and early 80s demonstrated the inhibitory effects of prostaglandins and epoxygenase products on Na^+ transport in this segment. This was followed by proof of the inhibitory effects of bradykinin and atrial natriuretic peptide, the latter being particularly targeted to the inner medullary collecting duct. Recently, considerable interest has developed about the relationships between G-proteins as possible regulators of ion conductances in both luminal and basolateral membranes and the role and innerplay of the inositol phosphates and adenylate cyclase systems in regulating these processes.

Vasopressin-Sensitive Water Transport in the Collecting Duct

The rapid development of our understanding of the mechanism by which vasopressin induces an increase in water permeability of the luminal membrane of the cortical collecting duct is beautifully documented throughout the meetings of the Society. The basic phenomenon of the water permeability increase produced by vasopressin had been thoroughly studied from the late 50s through the 60s, using the frog skin and toad bladder models. These approaches had led to identifying the luminal membrane as a rate-limiting barrier acted upon by vasopressin; investigators envisioned a dual barrier model (presented in Fig. 11.12) involving a diffusion barrier to limit solute access to an underlying porous barrier that was a primary target of vasopressin action.

The toad bladder has continued to be used as a primary experimental model for vasopressin-regulated water permeability until the present time. However, applying the isolated perfused tubule technique to the cortical collecting duct in the late 1960s helped determine the nature of the permeability change induced by vasopressin. Because the cortical collecting duct had only a single-cell layer and lacked the diffusion barrier present in thicker serosal layers and the unstirred regions inherent in the toad bladder, it was possible to examine the vasopressin-sensitive luminal membrane more directly. At ASN meetings in the early 1970s J. A. Schafer and T. E. Andreoli reported that the epithelium itself provided a significant constraint to the diffusion of water and accounted for much of the disparity between osmotically and diffusionally measured water permeabilities that had served as the basis of the pore enlargement hypothesis for vasopressin action. Additional experiments established that the effect of vasopressin in increasing water, urea, and Na^+ permeability in the toad bladder and cortical collecting duct were independent processes. In fact, in the cortical collecting duct, the reflection coefficients for all ions and urea were 1.0, which established that the water permeation pathway induced by vasopressin had to be restrictive enough to exclude solutes as small as Na^+ and urea. By the late 1970s the site of vasopressin-induced water permeability was well recognized as a water channel, rather than a true hydrodynamic pore, permitting only single-file movement of water.

At the same time, the intracellular events responsible for regulating the number of effective water channels were established. A 1974 ASN symposium, "Microtubules and the Effect of Vasopressin," suggested that the cytoskeleton was involved somehow in causing these permeability changes. In 1975, the first freeze-fracture micrographs of intramembrane particles that might be the water channels were presented at the ASN. The 5 investigators involved in this work, William Kachadorian, Sherman Levine, James Wade, Richard Hays, and Vincent DiScala, remained, throughout the 70s and 80s, at the forefront of investigation into this water channel and its regulation in the cortical collecting duct and toad bladder. Within the next 2 years intramembranous particle aggregates, referred to as intramembrane particles (IMPs), were observed in freeze-fracture electron micrographs. Their appearance in the luminal membrane was found to coincide temporally with the increased water permeability induced by vasopressin and to be inhibited by inhibitors of cytoskeletal organization such as colchicine. A symposium at the 1977 ASN meeting, addressing the mechanism of vasopressin (AVP) action, in relation to the intracellular events associated with the increased water permeability, summarized these rapid advances. Thomas Andreoli chaired the symposium, with presentations by Thomas Dousa, Richard Hays and James Wade.

From 1978 through the early 1980s further morphologic evidence suggested that the IMPs were transferred from subapical membrane vesicles in the cytoplasm to the luminal membrane by a process of membrane fusion. Membrane fusion was displayed in beautiful scanning electron micrographs during the same time. The presence of IMPs correlated with vasopressin action were also found in rat and rabbit cortical collecting ducts. The series of events beginning with vasopressin combination with its receptor and the activation of adenylate cyclase, through the insertion and retrieval of water channels in the luminal membrane of the toad bladder and cortical collecting duct, were elegantly summarized in Joseph Handler's 1987 Homer Smith award lecture entitled "ADH Moves Membranes."

During the last few years, increasing attention has been directed at isolating, purifying, and characterizing the proteins that comprise the aggrephores, that is, the IMPs and their associated vesicles. In the mid-1980s the development of extracellular phase fluorescent markers permitted the retrieval of endocytosed aggrephores. By 1986 the physical properties of some of the proteins that comprised these aggrephores were presented. In each of the subsequent years, sessions addressed the identification of candidate water channel proteins on the molecular events that resulted in their sorting and insertion and their fate after endocytosis. It seems likely that within the next few years the water channel itself will be identified, cloned, and sequenced.

Throughout the years, attention was also paid to other intracellular events that modified the actions of vasopressin to increase the water permeability of the luminal membrane. In particular, during the late 1970s the effects of changes in extracellular Na^+ were found to be associated with inverse changes in intracellular calcium, which was demonstrated to be an inhibitor of the water permeability response. At a symposium at the 1982 ASN meeting, Eric Windhager and Ann Taylor presented evidence of the role of intracellular calcium as a regulator of the water permeability response. In subsequent years, it was shown that α_2 adrenergic agents, bradykinin, prostaglandins, and the phosphoinositide system were also regulators of the water permeability response. Numerous abstracts at various ASN meetings have also demonstrated the relation of these regulatory pathways to the effects of changes in systemic ion balance, diabetes insipidus, and drug actions in the pathophysiology of the water permeability response to vasopressin.

Other Advances in The Physiology of Renal Salt and Water Handling

The Third Factor. An important focus of attention since the earliest ASN meeting has been the presence of a natriuretic hormone or "third factor."

Information derived from the early studies of Hugh DeWardener and his associates appeared to indicate that volume expansion released a natriuretic hormone that increased salt excretion. Reports delivered at the first 5 annual ASN meetings argued both in favor of and against the presence of circulating natriuretic hormones and hypotheses about the site of origin and the site of action of this hormone. By the late 1970s it appeared that the natriuretic hormone might be found, when atrial natriuretic peptide was identified, cloned, and sequenced, in rapid fashion. However, later presentations raised doubt about whether atrial natriuretic peptide was, in fact, the natriuretic factor responsible for the results observed in experiments such as DeWardener's.

Subsequent investigations have yielded evidence of another type of natriuretic factor, possibly deriving from the adrenal cortex and/or the hypothalamus. This natriuretic factor has remained as elusive as the original third factor, although current presentations suggest that it is ouabain-like factor that acts to inhibit ($Na^+ + K^+$)-ATPase. It is likely that this will continue to be an area of very active investigation.

Urea Transport along the Nephron. With the development of the passive model for countercurrent multiplication in the inner medulla, it became increasingly important to identify the urea transport characteristics of components of the loop of Henle. During the early 1970s reports at ASN meetings assigned the basic urea permeability properties of the proximal straight tubule and cortical collecting duct. During the 1980s increased attention was paid to urea transport in the thick ascending limb, the inner medullary collecting duct, and the papillary surface epithelium. This information has facilitated the development of a fairly comprehensive picture of urea transport along the nephron and has generally supported the model of passive countercurrent multiplication in the inner medulla.

Cell Volume Regulation. Throughout the 1980s the maintenance of cell volume became a very important topic. It was recognized that renal epithelial cells had to regulate their intracellular environment and volume in spite of rapid and often massive transcellular solute and water fluxes. Several transport pathways were identified which were activated and regulated by changes in cell volume in the proximal tubule, the cortical collecting duct, and the thick ascending limb; by the late 1980s numerous papers concerning the structure of these transporters appeared.

At about the same time, it was also recognized that cells in the inner medullary region had to withstand large changes in osmolality from diuresis to antidiuresis; much of the accommodation was achieved by the dumping or production of intracellular osmolytes in inner medullary cells. During the late 1980s many papers concentrated on the role of osmolytes in maintaining intracellular osmolality and on osmotic regulation. The expression and regulation of the synthesis of intracellular osmolytes and osmolyte transporters were the focus of considerable attention. For example, a free communication at the 1990 meeting presented evidence for the cloning and structure of the aldose reductase gene, an important enzyme in osmolyte production.

Summary

From its inception in 1968, the annual ASN meeting provided an important forum for the presentation of significant new findings regarding the mechanisms and regulation of salt and water transport along the nephron. Starting from the sketchy models of transepithelial ion transport in the proximal and distal tubule that were available in the late 1960s, we now know the primary ion transport mechanisms in both luminal and basolateral membranes of almost every nephron segment. Renal physiologists have been, in fact, on the forefront of the burgeoning field of epithelial transport physiology, and superb symposia and state-of-the-art lectures in this area characterized most ASN meetings.

During the late 1970s the emphasis began to shift toward the kinetic and molecular characterization of the identified transporters. Basic information about various hormones and autacoids and the specific effects they had on transport in different nephron segments developed rapidly. And the intracellular regulatory processes coupling extracellular receptors to membrane transporters became the focus of active investigation. By the late 1980s renal physiology had fully embraced the powerful new methodologies of cell and molecular biology. As we proceed into this new era, numerous investigators are studying the molecular structure-function relation of membrane transporters with expression, cloning, sequencing, and mutagenesis techniques. It seems likely that the next decade of ASN meetings will witness the presentation of the molecular details of the operation and regulation of many transporters involved in salt and water transport, as well as the genetic regulation of their expression.

12

Potassium

Gerhard H. Giebisch and Richard L. Tannen

Introduction

A Quarter Century

Potassium was an important topic for renal physiologists well before the establishment of the ASN, and this tradition has continued throughout the society's first quarter century. These topics are considered here under the general categories of renal potassium excretion, potassium acid-base interrelationships, extrarenal K^+ homeostasis, and the impact of alterations in potassium on other functions.

Renal Potassium Excretion

Status of Renal Potassium Handling Prior to 1967

The advances in our understanding of the renal handling of potassium have been truly impressive. In this brief historical overview of potassium transport we shall follow developments over a 25-year period. From a stage where knowledge was based almost exclusively on indirect and noninvasive approaches we have achieved comprehensive grasp of potassium transport in the kidney. We reached this point by combining whole kidney experiments with single nephron studies and with cell- as well as membrane-oriented investigations.

By the first ASN meeting in 1967 the foundations of our present knowledge of potassium transport by the kidney were based largely on whole kidney experiments. Renal clearance experiments by MacCance and Widdowson, and by Wirz, had demonstrated that under special circumstances the kidney excreted potassium at a rate significantly in excess of the amount filtered. The notion that filtration, reabsorption, *and* secretion participate in the renal control of potassium excretion reached firm ground through the incisive experiments of Berliner, Kennedy, and Orloff and of Mudge, Foulks, and Gilman, based on a series of classical clearance experiments. Berliner and his colleagues proposed that filtered potassium is largely reabsorbed in a "proximal" nephron region and secreted "distally" at a nephron site that also responded to those stimuli known to modulate potassium excretion. They also suggested that sodium reabsorption and potassium secretion were tightly coupled, and that acid-base disturbances and diuretics had profound and predictable effects on renal potassium secretion.

The proposal that a distal nephron site played a key role in the process of potassium excretion received further support from experiments by Morel, who infused radioactive potassium into rats and followed its urinary excretion. He observed that the specific activity of potassium quickly attained that of the renal cortex but differed sharply from that in plasma. He concluded that cell potassium must have contributed importantly to urinary potassium and that filtration and reabsorption could not account for potassium excretion.

The introduction of the stop-flow technique in the late 1950s by Malvin, Vander, and Wilde also provided an approach to localizing potassium transport within the nephron. Evidence supporting an important distal site of potassium secretion was presented in a paper by Sullivan, Wilde, and Malvin in 1960.

The renaissance of applying micropuncture techniques to the study of ion transport in successive tubule segments, and the development of a novel ultramicro-flamephotometer which permitted the accurate measurements of potassium and sodium ions in nanoliter samples, provided investigators with the necessary tools for evaluating potassium transport at the single-nephron level. Such experiments, carried out in rats in the early 1960s by Marsh, Rumrich, and Ullrich and by Malnic, Klose, and Giebisch, firmly established that extensive potassium reabsorption took place along the proximal tubule and the loop of Henle and that a powerful secretory mechanism was present in the "late" distal tubule (initial cortical collecting tubule). Additional studies by Malnic, Klose, and Giebisch included measurements of transepithelial electrical potential differences during the establishment of steady-state concentration gradients and demonstrated the active nature of potassium secretion. Several colleagues, including Windhager, Hierholzer, Wright, Strieder, Khuri, De Mello-Aires, Chomety, and Duarte, collaborated with Giebisch in an extensive series of micropuncture studies which demonstrated that distal potassium secretion was significantly modulated by potassium intake, acid-base disturbances, distal tubule flow rate, several diuretics, and adrenal steroids.

Potassium Transport Along The Nephron

Interest in problems related to renal tubule potassium transport grew continuously from 1968. An important presentation by Morgan and Berliner in 1968 dealt with potassium transport along the loop of Henle. They confirmed extensive net potassium absorption, but inhibition of transport, even net secretion, in some instances, following addition of furosemide to the perfusion fluid.

The introduction of the in vitro tubule perfusion method by Burg, Grantham, and Orloff extended the study of potassium transport to several nephron segments not accessible to micropuncture from the kidney surface. In 1969 Grantham, Burg, and Orloff presented their first paper on sodium and potassium transport and demonstrated the ability of isolated cortical collecting tubules to generate steep potassium concentration gradients that increased with reduction of flow rate and showed marked sodium dependence. The inclusion of transepithelial potential differences enabled the direct comparison of transepithelial chemical with electrical potential differences. Hellman and O'Neil also used the isolated cortical collecting duct in their investigation of the effects of desoxycorticosterone acetate (DOCA) upon electrical conductances. In 1976 they reported an increase of transepithelial resistance after DOCA which was largely accounted for by a fall of the paracellular conductance. They argued that backflux of ions would thus decline after hormone treatment and facilitate the establishment of steeper transepithelial gradients of both sodium and potassium. In an earlier study these authors had reported that cortical collecting tubules, harvested from DOCA-treated rabbits, absorbed sodium and secreted potassium ions at a much faster rate than control tubules.

A paper by Battalina, Bhattacharya, Lacy, and Jamison, also reported in 1976, drew attention to their finding that potassium ions accumulated at strikingly high concentrations along the descending limb of juxtamedullary loops of Henle. Calculations indicated that potassium ions must have been secreted into these tubule segments. Based on these findings, and several additional studies in which potassium accumulation at the tip of Henle's loop of juxtamedullary nephrons was found to vary with the state of potassium balance, the authors developed the concept of *potassium recycling*. According to their view, potassium ions normally leak out of the medullary and papillary collecting duct, enter the interstitium, and diffuse into the descending limb of Henle's loop. It is the potassium secreted by the late distal tubule (initial collecting duct) and cortical collecting duct that represents the source of the recycled potassium. Potassium recycling explains the high medullary and papillary potassium concentrations and the observation that the amount of potassium that accumulates in the medullary interspaces depends critically upon the rate of potassium secretion in the renal cortex.

In 1977 Good and Wright reported interesting observations on the relationship between distal tubule flow rate and distal tubule potassium secretion. Elaborating on earlier observations by Khuri, Strieder, and Giebisch, in which the strong flow-dependence of distal tubule potassium secretion had been established, Good and Wright demonstrated that flow-dependent enhancement of potassium secretion could also occur when sodium reabsorption failed to increase as it does normally under free flow conditions. In Good and Wright's experiments, enhanced potassium secretion was, however, associated with a fall of lumen potassium concentration and the generation of steeper potassium concentration gradients between tubule cells and lumen. These experiments demonstrated that 2 parallel mechanisms exist for potassium secretion. One depends on the coupled exchange of potassium for sodium, the other, relatively uncoupled from sodium, on the establishment of steeper concentration gradients that drive potassium from cell to lumen.

Stanton and Giebisch reported in 1979 on microperfusion studies in which a direct inhibitory effect of systemic metabolic acidosis on distal tubule potassium secretion was demonstrated. Of interest was their finding that at the time of reduced distal secretion, potassium excretion in the whole kidney was significantly elevated. This kaliuresis was explained by the enhanced distal flow rate that follows induction of metabolic acidosis by sodium transport inhibition in proximal tubules. Since flow rate was kept constant in perfused tubules, the *direct* inhibition of potassium secretion by acidosis could be unmasked.

The importance of the interrelationship between sodium and potassium transport was emphasized in 1979 by a symposium entitled "Sodium and Potassium Transport by the Collecting Ducts." Transport was studied by micropuncture in vivo (Reineck), microcatheterization (Sonnenberg), and in vitro microperfusion (Grantham). An interesting presentation by Fine reported on the adaptive and stimulating effects on potassium secretion of uremia. A separate session on potassium transport covered the topics of potassium adaptation (Doucet and Katz; Hayslett, Myketey, Binder, and Aronson), and loss of potassium by magnesium deficiency (Francisco and DiBona). In 1979, Cemericic, Wilcox, and Giebisch reported results of experiments that demonstrated the depressing effects on intracellular potentials and potassium activities by metabolic and respiratory acidosis in proximal tubule cells of rats. These experiments were among the first demonstrating the possibility of measuring both cell potentials and potassium activity in single tubule cells.

Potassium transport in perfused proximal tubules was also investigated by Wasserstein and Agus, and by Work, Troutman, and Schafer. Their reports at the ASN meeting in 1980 demonstrated the ability of proximal straight tubules to secrete potassium, observations that supported participation of these nephron segments in potassium recycling.

A symposium, held in 1987, discussed the function of the *papillary collecting duct*, a nephron segment that had been long neglected. The presentations included a report by Stanton who defined the ion transport functions of this tubule segment and described its capability of bidirectional potassium transport by an amiloride-sensitive, cation-unselective channel in the apical cell membrane.

The development of tissue culture techniques for growing renal tubule cells in vivo, including those of the cortical collecting tubule, provided yet another preparation for the study of potassium transport. A novel primary tissue culture preparation, largely consisting of principal cells, was developed in 1984 by Minuth, Gross, and Frömter and used for electrophysiological characterization of cell properties. In 1985 Bello-Reuss and Webber reported on the electrophysiological properties of a novel renal cell culture preparation in which they characterized the properties of principal cells in vitro by electrophysiological techniques. In 1987 Schmidlin-Ren, N. Fejes-Toth, and G. Fejes-Toth described the effects of vasopressin and luminal pH changes on potassium transport in a tissue culture preparation of collecting tubule cells. The development of cell cultures composed predominantly of principal or intercalated cells constitutes a real advance, not only because now it permits the study of potassium transport in vitro under carefully controlled conditions, but also because it provides enough material for the isolation and analysis of membrane proteins (channels and pumps) which are an integral part of potassium transport systems.

Cell Models of Potassium Transport

Knowledge of the driving forces that act on potassium ions during their translocation across the tubule epithelium provided the information necessary for the construction of cell models of potassium transport along the nephron. From these models researchers gained significant insight into the mechanisms by which potassium ions traverse the apical and basolateral cell membranes of the cells lining the proximal tubule, the thick ascending limb, and the collecting ducts. All these cell models are based on the 2 membrane transport model of Ussing and Koeffoed-Johnsen in which the asymmetrical distribution of pumps and channels infers vectorial transport properties to epithelial cells.

The transport model for *potassium secretion*, originally proposed by Malnic, Klose, and Giebisch in 1964 and 1967, envisaged potassium secretion as a 2-step process, involving active uptake of potassium across the basolateral membrane by the Na-K ATP-ase, and passive diffusion of potassium from cell to lumen across the apical membrane. Such passive egress of potassium was thought to be favored by a significant sodium permeability, selectively localized in the apical membrane, that depolarizes the membrane potential and thus lowers the energy barrier for potassium diffusion. This cell model is a modification of Berliner's original model (1961) in which emphasis was also placed on the coupling between potassium secretion and sodium reabsorption by the basolateral Na-K ATP-ase; it has been confirmed and extended since its inception (Fig. 12.1).

The use of the perfused, isolated kidney enabled Silva, Solomon, Besarab, and Epstein to study potassium excretion and its dependence on metabolic substrates. In 1974 they provided evidence that glucose is a requirement for adequate rates of potassium secretion by the isolated kidney, and in 1975 they showed that the presence of specific metabolic fuel is required for the adequate expression of the stimulatory effect of aldosterone upon potassium

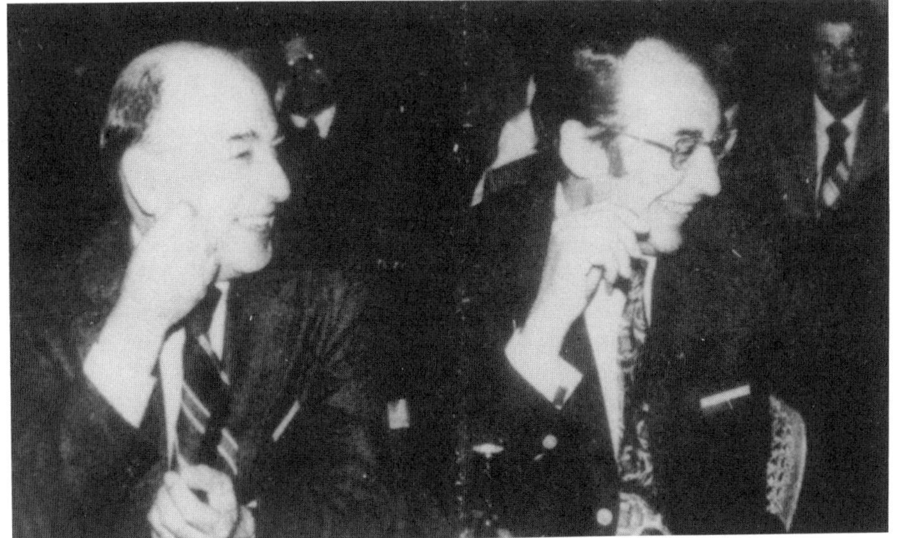

Figure 12.1. Robert Berliner (left) and Gerhard Giebisch at a meeting in 1975.

excretion by the isolated kidney. Both studies underscore the participation of an active component of transport in the overall process of potassium secretion.

Several studies provided support for the proposed two-membrane model of distal potassium secretion. In 1976, Garcia, Malnic and Giebisch disclosed evidence that an externally applied current which changed the transepithelial electrical potential difference across the late distal tubule also altered potassium secretion in a predictable way, that is, increasing the lumen-negative potential accelerated potassium secretion. A microelectrode study of the rabbit cortical collecting tubule in which apical and basolateral membrane potentials were directly assessed confirmed the localization of significant sodium and potassium conductances in the apical membrane of collecting duct cells. This study by Koeppen and Giebisch in 1981 provided additional electrical characterization of the majority of collecting duct cells.

The cell model of potassium secretion was refined by the observation of Velazquez and Wright, who presented evidence in 1981 in support of an additional apical transport pathway for potassium secretion. They suggested the presence of electroneutral potassium-chloride cotransport in distal tubule cells, basing their proposal on distal tubule perfusion studies in which they identified a component of potassium secretion that was voltage- and barium-independent. In 1981 O'Neil demonstrated barium's ability to block the apical cell membrane potassium conductance. Through distal tubule perfusion experiments Wright and his associates demonstrated that the putative potassium chloride cotransporter could be activated whenever the lumen chloride concentration fell to low levels. They argued that such potassium secretion could occur during states of chloride depletion or replacement of distal tubule chloride by other anions such as bicarbonate.

Two important advances in our understanding of distal nephron potassium transport dealt with the resolution of the problem of *distal cell heterogeneity*. Progress in unraveling the mechanisms underlying the process of potassium reabsorption was also important.

Strong evidence supporting the notion of functional cell heterogeneity was forthcoming from morphological studies in which exogenous potassium loading induced significant basolateral membrane amplification in principal cells. Dietary potassium deprivation, on the other hand, led to morphological alterations confined to the apical membrane of intercalated cells. In 1984 the results of such studies were summarized at a symposium, "Morphological Insights into Transport Mechanisms." Emphasis was placed on the morphological changes of principal and intercalated cells following a wide variety of changes in potassium metabolism.

Further support for functional cell heterogeneity was also furnished by studies in which electrical potentials and cell conductances demonstrated marked differences between 2 cell populations. Significant conductances for sodium and potassium are present in principal cells (see reports by Koeppen, 1981, 1982; O'Neil and Sansom, 1983, 1984; Sansom, Muto, and Giebisch, 1985; and Bello-Reuss, 1988), whereas lack of significant ionic conductances has been found consistently in the apical membrane of intercalated cells.

Hayhurst and O'Neil provided additional evidence for functional differences between principal and intercalated cells with observations of differential volume changes in the 2 cell types following lumen perfusion with solutions containing high concentrations of potassium and sodium. Extensive cell swelling was limited to principal cells, but absent in intercalated cells.

The fact that principal and intercalated cells serve different roles in sodium and potassium transport was also observed by Beck, Dörge, Giebisch, and Thurau in electron-probe studies in which the time-dependent uptake of rubidium could be followed in individual cells of superficial distal tubules in the rat. A bolus injection of rubidium led to rapid uptake in principal cells, but only to a low rate of accumulation in intercalated cells. When sodium and potassium transport were stimulated, principal cells responded with acceleration of basolateral rubidium uptake whereas intercalated cells remained quiescent. These studies support the functional "division of labor" in the distal nephron: principal cells secrete potassium and reabsorb sodium and display a high turnover rate of basolateral ATPase-dependent sodium-potassium exchange. In contrast, intercalated cells are thought to subserve hydrogen ion secretion and potassium reabsorption. Accordingly, their basolateral ATPase turnover rate is low.

The process of *potassium reabsorption* by the kidney is less well understood than that of potassium secretion. This occurs, partly, because net potassium reabsorption is difficult to demonstrate and can thus be studied only indirectly or under very special experimental conditions. Giebisch, Klose, and Malnic had already postulated in 1962 and 1964 that an element of potassium reabsorption was present in distal tubules even in the presence of net secretion.

They argued that the magnitude of the transepithelial electrical potential across the distal tubule would predict a much higher lumen potassium concentration than was uniformly observed. To account for the observed lower potassium concentrations, potassium reabsorption must have been present and reduced luminal potassium to levels well below those expected from the electrical potential.

Significant advances occurred in the late 1980s when Doucet, Garg, and Wingo, together with their respective associates, discovered a ouabain-insensitive, K-activated ATPase in isolated tubule segments of the collecting tubule. Enzyme activity was sharply elevated during dietary potassium deprivation, suggesting an adaptive increase of enzyme activity in states of enhanced potassium conservation. Observations by Wingo and Okusa, and their colleagues, confirmed that potassium absorption and hydrogen ion secretion could be inhibited across both the late distal tubule and the medullary collecting duct by gastric potassium-hydrogen ATP-ase inhibitors in animals deprived of potassium. These investigations suggested that potassium reabsorption was activated in states of potassium deprivation and may even totally replace potassium secretion. It is likely that both secretion and reabsorption are active even under conditions of adequate potassium intake so that, at any given time, net potassium transport is the sum of 2 opposing transport events.

Cell models of potassium transport in the *thick ascending limb* of Henle's loop have emphasized the importance of a coupled transport mechanism for sodium, 2 chloride, and potassium ions. The mechanism has been explored both in mammalian tubules and in the amphibian diluting segment which shares many transport properties with its mammalian counterpart in the loop of Henle. In 1981 Greger and Schlatter reported their electrophysiological explorations that firmly supported the cotransport model. The reports by Andreoli, Hebert, and Friedman also provided evidence for a cotransport mechanism in the thick ascending limb of Henle that reabsorbed sodium, 2 chloride, and 1 potassium ions in an electroneutral fashion. Oberleithner and his associates had also observed that the same cotransporter for sodium, 2 chloride, and potassium ions was present in the amphibian diluting segment. Their conclusions were based both on electrophysiological data and on cell sodium activity measurements, the latter providing strong evidence for tight coupling between the countertransported ions. The studies of Greger and his associates, of Hebert, Andreoli, and Friedman, as well as those of Oberleithner, Guggino, and their colleagues demonstrated that loop diuretics act by inhibition of the apical cotransport mechanism. Experiments on vesicle preparation from medullary tissue, reported by Hannafin, Kinne-Safran, and Kinne in 1983, provided independent and further evidence supporting the electroneutral cotransport mechanism in the mammalian thick ascending limb.

All investigators of the mechanism of ion transport in the thick ascending limb of Henle consistently found a significant potassium conductance in the apical cell membrane. This potassium channel, later defined both by Wang and his associates as well as by Greger and his colleagues, serves to supply potassium ions for the cotransport of sodium and chloride the luminal supply would be inadequate in view of the low concentrations of potassium in the tubule fluid entering the loop of Henle. The state of the field was thoroughly reviewed by Stokes in 1985 in an invited lecture, "Perspectives on the Na, K, Cl Cotransport System."

Compared with the potassium transport mechanisms in the *distal nephron* and the loop of Henle, potassium transport in the *proximal tubule* has been less thoroughly investigated. It had been generally assumed that proximal potassium reabsorption was functionally closely linked to sodium-induced fluid transport, but direct evidence had been slow in forthcoming. Bomsztyk and Wright carefully investigated this problem and communicated their results in 1981. In a proximal microperfusion study they demonstrated entrainment of potassium with fluid movement, thus providing strong evidence in support of the view that proximal tubule potassium reabsorption was a secondary active transport that depended on sodium translocation. More recently (1988), A. Weinstein has provided an extensive theoretical study of proximal tubule potassium transport in which the individual components of proximal potassium transport (diffusion, solvent drag, and "active" movement) are derived.

Potassium Transport Across Tubule Cell Membranes

Electrophysiology—Membrane Currents and Conductances. Since the early studies defining the electrical profile of proximal and distal tubule cells, considerable advances have been made in our understanding of the active and passive transport components of apical and basolateral membranes of specific tubule segments. In a major way these studies have also helped to understand the mechanisms by which potassium ions are transported in the kidney. The methods used for the exploration of membrane transport properties have involved tracer flux measurements and electrophysiological approaches which have more recently included also the application of patch-clamp methods for the definition of single potassium channel properties.

The basic models of potassium transport in the proximal tubule, thick ascending limb of Henle, and collecting duct all had in common the presence of a sodium-potassium ATP-ase in the basolateral membrane, yet were distinguished by different transport mechanisms in the apical membrane. Although the apical membrane of proximal tubule cells is only sparingly permeant for potassium ions, the apical membrane cells of the thick ascending limb and of initial and cortical collecting duct cells has a distinct apical potassium permeability subject to regulation by physiological and pathological factors.

In 1980 Biagi reported the first measurements of cell potentials and potassium activities in isolated mammalian perfused tubules. This method, which opened the way to direct exploration of the driving forces acting across the apical and basolateral membrane, was used by a few investigators to explore the conductance properties of single potassium secretory cells. The studies of Horisberger (1986), Koeppen and Giebisch (1981), O'Neil and Sansom (1984), Sansom, Muto, and Giebisch (1985), and Schlatter and Schafer (1986) are examples of studies in which the conductance properties (and in some instances the cell potassium activity) of single collecting duct cells were evaluated. These investigations have contributed significantly to our present concepts of potassium transport mechanisms. In particular, these experiments, carried out in mammalian and amphibian collecting duct cells, yielded information on the complex interaction between potassium and sodium transport operations in the apical and basolateral cell membranes and defined the effects of mineralocorticoids, changes in potassium balance, and acid-base parameters.

Patch-Clamp Techniques. Additional advances were made when the patch-clamp technique was applied to the exploration of potassium and sodium channels in renal tubule cells. During the early 1980s the patch clamp technique, originally introduced by Sackman and Neher in 1976 and described in detail in 1978 and 1981, was adapted to the exploration of channel activity in several tubule preparations. These explorations included the reports by Hunter, Giebisch, Boulpaep, and Kawahara; Palmer, Frindt, Sackin, and their associates; Guggino and his colleagues; Eaton and his associates; and Greger, Schlatter, and Bleich, as well as Frömter and his colleagues. Following the identification of specific potassium channels in apical and basolateral cell membranes, work has continued with studies focusing on the regulation of potassium channels, including the exploration of the effects of cell messengers, hormones, cell volume alterations, and acid-base disorders. Beginning in 1983 the reports of the following researchers and their associates testify to the continued interest of renal electrophysiologists in the exploration of ion channels in tubule membranes: Hunter, Guggino, Kawahara, Palmer, Sackin, Eaton, Parent, Teulon, Stanton, Wang, Schlatter, Greger, Gross, and Frömter. Palmer presented an overview of the techniques and its application to the renal tubule in 1984.

The numerous studies on renal ion channels established the general properties of potassium channels. It soon became clear that several potassium channels are present in renal tissue. Maxipotassium channels (single channel conductance $\approx$ 100 ps) are present in apical membranes of the cells of proximal tubules, thick ascending limb, and cortical collecting tubule. They are calcium-sensitive, activate with depolarization, and are normally in a state of low open probability, but can be made to open with cell swelling. Most likely they play an important role in cell volume regulation; evidence indicates that calcium ions are involved in their activation. Low-conductance potassium channels with a high open probability, sensitive to pH changes (acidosis diminishes and alkalosis enhances channel activity), but not affected by calcium ions, are located in the apical membrane of the cells lining the thick ascending limb and the cortical collecting tubule. They are thought to mediate potassium recycling (thick ascending limb) and potassium secretion (cortical collecting tubule). These channels are under the control of protein-kinase A (stimulation) and protein-kinase C (inhibition), and they are also depressed by ATP.

Potassium channels in the basolateral membrane of tubule cells have also been observed. They are more difficult to study because the removal of the basement membrane poses problems, and enzymatic treatment to facilitate access may affect channel properties. Nevertheless, progress has been made in the identification and characterization of basolateral, potassium channels. They belong to a family of channels with medium conductance (30–50 ps), demonstrate different voltage gating than apical potassium channels (many basolateral potassium channels increase channel activity with cell hyperpolarization), and are calcium-insensitive. These potassium channels are the substrate of the basolateral potassium permeability and thus contribute to the cell potential. Sackin and his colleagues have found that in the proximal tubule these channels participate in the increase of cell potassium permeability that occurs during cell swelling.

Modulation of Potassium Transport

Since 1967 ASN meetings have issued reports of the large number of studies focusing on the regulation of potassium transport. These studies have explored the effects of hormones, changes in acid-base balance, tubule flow rate, and cell messengers on potassium transport. The adaptation of the renal tubule to alterations of potassium metabolism have also been the topic of numerous investigations. A symposium entitled "Potassium Metabolism—The Role of Adaptation" was held in 1980.

Starting with a report by Boyd and Mulrow in 1970 discussing the interesting observation that changes in sodium balance may be critically involved in the release of aldosterone that follow alterations in potassium balance, many studies have concentrated on the definition of the effects of adrenal steroids on potassium metabolism. A recurrent theme was the analysis of the effects of mineralocorticoids and glucocorticoids on renal potassium transport. Wingo reported in 1980 that potassium secretion could still take place through an active process even in tubules of adrenalectomized rabbits, and several reports (Bia and De Fronzo, 1981 and 1982; Field and colleagues, 1983) affirmed that mineralocorticoids directly affect potassium secretion in the distal tubule, whereas glucocorticoids administered at physiological concentrations, stimulated potassium secretion indirectly by enhancing distal flow rate. The direct stimulating effect of vasopressin upon distal tubule potassium secretion was reported by Field and colleagues in 1982 and later confirmed by Schafer and Troutman, in the cortical collecting duct, in 1984. Stanton defined the direct effects of systemic acid-base disturbances on distal tubule potassium secretion in 1980 and a stimulating effect on potassium reabsorption in the loop of Henle by aldosterone in 1985. Inhibitory effects of bradykinin and protein-kinase C inhibitors were detected by Tomita and colleagues in 1984 and by Hays and associates in 1987. The inhibitory effect of phorbol esters on potassium secretion in the perfused cortical collecting tubule was reported by Hays, Baum, and Kokko in 1986.

The effects of flow rate on distal tubule potassium transport had been defined earlier by Khuri and his colleagues and further defined by Good and Wright (see "Potassium Transport along the Nephron" above); in 1980 Stokes also explored the effects of flow rate in the cortical collecting tubule. In this study, Stokes assessed the dependence of potassium secretion on flow rate and sodium transport, defining the concentration range over which sodium ions stimulated potassium secretion.

The dependence of the stimulating effect of aldosterone on distal potassium secretion was the topic of an investigation by Hayhurst and O'Neil in 1985. The authors disclosed strong evidence for a permissive role of luminal sodium supply for the expression of high ATPase levels in cortical collecting ducts. These observations confirmed earlier studies by Petty, Marver, and Kokko. Several studies explored the factors responsible for the insertion of ATP-ase into distal and collecting duct cells (Katz, Garg, and Doucet). The adaptive response of the distal tubule to prolonged exposure of large diuretic-induced sodium loads was the topic of functional and morphological investigations by Stanton and Kaissling (1986). Chronic furosemide administration was found to stimulate both sodium absorption and potassium secretion in perfused tubules at a time when the diuretic effect had been fully dissipated. At the same time, marked amplification of the basolateral membranes of principal cells was observed. These results are of interest because they demonstrate the modifying secondary effects on "downstream" tubule segments in the response to diuretics.

Potassium—Acid Base Interrelationships

Although the issues of potassium effects on acid-base homeostasis and the influence of acid-base perturbations on potassium regulation had captured the interest of renal physiologists for several decades prior to the first ASN meeting in 1967, presentations on this topic during the first decade of meetings were sparse.

In 1968 Sebastian, Morris, and their co-workers from San Francisco presented data on K^+ wasting with renal tubular acidosis (RTA), which indicated that the defect could persist in some patients with distal RTA despite correction of the acidosis and that K^+ wasting was secondary to increased distal delivery of sodium and bicarbonate in patients with the proximal form of the disorder.

In 1975 Fraley and Adler reported that bicarbonate administration could reduce plasma K^+ concentration independent of changes in pH. The effectiveness of bicarbonate therapy has recently grown controversial, reappearing on the program of the 1989 meeting.

The effect of pH homeostasis on renal potassium handling initially appeared on the program in 1979. Using in vivo microperfusion, Stanton and Giebisch elegantly demonstrated that acidosis directly inhibits, whereas alkalosis stimulates, K^+ secretion by the distal tubule. Subsequent studies throughout the 1980s, utilizing this technique as well as in vitro microperfusion, suggested, for the most part, that a low intraluminal pH could impair K^+ secretion. In an attempt to define the cellular events responsible for changes in K^+ secretion, Giebisch and co-workers also used intracellular electrodes both in vivo and in vitro to ascertain the voltage profile and intracellular K^+ activity of cells in response to pH manipulations.

Reports on the effects of both a high potassium and potassium depletion on renal acidification have appeared on the program with regularity since the late 1970s. In 1977 micropuncture studies carried out at Yale examined the mechanism for the decrease in ammonium excretion produced by a high potassium diet. In the late 1980s Good and his co-workers demonstrated that a high potassium concentration impaired ammonium absorption by the thick ascending limb of Henle, suggesting that it could also impair ammonia secretion into the collecting duct. They also directly confirmed in vivo that a high potassium level decreases renal ammonia production. Studies reported in 1979 on the isolated perfused kidney demonstrated that increased ammonium production and excretion could reduce potassium excretion.

A variety of technologies, including the perfused kidney, brush border membrane vesicles, micropuncture, and in vitro microperfusion, were employed during the 1980s to demonstrate that K^+ depletion increases proton secretion by both the proximal and distal portions of the nephron. Beginning in 1988 considerable attention was focused on the role of the gastric H-K-ATPase in the kidney. Molecular biology techniques demonstrated the presence of gastric H-K-ATPase; Wingo's in vitro microperfusion studies, utilizing the H-K-ATPase inhibitor omeprazole, demonstrated inhibition of both proton secretion and K^+ reabsorption in outer medullary collecting ducts of K^+-depleted rabbits; and microscopic techniques by the Florida group indicated that the H-K-ATPase was translocated to the apical border of intercalated cells in response to K^+ depletion. In 1990 it was suggested that a defect in this transport system might account for some forms of distal RTA.

An important experimental observation was made in potassium-depleted normal human volunteers in 1983 by Sebastian and his co-workers from San Francisco. They found that sodium chloride restriction markedly increased plasma bicarbonate concentration produced by modest K^+ depletion; they thereby firmly established that K^+ depletion produces alkalosis in humans and also uncovered an interplay between sodium chloride retention and the induction of alkalosis.

Extrarenal K^+ Homeostasis

In 1974 Hayslett, Binder, and their co-workers reported that the colon adapted to chronic K^+ loading in a fashion analogous to the distal nephron with increased K^+ secretion and an increase in NaK ATPase.

Beginning in 1977 the mediators of cellular potassium uptake appeared as a topic at ASN programs, with regularity. DeFronzo and his Yale colleagues and Sterns and his Rochester co-workers addressed the role of insulin in mediating cellular K^+ uptake as well as whether an increase in potassium directly stimulated pancreatic insulin release. Several reports by these groups, from Beth Israel Hospital in Boston and other research centers, addressed the role of catecholamines in K^+ homeostasis. These reports demonstrated that beta 2 agonists increase cellular uptake of potassium, that their blockade can impede K^+ tolerance and cause hyperkalemia in certain clinical settings, and that their administration might be valuable for the therapy of hyperkalemia but in other settings can provoke pathologic hypokalemia. The reports also suggested that potassium regulation of catecholamine release might serve as a feedback control mechanism for K^+ homeostasis. This topic was of sufficient interest to merit an invited presentation by DeFronzo at a 1987 grand rounds discussion of a hyperkalemic patient with metabolic acidosis.

Several interesting abstracts also addressed the potential impairment of extrarenal K^+ homeostasis in patients with chronic renal failure (CRF): an abstract discussing impaired uptake of potassium by erythrocytes from patients with CRF was reported in 1977; a second, on an impaired response to beta 2 agonists, appeared in 1986; and a third, discussing an impaired response of pancreatic insulin release which was corrected by parathyroidectomy, appeared in 1990.

The Impact of Alterations in Potassium on Other Functions

Throughout the history of the ASN the impact of both a high K^+ intake and of K^+ depletion on a variety of both renal and extrarenal functions has generated considerable interest.

The earliest abstracts presented in the 1970s explored the effects of potassium on aldosterone and renin secretion; the latter still remains somewhat controversial—in 1987 a report suggested that PRA levels in humans correlated directly rather than inversely with plasma potassium concentration.

The abnormality in urinary concentration that accompanies K^+ depletion had been appreciated for several decades before the first ASN meeting, but its pathophysiology had eluded delineation. In 1976 Ferris and his co-workers presented evidence suggesting the concentrating defect might be secondary to an increase in prostaglandin synthesis. Subsequent abstracts throughout the late 70s and early 80s utilizing newly developed microanalytical techniques documented a decrease in papillary solute accumulation, defective chloride transport by the thick ascending limb, and an impaired cyclic adenosine monophosphate (cAMP) response to vasopressin by the cortical and papillary collecting duct. Berl considered this topic in an invited lecture during a symposium on water balance at the 1978 meeting. The accumulation of data suggests that the concentrating abnormality may result from the summation of a variety of K^+-depletion-induced abnormalities.

Pathologic changes in phospholipid metabolism and cell growth induced by K^+ depletion were presented in the mid-1970s by Toback and his co-workers and represent some of the earliest interest by the ASN membership in the topic of growth regulation.

Potassium adaptation by the exercised muscle was reviewed in 1980 by Knochel at a symposium on K^+ metabolism, and the impact of K^+ depletion on muscle metabolism appeared on the program in 1990.

Several novel effects of potassium on renal electrolyte handling were presented during the 1980s. In 1981 Stokes reported that a high potassium concentration impairs sodium absorption by the thick ascending limb and suggested that this might provide a mechanism whereby medullary K^+ recycling increases K^+ secretion. In the past few years Lemann and his co-workers from Milwaukee have reported that a high potassium intake diminishes, whereas K^+ restriction increases, urinary calcium and phosphate excretion. The underlying mechanism remains to be clarified.

Starting in 1981 a substantial number of presentations have addressed the relationship between K^+ homeostasis and hemodynamics, including the issues of hypertension and vascular damage.

In 1981 Linas reported that the decrease in renal blood flow found with K^+ depletion is mediated by both increased angiotensin II and thromboxane; in 1986 it was reported that hyperkalemia both increases renal blood flow and impairs renal autoregulation.

The role of a high potassium intake in hypertension first appeared as a topic at an ASN meeting in 1983, when Tobian and his co-workers reported that a high potassium diet could minimize renal vascular and tubular pathology independent of potassium's capacity to decrease blood pressure. Later presentations from this group expanded this hypothesis to include protection against stroke and left ventricular hypertrophy and provided some pathophysiologic insight into the mechanism of the vascular protective effects of a high K^+ diet. The capacity of a high potassium diet to protect from stroke has been confirmed by other investigators; data also indicate that a high K^+ diet stimulates release of endothelium-dependent relaxing factor which, as Moncado's state-of-the-art address in 1990 summarized, represents the L-arginine:nitric oxide pathway. Tobian was invited to review his studies as a speaker at a 1988 symposium on antihypertensive therapy.

From 1983 to 1985 Linas and his co-workers from Denver reported that potassium depletion was antihypertensive in both genetic and secondary models of hypertension in the rat, and provided some insight into the potential mechanism. In 1985 Krishna confirmed earlier observations that mild potassium depletion resulted in sodium retention; subsequently, he reported that mild potassium depletion also increased blood pressure in both normotensive and hypertensive men, a subject he was invited to discuss in 1989. Lawton and co-workers also suggested recently that a low K^+ diet can exert hypertensive effects. The disparity between the animal and human studies concerning the role of K^+ depletion in hypertension is currently unexplained.

13

Renal Acid-Base Physiology

Philip R. Steinmetz, David Z. Levine, and Gerhard H. Giebisch

Introduction

A Quarter Century

The role of the kidney in regulating systemic acid-base balance and the mechanisms for urinary acidification were major areas of investigation in the 1940s and 1950s, an early growth period for renal physiology. The studies of Robert Pitts and his associates at Syracuse University and Cornell University Medical College defined the overall operations of urine acidification by the intact kidney. Robert Berliner and his coworkers at the laboratory of kidney and electrolyte metabolism at the National Heart Institute characterized the ion exchange mechanisms along the nephron. They studied the renal secretion of hydrogen ions as it related to potassium secretion and sodium reabsorption from the overall behavior of electrolyte excretion by the kidney. The advent of new techniques for the examination of acid-base events in individual renal tubules permitted the field to expand and investigators to explore a wide range of new questions about the functions of the major tubule segments that were accessible to micropuncture. As a result, renal acid-base physiology gathered considerable momentum during the 1960s and contributed to the flourishing of the larger field of nephrology which was preparing for organizing its own Society in 1967.

In this chapter we shall first attempt to set the stage for renal acid-base physiology in the mid-1960s. The field was full of "élan vital" and was already differentiated in a number of subdisciplines. Then, we shall follow these disciplines, that is, the ones dealing with renal acid-base physiology over the 25-year period leading up to the anniversary of 1992. Rather than presenting an exhaustive review of all things "acid-base," we shall follow the major trend that can be discerned in the shifts of focus in the activities of the members of the society and the research programs of the annual meetings. We plan to highlight the advances which constitute this trend somewhat selectively according to our perceptions of how they came about. The constraints of the format shall not permit us to be as complete as we might have been for a more encyclopedic review of renal acid-base history. We apologize for the inevitable shortcomings of this approach. The shift in the focus of research over the years has been from the overall renal mechanisms to ever smaller scales of structure and function, reflecting the most fundamental events we can reach with our experimental tools. The period covers a great many in vivo and in vitro studies of different tubule segments; it witnessed a variety of approaches to the study of individual epithelial cells and to the appropriate cellular models. Once satisfactory double membrane models were established, the attention shifted to the single membrane, apical or basolateral, and to the individual transport molecules that do the work in the epithelial cell.

This trend of our studies toward the cellular and molecular levels has been a major force over the first 25 years of the Society, yet the spectrum of activities has been diverse. In some complex areas of investigation the initial approaches and interpretations were inadequate. Progress in understanding could only be made after comprehensive and painstaking efforts of a few dedicated investigators with the courage to avoid band-wagon conclusions. Where progress depended on patience and precision and the focus remained steady on *one* level of organization. In other endeavors physiologic discoveries were applied to the understanding and improved recognition of renal disorders of hydrogen ion secretion or were applied to the better integration of acid-base factors on a larger scale. We shall include several of theses contributions as we develop our theme and we shall devote the last section to new endeavors to apply the knowledge of molecular biology to an understanding of large complex systems and of clinical disorders of acid-base balance.

State of Renal Acid-Base Physiology in the 1960s

In the mid-60s many of the nephrologists working at university hospitals were well trained in clearance and balance studies. In the field of acid-base balance, especially, there was a strong tradition for workmanship in conducting physiologic studies in whole animals and in human subjects. High standards had been established by the associates and trainees of Homer Smith at New York University Medical School, of John Peters at Yale University, and of Robert Pitts at Cornell University College of Medicine, to mention a few of the leaders. The renal responses to hypo- and hypercapnia and to the administration of acid or alkali loads were studied extensively and interpreted in a sophisticated manner in terms of renal mechanisms in either the proximal or distal nephron. Arnold Relman, at the time at Boston University School of Medicine, and William Schwartz at Tufts University had developed a following of young nephrologists in Boston interested in the role of anions in acid-base balance and in clinical acid-base disorders. They were able to distinguish between distal mechanisms involving changes in the rate of Na/H exchange and proximal mechanisms involving changes in HCO_3^- reabsorption by the proximal tubule by precisely defining the overall operations of the kidney under control and under experimental conditions. Although by present standards these mechanisms included a variety of transport processes lumped together, they were useful simplifications not only for understanding acid-base disorders, but also for providing a rationale in their management. The principals of electroneutrality and the reciprocal behavior of individual anions like Cl^- and HCO_3^- or individual cations like Na^+, K^+, and H^+ within the total anion or cation concentrations in body fluids were themes that were applied widely. During the first decade of the society's existence these themes were explored further and precise distinctions were made between overall ion exchange operations at the levels of the kidney and the tubule and direct coupling of ion flows in transport systems at specific cell membranes. At a smaller scale the transport physiologists again tried to account for the balance of charge, first across the membranes of epithelial cells and later across each of the transport molecules involved in acid-base transport.

In the mid-60s in vivo micropuncture studies had already made significant contributions to the understanding of tubular acidification. The first micropuncture studies had been carried out in amphibia by Montgomery and Pierce in 1937 in the laboratory of Richards in Philadelphia. These and subsequent studies in 1956 by Gerhard Giebisch at the Department of Physiology, Cornell had demonstrated that in the amphibian tubule the fluid remains isohydric in the proximal segment and first becomes acidified in the distal segment. These studies, which had influenced the assumptions of classic renal physiologists for many years, were superceded in 1960 by a micropuncture study of the rat kidney by Carl Gottschalk, William Lassiter, and Margaret Mylle at the University of North Carolina. Their study indicated that in the mammalian kidney acidification does begin in the proximal tubule as judged from the pH of tubular fluid samples measured with the quinhydrone microelectrode. In the proximal tubule the pH fell about half a pH unit and progressive acidification appeared to occur in the distal convoluted tubule and collecting duct. The mechanism of acidification of the proximal tubule was explored in 1965 by Floyd Rector, Norman Carter, and Donald Seldin (Fig. 13.1) at the University of Texas Southwestern Medical School by means of newly developed pH-sensitive glass microelectrodes. In an important contribution to the understanding of proximal HCO_3^- reabsorption,, they convincingly demonstrated that the filtered HCO_3^- is converted to H_2CO_3 by the secretion of H^+ into the tubular lumen. They measured the in situ pH in the lumen of the proximal tubule and demonstrated that during carbonic anhydrase inhibition this in situ pH is lower than that of a fluid sample in which the H_2CO_3 has reached equilibrium with the CO_2 tension of plasma. Hence, the rate of H_2CO_3 formation from HCO_3^- and secreted H^+ exceeds the rate at which H_2CO_3 can be dehydrated to CO_2 by the uncatalyzed reaction. The existence of a disequilibrium pH had been suggested

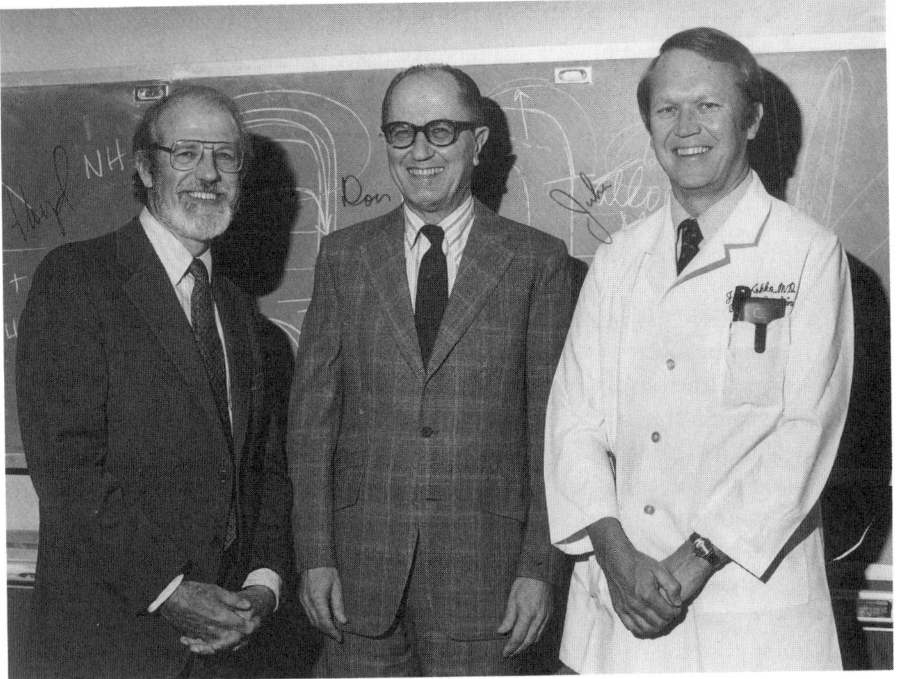

Figure 13.1. (From left to right) Floyd Rector, Donald Seldin, and Juha Kokko taken at the University of Texas Southwestern Medical School.

a few years earlier by Mackenzie Walser and Gilbert Mudge at Johns Hopkins School of Medicine on the basis of estimates of the uncatalyzed rate of dehydration of H_2CO_3 and the observed rate of HCO_3^- reabsorption. The studies by Rector and associates strongly indicated that in the proximal tubule HCO_3^- is reabsorbed by a mechanism of H^+ secretion and that carbonic anhydrase is normally available to the luminal fluid. These studies were extended in a number of new directions and led to a great many presentations on the role of the CO_2 tension and luminal carbonic anhydrase during the annual meetings of the Society.

Another major subject of study in the 1960s was the renal production and excretion of ammonia. The adaptive responses of the kidney to acid-base changes were being examined systematically in the laboratory of Pitts and his associates in New York and in the E. P. Joslin Research Laboratory of Cahill and his associates at Harvard Medical School. The importance of the proximal tubule for ammonia secretion was recognized by Giebisch and his associates working next door to Pitts at Cornell. The developments in our understanding of the metabolism and handling of ammonia by the kidney are reviewed in the chapter on renal metabolism.

The introduction of the turtle urinary bladder as a model preparation for the study of anion transport by William Brodsky and Theodore Schilb at the University of Louisville School of Medicine and the initial studies on the cellular mechanisms of urinary acidification in this preparation by Philip Steinmetz and Howard Frazier at Harvard also took place in the mid-60s just before the Society was established.

Shift of Focus to the Tubular Level

The Convoluted Tubules

With the success of micropuncture studies and the realization that many of the major questions in renal acid-base handling were not approachable by refinements in micromeasurements and perfusion techniques, more and more laboratories dedicated their efforts to the study of individual tubules. The work by Floyd Rector and his associates on the dependence of bicarbonate reabsorption in the proximal tubule on luminal carbonic anhydrase and its implications for mechanisms of hydrogen secretion stimulated new investigations of acid-base transport in the segments of the proximal and distal tubule that were accessible to micropuncture in vivo. Gerhard Malnic and his associates Frederico Vieira and Marguerida De Mello-Aires in the department of physiology at the University of Sao Paulo used a pH sensitive antimony microelectrode to explore the acidification processes in both the proximal and distal tubules. They confirmed the major observations on the disequilibrium pH after carbonic anhydrase inhibition of Rector's group. As Rector had done, they assumed that the tubule CO_2 tension used to calculate the equilibrium pH was the same as that of systemic arterial blood. It is of interest that subsequent micropuncture studies in which the PCO_2 of the tubular fluid was measured directly in situ have yielded a range of values most of which have been higher than arterial blood. Thus, Morgan Sohtell and Bertil Karlmark at the University of Uppsala developed a microelectrode designed for measuring PCO_2 in small tissue compartments and found an elevated PCO_2 in situ in the proximal tubule. Thomas DuBose and his associates working at the time in the laboratory of Juha Kokko in Dallas with an electrode adapted from an earlier model of Caflish and Carter, also reported values above arterial PCO_2. Similarly, John Gennari and his associates at the University of Vermont School of Medicine found somewhat elevated values. In contrast, in his most recent studies, Malnic finds that the PCO_2 values are the same as in arterial blood if CO_2 diffusion problems are avoided in the inner reference solution of the microelectrode. All studies, however, have supported the existence of an acid disequilibrium pH after carbonic anhydrase inhibition.

Despite the acceptance of hydrogen ion secretion as the major mechanism of bicarbonate reabsorption in the proximal tubule at the meetings of the Society during the 1970s, investigators were aware of the fact that a fraction of bicarbonate reabsorption remained to be explained. Thomas Maren, of the department of pharmacology and therapeutics at the University of Florida

College of Medicine, kept investigators on their toes by pointing out that carbonic anhydrase inhibitors failed to inhibit some 60 to 70% of filtered bicarbonate in whole kidney studies and, hence, that proximal bicarbonate reabsorption persisted to a significant extent after acetazolamide. He continued to make the case for the existence of a major component of bicarbonate reabsorption in the ionic form. It was not until the end of the 1970s that investigators had completed enough studies to account for the apparent discrepancies between the effects of the inhibitors on bicarbonate reabsorption in the proximal tubule and in the whole kidney. Martin Cogan, David Maddox, and David Warnock, working with Rector in San Francisco, demonstrated near-complete inhibition of bicarbonate reabsorption in proximal tubules during free-flow conditions. Similarly, Maurice Burg at NIH demonstrated virtually complete inhibition in the isolated perfused rabbit proximal tubule (see below). Their studies and studies from several other laboratories provided the required explanations. Some of the bicarbonate that escapes reabsorption in the proximal tubule is reabsorbed at more distal sites despite carbonic anhydrase inhibition. Some reabsorption occurs in the deep nephrons not accessible to micropuncture; finally, the small portion that continues to be reabsorbed in the proximal tubule can be accounted for by the recycling of carbonic acid.

The cortical tubules accessible to micropuncture were explored not only during free-flow conditions, but also by microperfusion techniques. Malnic and coworkers explored the kinetics of bicarbonate reabsorption by stopped flow microperfusion by the continuous monitoring of luminal pH in split droplets containing bicarbonate. They also went a step further in controlling the peritubular as well as the luminal environment by introducing methods for peritubular capillary perfusion. This approach enabled them to explore the effects of tubular buffer load and peritubular pH and PCO_2 on the rate of acidification independently of systemic changes in extracellular volume and composition. This attempt to exclude volume factors was quite compelling at the time because of the recognition that extracellular fluid volume expansion caused substantial inhibition of bicarbonate reabsorption in the rat, by Mabel Purkerson and her associates working with Neil Bricker at Washington University, and in the dog, by Neil Kurtzman serving a tour of duty at Brooke Army Medical Center. Malnic's perfusion experiments demonstrated that the luminal bicarbonate load and the peritubular pH were more important in the regulation of bicarbonate reabsorption that the peritubular CO_2 tension per se. Much of the evidence for increased bicarbonate reabsorption during acute hypercapnia had been developed originally during whole animal studies in the 1950s. David Levine from the University of Ottawa Medical School was one of the early investigators to attempt to account for the role of the individual components of systemic acid-base balance. His micropuncture studies indicated that hypercapnia stimulated proximal bicarbonate reabsorption only if the extracellular fluid bicarbonate levels were allowed to rise. Subsequent studies under free-flow conditions by Marty Cogan and in isolated perfused proximal tubules by Sei Sasaki, Christine Berry, and Floyd Rector in San Francisco have further defined the importance of the bicarbonate concentrations on the two sides of the epithelium. They have also indicated, consistent with Levine's results, that increases in pCO_2 are less effective in increasing the rate of proximal HCO_3 reabsorption than decreases are in reducing it.

With the development of microcalorimetry for the measurement of total CO_2 by Gerald Vurek and coworkers at the National Institutes of Health, studies of bicarbonate transport were facilitated through free-flow micropuncture studies as well as through studies of isolated perfused tubule segments. The load dependence of bicarbonate reabsorption by the proximal tubule was characterized further by David Maddox and John Gennari, University of Vermont, in Munich-Wistar rats. They reported a strong dependence of the H^+ secretion rate on the bicarbonate load in the early proximal tubule.

As the 1970s advanced, many of the renal laboratories expanded their methodologies to include microperfusion studies of isolated perfused tubule segments. Segments that had been inaccessible to in vivo micropuncture could now be isolated, perfused, and studied by the methods introduced by Maurice Burg and his associates at NIH. The permeabilities and the characteristics of bicarbonate transport were examined in the different segments of the proximal tubule as well as in thick ascending limb, distal tubule, cortical collecting duct (CCD), and outer medullary collecting duct (OMCD). Some of these studies were included in Burg's Homer Smith award lecture at the 1977 annual meeting of the Society.

One interesting issue during this period was the sodium dependence of proximal bicarbonate reabsorption, because several major transporters responsible for H^+ secretion in the proximal tubule have proved to be sodium dependent, that is, an apical Na/H antiporter and a basolateral Na-3 (HCO_3) symporter (see section below, under Focus on the Membrane Level). The initial in vivo micropuncture studies of rat proximal tubules by Malnic, Giebisch, and Ullrich and their respective coworkers revealed no strict dependence on HCO_3^- reabsorption on luminal sodium. Later more elaborate studies by Chan and Giebisch demonstrated that HCO_3^- reabsorption was reduced but not abolished, by sodium removal. The in vitro preparation of the perfused rabbit proximal tubule had the advantage of permitting greater control over the composition of the luminal and bath solutions and enabling Maurice Burg and Dwight McKinney at Bethesda to demonstrate that inhibition of sodium transport by either sodium removal or ouabain addition caused a marked inhibition of HCO_3^- reabsorption.

Before the new technique (see section, Focus on the Membrane Level) for continuous monitoring of intracellular pH by means of fluorescent dyes were developed, intracellular pH estimates were made on the basis of the distribution of the weak acid indicator dimethyloxaxolidinedione (DMO). Albert Struyvenberg, working in Arnold Relman's laboratory at Boston University, reported in 1968 that the intracellular pH of separated canine tubules was relatively alkaline. These initial studies and subsequent studies in 1980 by Jack Kleinman and his associates at the Medical College of Wisconsin demonstrated that acetazolamide made the cells more alkaline, whereas ouabain caused acidification of the cells. Maurice Bichara and Michel Paillard and several associates working in Paris, in affiliation with the Institut National de la Santé et de la Recherche Medicale, observed cell acidification following ouabain and following removal of external sodium. Another line of evidence for the existence of a Na/H antiporter was reported the following year in the isolated perfused preparation of proximal tubule. George Schwartz at the Albert Einstein College of Medicine was able to reverse the usual direction of transport by the Na/H antiporter by acidifying the luminal perfusate or by increasing the cell sodium concentration. These studies all demonstrated the importance of the antiporter first characterized by Heini Mürer, Ullrich Hopfer, and Rolf Kinne at the Max Planck Institute in Frankfurt in brushborder vesicles.

The attractiveness of a simplified model calling for one mechanism for a major nephron segment like proximal tubule, however, did not match reality for long. As soon as the characteristics of the Na/H antiporter were better defined, new evidence began appearing indicating that the brush border contained a second H^+ secreting mechanism. In 1982 Eva Kinne-Saffran, Renaud Beauwens, and Rolf Kinne at the Max Planck Institute provided evidence for an ATP-driven proton pump in brush border membranes from rat cortical tubules. A variety of old and new studies has supported the importance of a sodium-independent primary active transport system in bicarbonate reabsorption by the proximal tubule. As discussed, the in vivo micropuncture studies allowed for a sodium-independent component of bicarbonate reabsorption. In 1985 Norman Bank and his associates at Montefiore Hospital in New York provided evidence for a DCCD (dicyclohexylcarbodiimide)-sensitive component of proximal bicarbonate reabsorption in perfused proximal tubules. Ira Kurtz at UCLA provided evidence for a role of a glycolysis-dependent H^+-ATPase in cell pH regulation and presumably bicarbonate reabsorption in rabbit S3 proximal tubule. Similarly, studies by Dennis Brown and his associates on the localization of antibodies against vacuolar H^+-ATPase indicate that the brush border membrane is a site for this ATPase (see section 6 under Focus on the Single Membrane Level).

From Distal Tubule to Collecting Duct

The classical clearance studies of the 1950s and early 1960s had yielded many useful concepts and a black box approach which was applied widely to the understanding of clinical acid-base disorders. With the advent of in vivo micropuncture techniques, investigators soon confirmed that the distal tubule participated in urinary acidification. However, it also soon became apparent that the processes of urinary acidification continued well beyond the late segments of distal tubule still accessible to puncture. What had been called the late distal tubule became the connecting tubule to the collecting duct. Considerable progress in the understanding of acid-base transport was made when segments of the rabbit collecting duct were isolated and perfused for study in vitro. Remarkable differences were found between the cortical collecting duct (CCD) and outer medullary collecting duct (OMCD) with its inner and outer stripes, as investigators learned to identify and separate each of the segments for study. At the same time microcatherization techniques were refined for study of the inner medullary collecting duct (IMCD). One of the first studies pertinent to distal urinary acidification was carried out in 1974 by Larry Stoner, Maurice Burg, and Jack Orloff at NIH. They observed in the perfused cortical collecting tubule that amiloride caused a reversal of the lumen negative to a lumen positive potential, and recognized that this lumen positive voltage might represent the electrical activity of an acidification process. They demonstrated that this positive voltage was abolished by acetazolamide and increased by increased CO_2 tension. A few years later Bruce Koeppen and Sandy Helman at the University of Illinois further characterized the mechanism of acidification in the rabbit CCD by demonstrating that it was an active process that could generate a pH gradient when HCO_3^- was omitted from the luminal perfusion solution. These studies in the CCD suggested that the process of urinary acidification represented an electrogenic mechanism of H^+ secretion comparable to that observed in turtle urinary bladder (see section under Focus on the Cellular Level). The acid-base behavior of the CCD, however, proved to be surprising: in the rabbit this segment was shown to be capable of either net acid or net alkali secretion depending on dietary intake. In 1977 and 1978 Dwight McKinney and Maurice Burg demonstrated in an interesting series of studies at NIH that cortical tubule segments dissected from alkali-loaded rabbits would secrete HCO_3^-, whereas segments from acid-loaded rabbits reabsorb HCO_3^-. Bicarbonate secretion has also been observed in isolated perfused rat collecting ducts by James Atkins working with Burg and in rat distal tubules studied in vivo by David Levine and his associates at Ottawa. The characteristics of the bicarbonate secreting transport systems and the studies attempting to identify the cells responsible for bicarbonate secretion are reviewed in the sections on cellular level and single membrane level. The remarkable conclusion from a great many studies is that the function of HCO_3^- secretion is limited to a small segment of the nephron, namely the late distal tubule, the connecting tubule, and the CCD. The OMCD is not involved in HCO_3^- secretion, even after alkali loading. The OMCD, on the other hand, has potent transport systems for H^+ secretion. William Lombard, Juha Kokko, and Harry Jacobson at the University of Texas Southwestern measured the rates of bicarbonate reabsorption in this segment by microcalorimetry and demonstrated that bicarbonate was reabsorbed at brisk rates in the OMCD. Studies by Victor Schuster and John Stokes at the University of Iowa have clarified some of the differences between CCD and OMCD and have indicated that the OMCD is not involved in HCO_3^- secretion (see sections referred to above). The characteristics of OMCD acidification were explored by Dennis Stone working with Donald Seldin, Juha Kokko, and Harry Jacobson. They demonstrated in 1983 that mineralocorticoid hormone stimulated HCO_3^- reabsorption in adrenalectomized rabbits and that this stimulation occurred independent of sodium transport, results similar to those reported for H^+ secretion in turtle and toad urinary bladder. Acidification by the OMCD, in addition to being stimulated by aldosterone, was found to be inhibited by the hormone PGE_2 in studies by Steven Hays working with the same group in Dallas.

The first evidence indicating that the IMCD contributed to H^+ secretion along the nephron was reported by Karl Ullrich and his associates in 1958 at the Physiologic Institute at the University of Göttingen. They demonstrated a progressive lowering of pH along the IMCD of the hamster by means of a microcatherization technique. Harold Sonnenberg at the University of Toronto applied this technique to the rat IMCD in 1974. During the 1980s several further studies of urinary acidification by the IMCD were undertaken by the associates of Edward Alexander and John Schwartz at Boston University. Howard Bengele, Mark Graber, and other associates played an important role in describing the acid-base behavior of this segment during acid-base disorders. In recent years this work was extended to the study of cell cultures of the IMCD which revealed the existence of a NEM-sensitive H^+-ATPase as well as a Na/H exchanger. The study of the precise distribution of these transporters among the segments of the IMCD and their regulation by second messengers continues into the 1990s by the Boston group, by Kleinman and his associates in Milwaukee, and by Susan Wall and Mark Knepper and their associates at NIH.

Focus on the Cellular Level

Urinary Acidification by Model Epithelia

Understanding of epithelial transport was greatly advanced by the introduction of isolated epithelial preparations such as frogskin and toad urinary bladder, which could be studied in vitro as flat sheets mounted in lucite chambers between two bulk solutions that could be sampled and monitored. Ussing and his associates in the laboratory of zoophysiology at the University of Copenhagen were the first to develop a double-membrane model for the description of transport across the apical and basolateral membranes of epithelial cells. They applied this analysis to the transport steps for sodium across the frogskin and demonstrated that the two steps were very different. The entry step represented downhill movement along an electrochemical sodium gradient, whereas the exit across the basolateral cell membrane occurred uphill and required the metabolic energy of ATP hydrolysis. Leaf and his associates at Massachusetts General Hospital reached similar conclusions for the toad urinary bladder. They observed that in toads originating from the Dominican Republic the net rate of sodium transport was equivalent to the short-circuit current and, hence, that sodium transport was the principal electrogenic active transport process. This made the toad bladder an attractive model for the study of sodium transport but less attractive to acid-base transport physiologists. Although it was later found that bladders of toads obtained from mainland South America did acidify the urine by an electrogenic mechanism, acid-base physiologists remained on the sidelines until the mid-1960s when Schilb and Brodsky, at the University of Louisville, made the interesting observation that the contents of a sac preparation of the urinary bladder of the fresh water turtle acidified with time. This observation, made during a study of the osmotic properties of the turtle bladder, led them to a new study of the mechanism of urinary acidification in this urinary epithelium. They postulated that the nature of the acidifying process could be uncovered from the way this process affects the transmural pH and CO_2 gradients in vitro. Brodsky had carried out theoretical and experimental studies a few years earlier in the intact kidney and had suggested that the reabsorption of HCO_3^- per se might play a major role in acidification by the renal tubules. Even if HCO_3^- was in short supply in the lumen, the diffusion of CO_2 into the tubular fluid could generate HCO_3^- by the hydroxylation of CO_2 and this HCO_3^- could be reabsorbed by a HCO_3^- transport system. Such a mechanism would lower the luminal pCO_2 and allow for urinary acidification without H^+ secretion. At the time, Thomas Maren also entertained a direct mechanism for reabsorptive HCO_3^- transport on the basis of observations that a significant portion of HCO_3^- reabsorption occurred independent of carbonic anhydrase. With this background Schilb and Brodsky approached the turtle bladder sac preparation as a possible model for the study of HCO_3^- reabsorption. Steinmetz and Frazier and their associates at Harvard, on the other hand, decided to study the turtle bladder as a flat epithelial sheet in the Ussing chamber to define the profile of active and passive steps across the epithelium. To do this they exploited greatly simplified conditions, that is, without exogenous CO_2 and HCO_3^- and without transepithelial electrochemical gradients, the condition of "level" secretion. They measured the rate of luminal acidification by a pH stat titration method and were able to demonstrate that it represented an active transport process that was not directly dependent on sodium transport and that was electrogenic. This work was presented in Los Angeles at the first annual meeting of the Society in 1967. One disagreement between Schilb and Brodsky and Steinmetz's group was the nature of the transported ion responsible for the acidification. Based on their measurements of transmural pH and total CO_2 gradients in the sac preparation, Schilb and Brodsky had calculated that the free CO_2 in the luminal solution was lowered consistent with outward HCO_3^- transport. This interpretation was supported by their initial finding that acetazolamide did not inhibit the transport process and by Maren's 1967 review which listed turtle bladder as a tissue not containing carbonic anhydrase. In contrast,

Steinmetz demonstrated H^+ addition to the luminal solution under conditions under which only metabolic CO_2 and HCO_3^- were present and observed inhibition of H^+ secretion by the carbonic anhydrase inhibitor acetazolamide. The controversy of the transported ion in urinary acidification led to detailed studies of the CO_2 profiles across the epithelium in both the sac and the sheet preparation and to further studies showing that carbonic anhydrase was present in a minority population of epithelial cells. Green and Frazier and, later, John Schwartz working with Steinmetz measured the PCO_2 of the sac preparation with a PCO_2 electrode and observed PCO_2 elevations within the sac consistent with a process of H^+ secretion. They also measured the metabolic CO_2 production with a conductivity meter and profiled the metabolic CO_2 concentrations across the epithelium in the Ussing chamber in the absence of exogenous CO_2. Schilb and Brodsky recalculated their free CO_2 values and perfected their methods of CO_2 sampling from the sac preparation. They agreed that a lowering of the PCO_2 in the sac preparation could not be demonstrated consistently in experiments of the kind they had initially reported, that is, in turtles kept at room temperature, but they took the position that the PCO_2 elevations reported by Green and Schwartz and their coworkers in Boston were not conclusive evidence for H^+ secretion because of the possible contribution of metabolic CO_2 production. At the same time Schwartz and Steinmetz agreed that the evidence for H^+ secretion should not be based on PCO_2 results alone. The outcome of this particular experimental approach was never completely resolved. During the 1980s Schilb and Brodsky returned to the CO_2 gradient analysis and applied it to bladder sacs of turtles that had been adapted in vivo to a hot environment of 32°C and reported that the process of acidification of the luminal solution was associated with lowering of the PCO_2. By this time, however, investigators in the field had become involved in purification studies of a vacuolar H-ATPase which was thought to be the acidification pump and were not longer willing to tackle the issue by way of an analysis of the CO_2 gradient.

Cells Specialized in Acid-Base Transport

The second issue regarding the presence or absence of carbonic anhydrase in the turtle bladder turned out to be quite important for the understanding of the cell biology of urinary acidification. In 1970 Scott, Shamoo, and Brodsky at Mt. Sinai Medical School demonstrated that the mucosal cells of turtle bladder did contain carbonic anhydrase that could be distinguished from that from red cell contamination. In the same year Rosen, working in the department of pathology at Beth Israel Hospital in Boston, reported his first histochemical studies indicating that the carbonic anhydrase was confined to a minority population of epithelial cells. These cells are now called carbonic anhydrase-rich or intercalated cells; in several of the epithelia they are also mitochondria-rich. The discovery of a population and later certain subpopulations of carbonic anhydrase-rich cells became important in the 1980s when increasing evidence suggested that the different transport functions reside in different types of epithelial cells.

To return to the early 1970s, the initial simplicity of the turtle urinary bladder as a model epithelium for urinary acidification was disturbed by the discovery of an active transport system for urinary HCO_3^- secretion. This system was recognized by Schwartz and Steinmetz when they tried to add exogenous CO_2 and HCO_3^- to their formerly "CO_2-free" preparation. By first brining net H^+ secretion to zero by means of an opposing pH gradient, they were able to measure HCO_3^- secretion into the mucosal solution by pH stat titration. Bruce Leslie, a Harvard medical student, then elected to work on the mechanism of HCO_3^- secretion for a year, as a predoctoral research fellow. He defined the overall characteristics of this secretory system as a one-for-one Cl for HCO_3 exchange that operated independently of sodium transport, but was inhibited by acetazolamide. For several years, this transport system appeared to represent a reptilian peculiarity that diminished the usefulness of the model preparation. By 1978, however, this transport system received new attention when McKinney and Burg at laboratory of kidney and electrolyte metabolism, National Heart Institute, observed that the cortical collecting duct of the rabbit was capable of net HCO_3^- secretion. Burg and his

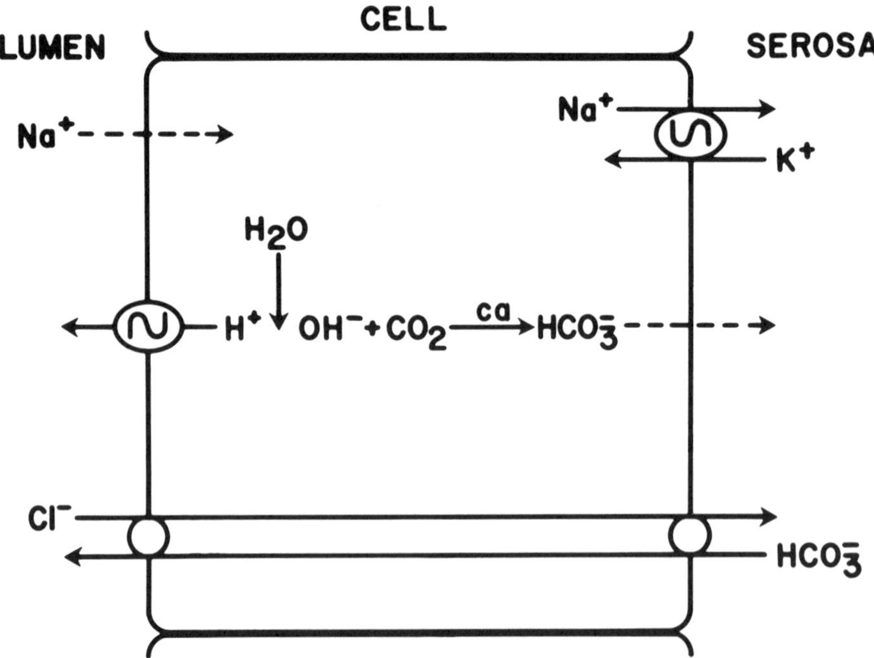

Figure 13.2. a. Black box model of early 1970s. Epithelial cell of turtle urinary bladder contains three transport systems. b. During the 1980s, the major transport functions are assigned to specialized cells, granular cells, and α and β type carbonic anhydrase (CA) cells. From Steinmetz PR. *Am. J. Physiol.* 251: F173, 1986.

associates—first, McKinney, and later, Garcia Austt, Good, Knepper, and Star—proceeded to characterize this HCO_3^- secretory system in the cortical collecting duct. The initial studies had suggested that the system was sodium dependent, but subsequent studies from the same laboratory as well as from the laboratory of Schuster at the University of Iowa School of Medicine suggested that HCO_3^- secretion was dependent on Cl^- rather than on Na^+ and that it was electroneutral comparable to that of turtle bladder.

To appreciate the recent developments in the understanding of the structure-function relationships of acid-base transport in α and β type intercalated cells, it is best to return to a study of the surface characteristics of turtle bladder before and after inhibition of H^+ secretion by the disulfonic stilbene SITS. In 1981 Russ Husted and his associates, at the University of

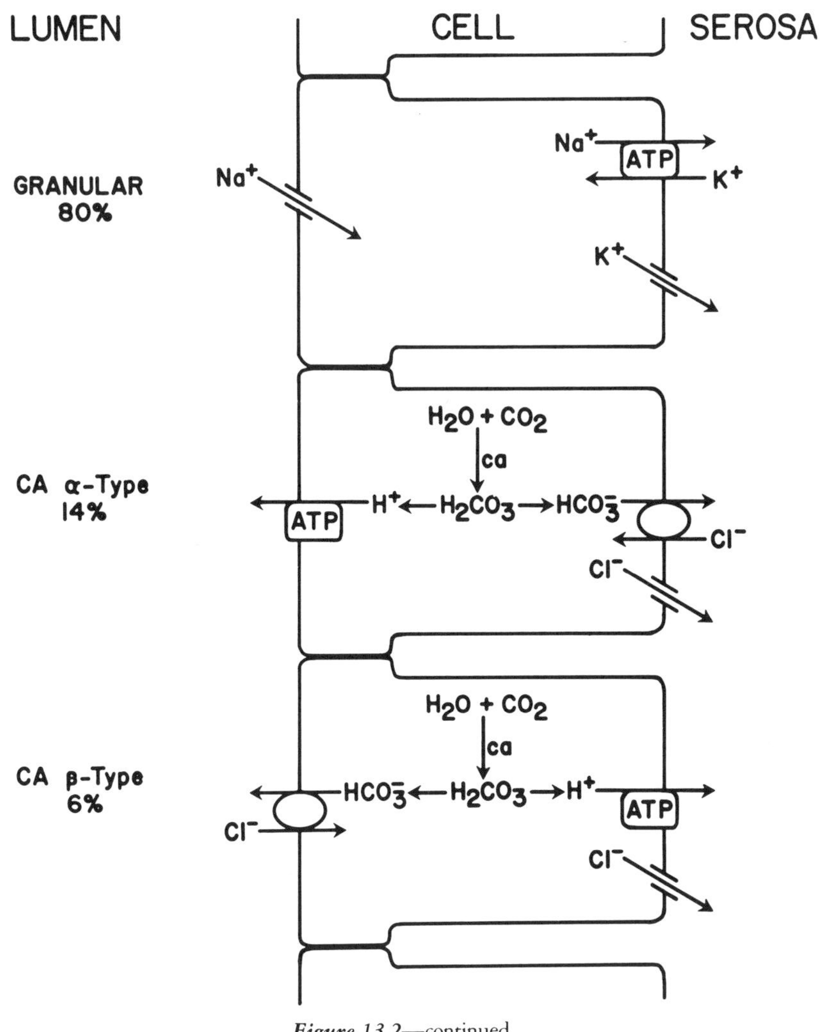

Figure 13.2—continued.

Iowa School of Medicine, reported that SITS caused a remarkable shrinkage in the apical membrane of the carbonic anhydrase-rich (CA) cells as judged from scanning electron microscopy and from histochemical studies for carbonic anhydrase. They were joined by David Stetson who began a series of morphometric and ultrastructural studies which would take several years and lead to the distinction of two subpopulations of carbonic anhydrase-rich cells. Husted's study on the virtual disappearance of cells with apical microplicae was followed by a fluorescence microscopy study demonstrating the dynamic behavior of the apical cell membrane of the CA cells. In an important study Stephen Gluck, Chris Cannon, and Qais Al-Awqati at Columbia University College of Physicians and Surgeons demonstrated that CO_2 addition to turtle bladder caused exocytosis of subapical membrane vesicles to the apical cell membrane. This study which was presented in November 1981 at the ASN meetings provided insight into the mechanisms by which the apical membrane area and, thereby, the number of H^+ pumps at the apical surface could be regulated. These structure-function studies of the CA cells were pursued further at the University of Connecticut School of Medicine, where it was discovered that the apical membrane changes of endo- and exocytosis occurred in only *one* type of CA cell, the so-called α type CA cell responsible for H^+ secretion. They recognized a subpopulation of β type CA cells whose apical membrane failed to respond to changes in CO_2 tension. The apical and basolateral membranes of these β cells had ultrastructural characteristics that were reversed from those of α cells. These studies along with the physiologic studies of HCO_3 secretion led to the interpretation that the β CA cells were responsible for HCO_3^- secretion (Fig. 13.2a and Fig. 13.2b). The interpretation that CA cells occur in two polarities was taken further by George Schwartz, Barasch, and Al Awqati who postulated that the intercalated cells of the rabbit cortical collecting duct could reverse their polarity in response to acid-base changes. Their conclusion was based on the intracellular pH response of these cells to unilateral Cl^- removal. These studies have stimulated many new investigations of the biology of intercalated cells (see sections under Shift of Focus to the Tubular Level and Focus on the Single Membrane Level).

Focus on the Single Membrane Level

Acid-Base Transporters and Intracellular pH of the Proximal Tubule

As the understanding of the function of the different segments of proximal and distal tubules and collecting ducts improved, renal physiologists shifted their focus to new kinds of experiments that became possible with the development of techniques for separating the apical and basolateral cell membranes of renal tubules. These studies have contributed most to our understanding of the apical and basolateral transport systems in the proximal tubule. Many of the early studies were carried out in the laboratories of Rolf

Kinne and his associates at the Max Planck Institute and presented at the 1978 meeting of the Society. Their techniques of differential centrifugation and free-flow electrophoresis allowed them to prepare vesicles of brush border and basolateral membranes and to study their transport characteristics separately. These studies directly demonstrated the existence of large differences in the transporters at the two cell membranes and supported the views that had been proposed in the double-membrane models for epithelial transport. Heini Mürer and Ullrich Hopfer working with Kinne first described the sodium/proton antiport in the brush border of the proximal tubule. The further characterization of this transporter in several laboratories became one of the major achievements of this early period in the Society's history. Although the existence of Na/H exchange had been postulated since Homer Smith's suggestion in the 1937 edition of *Principles of Renal Physiology* and although a sodium dependence of proximal bicarbonate reabsorption had been reported by several investigators, the existence of a sodium/proton antiport was first established in these brush border vesicles. The properties of the sodium/proton antiport were further defined by Burckhardt and his associates, also at the Max Planck Institute, and by Peter Aronson and his associates at Yale Medical School (Fig. 13.3). In 1985 Aronson received the Young Investigator Award of the American Society of Nephrology and presented a progress report on his work on the sodium/proton antiport and on several new anion exchangers that could induce bicarbonate transport in the proximal tubule. During the 1980s he and his associates at Yale proceeded to describe a diversity of anion exchangers that were inhibited by the disulfonic stilbenes, yet differed from the erythrocyte band 3 anion exchanger. These included a

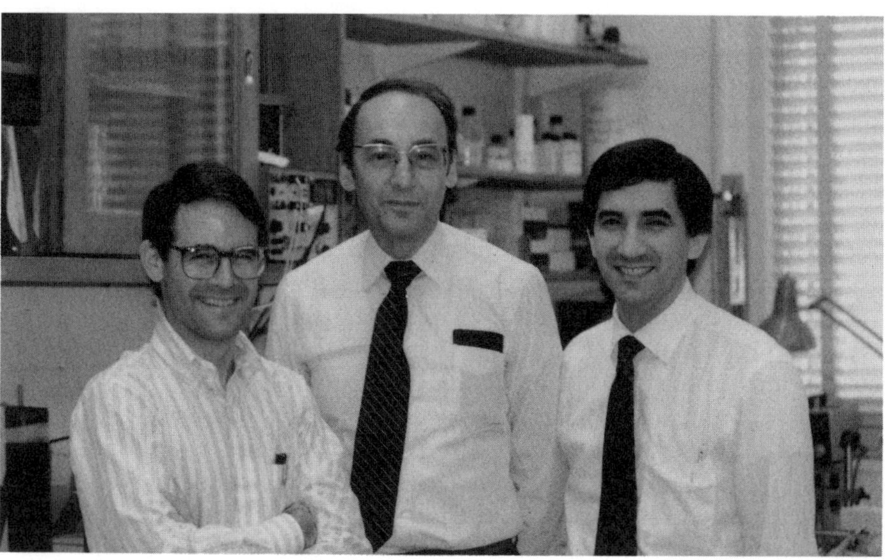

Figure 13.3. (From left to right) Peter Aronson, Gerhard Giebisch, and Walter Boron in the laboratory at Yale.

monocarboxylate-OH and a SO_4-HCO_3 exchanger as well as a Cl-formate exchanger in the brush border membrane. Although these transporters can bring about acid-base transport across the proximal tubule, they are quantitatively less important for vectorial transport than the basolateral Na-HCO_3 symporter first described in 1983 by Walter Boron and Emile Boulpaep, also at Yale, in amphibian proximal tubule. With respect to the symporter, Gerhard Burckhardt and Eberhard Fromter, with their associates Kenzo Sato and Koji Yoshitomi, demonstrated that bicarbonate transport across the basolateral cell membrane of rat proximal tubule was electrogenic. These electrophysiologic studies and studies by Biagi and Sohtell at Ohio State University indicated that this electrogenic bicarbonate flux was sodium-dependent. Robert Alpern and his associates at the University of California at San Francisco examined the bicarbonate exit step in microperfused proximal tubules by monitoring intracellular pH with a pH sensitive dye, BCECF, and found that it was a SITS-sensitive, Na-HCO_3 cotransport. Further studies in many laboratories have defined this cotransporter as an electrogenic system that translocates 3 HCO_3^- ions with one Na^+ ion across the basolateral cell membrane.

The regulation of proximal HCO_3^- reabsorption, which had been studied extensively at the whole tubule level by Malnic and his associates in Sao Paulo and by Rector and his associates in San Francisco (section under Shift of Focus to the Tubular Level), became the subject of new studies focused at the level of the individual membranes and transporters. Aronson had clarified the kinetic factors that regulate the transport rate of H^+ in brush border membrane vesicles and had described how the internal pH serves as an allosteric modifier of antiporter activity. He also explored the kinetics of the Na-3HCO_3 cotransporter in vesicles prepared from the basolateral cell membrane. In the mid-1980s, the development of pH-sensitive carboxyfluoresceins made it possible to study the regulation of intracellular pH across the apical and basolateral membranes of perfused tubules and thereby to explore acute regulatory as well as slower adaptive responses in acid-base transport. These approaches were used successfully by David Warnock and Robert Alpern, at the time at UCSF, by Walter Boron at Yale, and by a growing number of new investigators.

During this period interest in transepithelial acid transport and intracellular pH regulation converged. Intracellular pH regulation had its own separate and distinguished history. Much of it had taken place in nonpolar cells. Walter Boron played a major role in bringing these fields closer together and in applying intracellular pH methods to acid-base transport by the proximal tubule. For this work he received the Society's Young Investigator Award in 1986. Progress in the understanding of the regulation of proximal tubular bicarbonate transport and the role of intracellular messengers was rapid so that the 1988 Young Investigator Award went to Martin Cogan whose early work was reviewed above (section under Convoluted Tubules) and whose recent studies had focused on the potent stimulation of bicarbonate transport by angiotensin II. He showed how angiotensin II decreases adenylate cyclase activity and intracellular cAMP and thereby activates the apical Na/H antiporter. Edward Weinman and his associates at the University of Texas and Keith Hruska and Marc Hammerman and their respective associates at Washington University School of Medicine further clarified the roles of cAMP-dependent protein kinase, protein kinase C, and intracellular Ca in the regulation of this antiporter.

Acid-Base Transporters of Tight Urinary Epithelia

The tight urinary epithelia of the turtle and toad bladder and the mammalian collecting duct proved to be less suitable that the proximal tubule for the preparation of separated apical and basolateral cell membranes. The cellular heterogeneity of these epithelia made it nearly impossible to obtain pure preparations of either of these membranes for the minority cell populations involved in acid-base transport. The properties of the individual membranes, therefore, were characterized by other means. As discussed in the section on cellular level, the first approach was based on simplifying the sheet preparation of turtle bladder by eliminating the transport systems that were not of interest and by focusing on certain flows that were coupled and could be measured experimentally. For example, Renaud Beauwens and Qais Al Awqati explored the coupling between active H^+ transport and metabolism after they joined Steinmetz's group at the University of Iowa (Fig. 13.4).

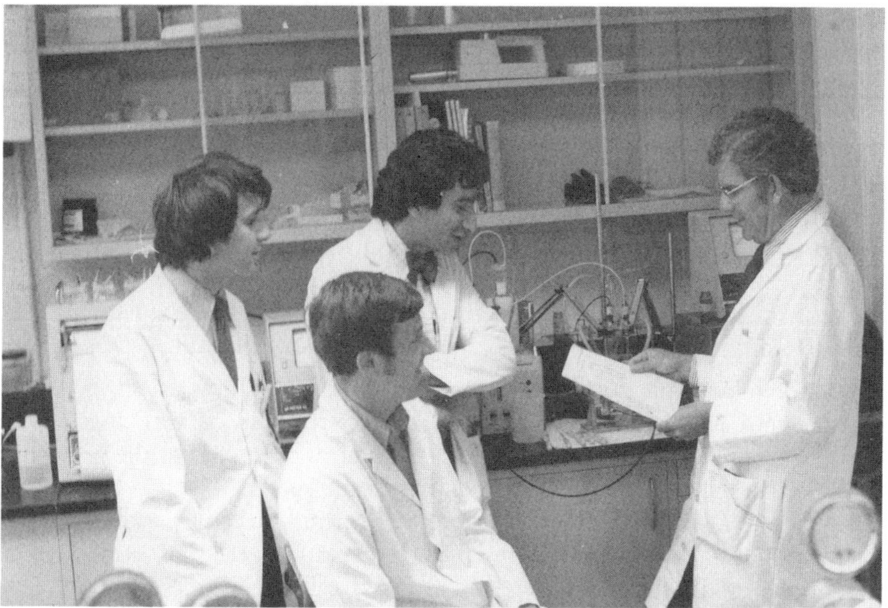

Figure 13.4. (From left to right, standing) Renaud Beauwens, Qais Al Awqati, Philip Steinmetz and a colleague at the University of Iowa.

They demonstrated in 1976 that the active transport rate was tightly coupled to the metabolic driving reaction measured as the rate of glucose oxidation. They used the formalisms of irreversible thermodynamics to describe the high degree of coupling and supported the interpretation of older studies by Steinmetz and Lawson indicating that the apical cell membrane was extremely tight to H^+ and HCO_3^- ions. A few years later Troy Dixon and Al Awqati took this line of thinking an important step further by attempting to reverse the direction of the proton flow through the acidification pump. They were able to show in Al Awqati's new laboratory at Columbia University that indeed the proton flow across the pump at the apical membrane could be reversed and that this reversal was associated with an increase in the ATP levels of the epithelial cells. Although their evidence for an H^+-translocating ATPase was developed in a complex experimental preparation, it was supported by several other lines of evidence. Studies at the University of Iowa showed that H^+ transport continued at substantial rates in the absence of O_2 and made the alternative possibility of a redox pump unlikely. During the 1980s several groups undertook biochemical studies in an attempt to purify the H^+-ATPase and to distinguish it from mitochondrial and other ATPases. A major advance was made by Stephen Gluck first as research fellow of Al Awqati in New York and later at the University of Chicago and Washington University. After initially characterizing an electrogenic, NEM-sensitive H^+-ATPase in turtle bladder, he obtained a similar ATPase in larger quantities from bovine kidney medulla. He was able to purify this ATPase with his coworkers Jerry Caldwell and John Hartwig and to characterize it as a vacuolar H^+-ATPase. Together with Dennis Brown at Massachusetts General he also showed by immunocytochemical techniques that the vacuolar H^+-ATPase is indeed distributed along the apical membranes of α type H^+-secreting cells in the collecting duct and that its distribution corresponds to that of the cytoplasmic studs coating the same membranes on thin section electron microscopy.

Another way of exploring the properties of the apical cell membrane of H^+ secreting cells was developed during the same period in the 1980s by Bruce Koeppen at the University of Connecticut. By applying refined electrophysiologic techniques to study individual epithelial cells in perfused segments of rabbit outer medullary collecting duct, he was able to distinguish two types of cells in the outer stripe of this segment. There was a common cell with an amiloride-inhibitable apical sodium conductance and a basolateral potassium conductance and a less common cell characterized by a very high apical resistance to all ions and a high chloride conductance instead of the potassium conductance in the basal membrane. The latter profile was also observed in all punctured cells of the inner stripe, a segment primarily involved in H^+ secretion. The electrophysiology of the inner stripe cell has served as an important model for the α type intercalated cell or H^+ secreting cell. The inner stripe cell is clearly unipolar in its acid-base transporting function in contrast to the intercalated cells of the cortical collecting duct. Furthermore, the intercalated cells of toad and turtle bladder have been difficult to impale for electrophysiologic study. Thus far, only the sodium-transporting cells have been explored successfully in these flat epithelia.

Still another way of examining the apical and basolateral transporters of intercalated cells was based on the monitoring of intracellular pH under conditions in which the transporters were manipulated experimentally. Mark Zeidel, Patricio Silva, and Julian Seifter at Harvard used this approach on separated and suspended outer medullary collecting duct cells. Matthew Breyer and Harry Jacobson, at the University of Texas Southwestern at the time studied individual cells of perfused rabbit OMCD segments by means of a pH sensitive carboxyfluorescein dye. These and similar studies enabled investigators to assess the roles of the apical H^+ pumps and the basolateral Cl/HCO_3 and Na/H exchangers in pH regulation and to distinguish between their roles in housekeeping functions and vectorial transport.

Early attempts to define the properties of the basolateral cell membrane of H^+ secreting cells were made in the late 1970s by Loren Cohen and Allan Mueller in Steinmetz's laboratory at the University of Iowa. They demonstrated that the basolateral cell membrane of turtle bladder epithelium possessed a very high permeability to HCO_3^- and that this permeability could be reduced markedly by the serosal addition of the disulfonic stilbene, SITS. Ehrenspeck and Brodsky at Mt. Sinai Medical School had demonstrated that serosal SITS inhibited the acidification current. Cohen found that this inhibition was associated with a transient increase in the DMO pH of the cell and suggested that SITS inhibited the exit step of HCO_3^- from the cell. The exit step was further defined subsequently by Fischer and associates who reported that it was chloride-dependent with a very high affinity for serosal chloride and postulated that the transport protein was a SITS-sensitive Cl-HCO_3 exchanger placed in parallel with a basolateral Cl^- conductance so that the negative charge could be transferred through a mechanism of recycling of Cl^-. In the mid-1980s several immunocytochemical studies were reported indicating localization of antibodies raised against components of the red cell band 3 protein at the basolateral cell membrane of intercalated cells in turtle bladder and collecting duct. Detley Drenckhahn and his associates at the University of Marburg, FRG, and Victor Schuster and Michael Jennings at the University of Iowa observed that the band-3 protein was co-localized with the structural protein ankyrin and spectrin. They also revealed that not all intercalated cells had immunoreactive basolateral membranes consistent with the existence of a subpopulation of HCO_3^- secreting intercalated cells.

Similarly, Jill Verlander working with Kirsten Madsen and Craig Tisher at the University of Florida localized the band 3 protein by an electron microscopic method at the basolateral cell membrane of rat intercalated cells.

Structure-function studies have played a major role not only in identifying the intercalated cells as responsible for vectorial acid-base transport, but also to explore the ultrastructure of the individual cell membranes. Thus, Stetson and Steinmetz based their distinction of α and β types of carbonic anhydrase-rich cells in turtle bladder not only on their response to CO_2, but more importantly, on the localization of rod-shaped intramembrane particles (on freeze fracture) and so-called studs (on this section electron microscopy) at either the apical or the basolateral cell membrane. These elements were only at the apical membrane of the CO_2-responsive H^+ secreting α cells, and only at the basolateral membrane of the minority population of cells they termed *β CA cells*. Once this distinction was made, it became possible to make closer comparisons of structure and function in the α CA cells. Thus, Steinmetz in his Homer Smith Award lecture and in subsequent studies with David Stetson was able to make an estimate of the H^+ transport rate per second per rod-shaped intramembrane particle in the apical cell membrane (Fig. 13.5). If a rod-shaped particle is a linear array of three globular particles and represents three studs on the cytoplasmic surface of the membrane, an interpretation that remains to be verified, then each pump would translocate about 60 protons per second. Similar analysis of morphometric and freeze-fracture

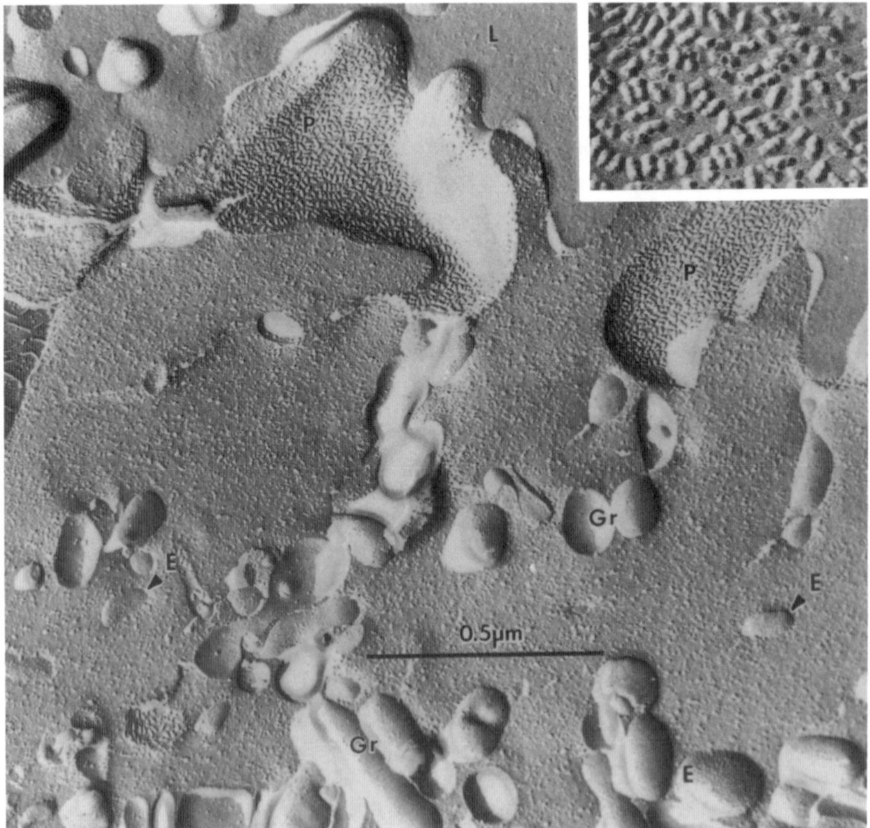

Figure 13.5. Freeze fracture study of the apical cell membrane of an O type cell of turtle bladder. Rod-shaped intramembrane particles on P face of apical membrane. Insert demonstrates that rod-shaped particles are composed of 2 or 3 globular units. See Stetson and Steinmetz. *Am. J. Physiol.* 249: F553, 1985.

studies before and after CO_2 stimulation suggest that a given α cell may increase the number of H^+ pumps in an apical transport position more than fourfold by recruitment of reserve pumps so that a stimulated α cell would have as many as seven million H^+ pumps at work. New studies by Dennis Brown and Stephen Gluck (section below) may well clarify the precise relationship between these ultrastructural elements and the specific subunits of the H^+-ATPase molecule.

Studies of the morphological consequences of acid-base disturbances in the distal tubule and collecting duct date back to the early 1970s when Hagège and Richet at Hopital Tenon in Paris reported that HCO_3^- loading and respiratory acidosis greatly increased the prominence of the intercalated cells in the rat collecting duct. The morphologic response of the collecting duct to acid-base disturbances were explored extensively by Craig Tisher and his associates Gary Hansen and Kirsten Madsen, first at Duke University and later at the University of Florida. They observed that the number of intercalated cells in the collecting duct was unaffected by respiratory acidosis and other acid base disturbances. In subsequent morphometric studies Madsen and Tisher reported that respiratory acidosis greatly increased the surface density of the apical plasma membrane in the intercalated cells of the outer medullary collecting duct. As in turtle bladder this membrane expansion could be accounted for by the addition of tubulovesicular membrane to the apical surface. Together with Verlander they also explored the cortical segment of the collecting duct and demonstrated two morphologically distinct types of intercalated cells corresponding to the α and β types of turtle bladder. Their studies supported the notion that intercalated cells occur in two polarities in this segment in both rat and rabbit. The intracellular pH studies of George Schwartz and his associates in New York had demonstrated that intercalated cells occurred in two functional polarities in rabbit CCD and had suggested that these functional polarities could be reversed as part of an adaptive response to an acid-base change.

Whether or not such a reversal of cell polarity constitutes an important adaptive response to external acid-base change remains an issue that is actively investigated. The mechanisms of endo- and exocytosis, however, became accepted as major factors in the regulation of the H^+ transport rate by α type intercalated cells. In addition to regulation of the number of H^+ pumps, investigators have looked at kinetic factors depending on the intrinsic properties of the H^+ pump and on possible activator and inhibitor mechanisms in the cytoplasm of the H^+ secreting cells. Olaf Andersen from Cornell's department of physiology developed a kinetic model of the regulation of H^+ transport in turtle bladder. Stephen Gluck and his associates presented studies at the 1990 meeting of the Society on the pH dependence of a cytoplasmic inhibitor and an activator which could play a role in regulating the H^+ transport rate. Similarly, electrophysiologic and intracellular pH studies are offering new insights into the messenger mechanisms and the possible role of activation of Cl^- channels in series or in parallel with acid-base transporters.

Entering the 1990s

By the end of the 1980s more of the topics on acid-base transport became grouped under the headings of cellular and molecular biology. The cloning and primary structure of membrane transport proteins became one field of activity for molecular biologists. As early as 1987 Jacques Pouyssegur and his associates at the University of Nice presented a symposium paper at the Society's annual meeting on the molecular genetics of the Na/H antiporter. They described new cloning strategies to elucidate the amino acid sequence of this transport molecule. As we enter the 1990s new collaborations have been undertaken to explore the expression and regulation of this antiporter. Peter Igarashi and Peter Aronson at Yale also have shifted their focus to such molecular studies, and several other laboratories have joined this direction of studies on the Na/H antiporter.

Considerable progress has been made also in the cloning and expression of band-3 related anion exchangers in the kidney by Seth Alper and his associates at Harvard. Similarly the localization of certain new and different anion transport proteins along the nephron are being explored in the hope of characterizing the apical transporters that have escaped detection with the original band-3 antibodies used by Drenckhahn and his associates at Marburg and by Schuster and Jennings, then at the University of Iowa (see above section).

As discussed above the proton pump at the apical membrane of the intercalated cells of collecting duct and turtle bladder was characterized by Stephen Gluck and his associates as a vacuolar H^+-ATPase that functions as an electrogenic pump. Over the last few years progress has been made in the cloning of several genes for this ATPase and it has become possible to determine some of the nucleotide sequences and predicted amino acid sequences of the messenger RNAs coding for subunits of the ATPase. Gluck's studies on the ATPase purified from bovine renal medulla and studies by Dennis Stone and Xiao-Song Xie in Dallas on the vacuolar H^+-ATPase from clathrin-coated vesicles of brain have provided a representation of the structure of this ATPase. It is a large protein with a molecular weight of about 580 kD and is composed of multiple subunits. The larger subunits form the cytoplasmic domain of the catalytic site where ATP hydrolysis and H^+ translocation are coupled (Fig. 13.6). This domain corresponds to the "studs" observed on this section electron microscopy by Dennis Brown and David Stetson and their respective coworkers in α type intercalated cells. Several of the smaller subunits comprise the transmembrane domain of the ATPase. The amino acid sequences of two of the subunits of the cytoplasmic domain are remarkably similar to subunits of the H^+ pump of the Archebacteria which are among the oldest organisms on earth.

Whether the vacuolar H^+-ATPase is the only H^+-ATPase responsible for proton secretion by the CCD and OMCD remains to be clarified. Recent studies suggest that a different P type ATPase may play a role in urinary

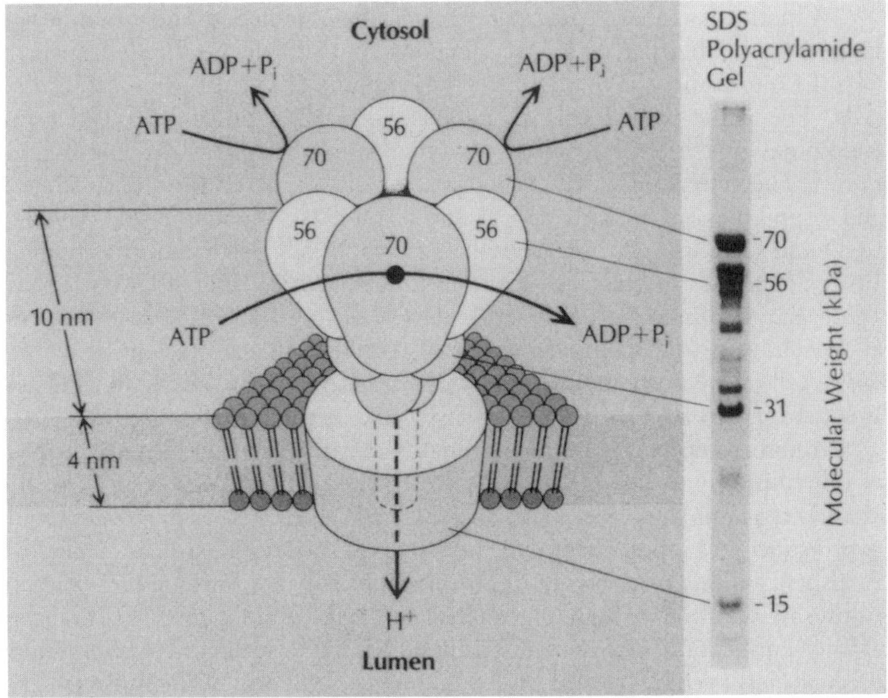

Figure 13.6. Recent model of the electrogenic proton pump for urinary acidification. The cytoplasmic domain of the V-type ATPase consists of tightly packed globular subunits and is involved in ATP hydrolysis. Smaller subunits are indicated based on electrophoresis of pump protein purified by its immunoaffinity for a monoclonal antibody (right). Reproduced from S. L. Gluck. Hosp. Pract. 24: 149, 1989.

acidification under conditions of potassium depletion. It has long been known that potassium depletion stimulates urinary acidification and causes morphological changes in the OMCD characterized by hypertrophy of cells and expansion of the luminal membrane area as described in 1980 by Stetson and his associates.

In the late 1980s Doucet and Marsy at the Collège de France and Lal Garg and Neelam Narang at the University of Florida found that potassium depletion stimulated an ouabain-insensitive K^+-ATPase. Charles Wingo and his associates, also at the University of Florida, observed that OMCD segments harvested from potassium-depleted rabbits demonstrated net potassium reabsorption not found in control rabbits. Omeprazole, the inhibitor of gastric H^+/K^+-ATPase caused comparable inhibition of the rates of bicarbonate and potassium reabsorption. Further evidence for a role of a H^+/K^+-ATPase was obtained by Wingo, Madsen, Smolka and Tisher who demonstrated H^+/K^+-ATPase immunoreactivity in the cytoplasm of a population of cells in the CCD and OMCD of rat and rabbit. The possible role and relative importance of the $H^+/K/$-ATPase in distal urinary acidification remains to be clarified during the 1990s.

Chloride channels participate in acid-base transport in a number of indirect ways. They permit the recycling of Cl in parallel with the electroneutral Cl/HCO_3 exchanger in the basolateral membrane of H^+ secreting intercalated cells. They also play a role in parallel with H^+ pumps in a variety of endosomes where they dissipate the charge generated by the electrogenic pump. The activation of Cl channels is usually regulated by protein kinases and second messengers. One approach to explore the function of H^+ secreting CCD and OMCD cells is to consider the whole cell patch clamp technique. Bruce Stanton and his associates at Dartmouth Medical School have used this approach to examine the regulation of the Cl channels, whereas Bruce Koeppen at the University of Connecticut has used this approach to characterize the whole cell pump currents with and without inhibition of the Na/K-ATPase. It is too early to attempt to give a perspective of this field.

Another approach gaining rapidly in the early 1990s is the development of cell culture lines capable of acid-base transport. Elsa Bello-Reuss and her coworkers at the University of Texas have been able to grow monolayers with two distinct cell types resembling principal and intercalated cells. Janet van Adelsberg and her associates at Columbia University are working on a primary culture of bicarbonate secreting intercalated cells, employing a technique of affinity purification. Another promising approach, a technique of immunodissection, has been developed by Arlyn Garcia-Perez and William Smith and by William Spielman and their associates at Michigan State University. Thus Chizuko Koseki, working with Hitoshi Endou at the University of Tokyo, isolated cells by means of monoclonal antibodies of intercalated cells. Similarly Gena Fejes-Toth and Aniko Naray-Fejes-Toth now at Dartmouth used monoclonal antibodies to recognize principal cells of the CCD and fluorescence-activated cell sorting to enrich their cultures of intercalated cells. They are also exploring the possibility, once raised by Hagège and Richet 20 years ago, that intercalated cells may be convertible into principal cells. These important and complex issues may well be sorted out during the 1990s.

The Overall System: Kidney Patient

The shifting of focus from kidney to tubule, to cell, to membrane, and to transport molecule has strained our ability to understand the overall system and to assess the precise role of the individual components elucidated at the cellular and molecular levels.

The principles we use for isolating and simplifying a system are not the same as the ones we need for integrating the parts. In real systems the parts interact with each other in various direct and indirect ways. The behavior of the overall system can not be derived in a simple way from adding all the parts. The process of integration often takes place at the bedside as house officers and fellows attempt to put together the varied data and points of view coming from bench researchers and clinical nephrologists. The meetings of the American Society of Nephrology have been able to capture this process of integration from their very beginning in 1967. Clinical acid-base disorders have served as themes for many communications, panels, and controversies. During the 1970s, for example, the pathophysiology of renal tubular acidosis (RTA) was often featured on the program. The different forms of RTA were regarded as experiments of nature designed to challenge renal physiologists. A somewhat different challenge was presented by the pathophysiology of metabolic alkalosis. Here the experimental attempts made aimed to attribute the disorder to a single ion deficit or to a single pathophysiologic alteration. To illustrate the importance of accounting for physiologic acid-base disturbances we mention these two disorders as examples.

During the early years of the Society, Curtis Morris and his associates Anthony Sebastian, Elizabeth McSherry, and Morris Schambelan at UCSF presented papers that contributed greatly to the classification of the different types of renal tubular acidosis and the associated disorders in potassium handling. Their studies also showed how alkali treatment could restore the growth of infants and children and could reduce the frequency of kidney-stone complications in adults. At the same time the work by Chester Edelmann and Rodriguez-Soriano at Albert Einstein clarified the distinction between proximal and distal renal tubular acidosis. In the mid-1970s Mitchell Halperin and Marc Goldstein at St. Michael's Hospital in Toronto and Bobby Stinebaugh at Methodist Hospital in Houston stimulated a new interest in the carbon dioxide tension of the urine. These and other investigators showed that the urinary CO_2 tension can provide information on the acidifying capacity of the distal nephron under specified conditions. This approach was used to distinguish between distal RTA caused by impaired H^+ secretion and RTA caused by increased back diffusion of H^+. Steinmetz and Lawson had demonstrated in 1970 in the turtle bladder that Amphotericin B can cause a defect in urinary acidification by dramatically increasing the passive permeability of the luminal cell membrane to H^+. Several observations made in vitro on the regulation of H^+ secretion proved applicable to clinical RTA. Thus Jose Arruda, Sandra Sabatini, and Daniel Batlle at the University of Illinois demonstrated how lithium, amiloride, and other factors reducing the lumen-negative voltage generated by sodium transport impaired urinary acidification in patients.

The interest in the pathophysiology of metabolic alkalosis dates back to the early 1960s when William Schwartz and his many associates at Tufts-New England Medical Center in Boston carried out a series of careful balance studies to demonstrate the critical role of chloride in the development, maintenance, and recovery of certain types of metabolic alkalosis. Norman Bank, Jerome Kassirer, Jordan Cohen, Howard Bleich, David Levine, and Richard Tannen were all associates of William Schwartz and subsequently dedicated much of their career to further acid-base studies (Fig. 13.7). Although chloride-depletion metabolic alkalosis has been recognized as a

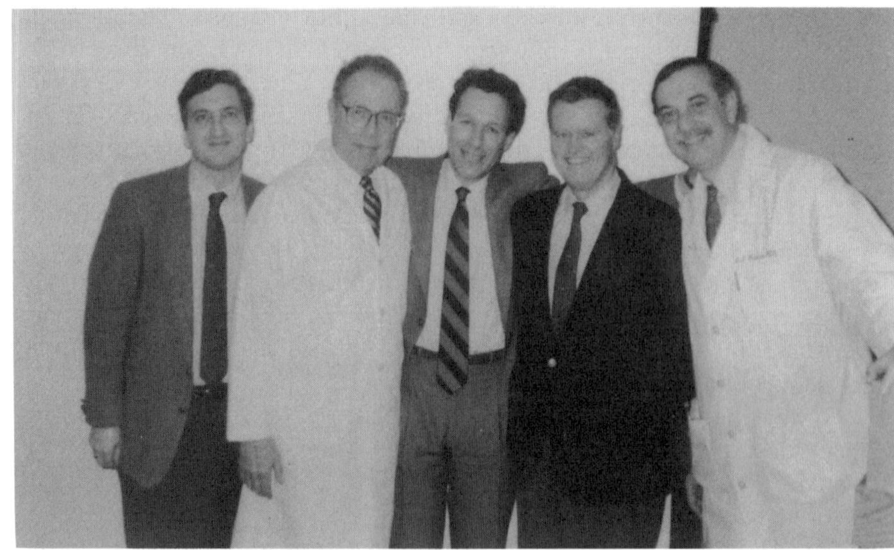

Figure 13.7. (From left to right) Nicolaos Madias, William Schwartz, David Levine, John Harrington, and Jerome Kassirer in the laboratory at New England Medical Center.

prototypic acid-base disorder, its pathophysiology has not been without controversy. Gastric fluid loss, for example, causes changes additional to changes in chloride depletion. Although it is theoretically possible to replace the lost chloride one for one with bicarbonate, associated losses of the cations, potassium, and sodium tend to occur in many clinical conditions. As a result, patients with a gastric alkalosis often sustain some potassium loss and some contraction of the extracellular fluid volume. Because of this complexity inherent in the clinical disorder, investigators have long attempted to distinguish between variables. Marty Cogan and his associates in San Francisco (see section on tubular level) have demonstrated that a decrease in glomerular filtration rate may contribute to the maintenance of the alkalosis by reducing the filtered load and renal excretion of bicarbonate. On the other hand, Robert Luke and John Galla at the University of Alabama were able to correct chloride-depletion alkalosis without volume expansion in the rat. They and others have made the case that chloride plays a unique intrarenal role in the correction of the alkalosis in accord with Bill Schwartz's original analysis. Neil Kurtzman, now at Texas Tech University Health Sciences Center and John Gennari at the University of Vermont think that other factors, such as slightly decreased filtered load of bicarbonate and most potassium depletion, can contribute significantly to the maintenance of the alkalosis. The interest in the intrarenal mechanisms that could play a role in the pathophysiology has been stimulated by the growing number of candidate transporters that link either chloride or potassium to acid-base transport in different nephron segments. The discovery of a chloride/bicarbonate antiporter first in turtle bladder and then in rabbit and rat CCD and connecting tubule has renewed work on the regulation of bicarbonate secretion by luminal chloride. David Levine and his associates at Ottawa observed that bicarbonate secretion in rats studied in vivo was regulated by luminal chloride. Similarly Daniel Gifford and his associates at Birmingham reported a chloride-dependence of bicarbonate secretion in CCD segments harvested from rats made alkalotic by peritoneal chloride/bicarbonate exchange. These authors feel that this anion antiporter can indeed contribute to the recovery from chloride-depletion alkalosis by secreting bicarbonate into the distal tubule and CCD in response to chloride administration.

These examples highlight how new discoveries at the level of the specialized cells and individual transport systems spurred new attempts to integrate the understanding at the level of the whole kidney.

Acknowledgment. This historical review was facilitated by research activities supported over the years by NIH. Steinmetz's research was supported by NIH grant DK-30693. Giebisch's research was supported by NIH grant DK-17433. Levine received support from the Medical Research Council of Canada.

14

Renal Hemodynamics

L. Gabriel Navar, Gerald F. DiBona, and Roland C. Blantz

Introduction

Recognition of renal hemodynamics as a specific area for study by nephrologists was not apparent during the formative years of the Society. This was thought to be the province of circulatory physiologists interested in the control of the renal circulation and associated phenomena such as renal blood flow autoregulation. Thus, the renal circulation was considered along with other vascular beds. For example, the American Heart Association had just sponsored a specific international symposium on "Autoregulation of Blood Flow," held in Indianapolis in 1963 (proceedings published as AHA monograph in 1964 Circ. Res. 14 Suppl 1). Several of the presentations addressed the renal circulation and a number of distinguished renal physiologists such as Carl Gottschalk, Ewald Selkurt, and Klaus Thurau participated. At that symposium, the existing concept related to the interaction between the macula densa segment of the distal tubule and the afferent arteriole was presented in a mathematical analysis by Arthur Guyton. This concept, had been developed by morphologists such as Goormaghtigh and others and was based on the well-known association among the structures of the juxtaglomerular complex. However, it had received little attention from renal physiologists and nephrologists with the notable exception of Laszlo Harsing from Budapest. In a series of papers published in 1957, Harsing and associates explained their physiological observations on the basis of a "tubuloglomerular equilibrium" by which "impulses coming from the macula densa play a role in the regulation of renal blood flow and glomerular filtration rate" (Acta Physiol Acad Scient Hung 12:342–349; 351–361; 363–371, 1957). The concept was of particular significance to investigators primarily interested in kidney physiology as opposed to circulatory physiology because it linked aspects of tubular transport function with circulatory control mechanisms. This increased interest was reflected at the 1966 International Congress of Nephrology where Klaus Thurau presented data supporting the macula densa feedback hypothesis as an explanation for the phenomenon of renal autoregulation. This seminal presentation sparked a great deal of interest which continues to this day on the mechanisms by which macula densa cells communicate with the glomerular vascular elements.

Among members of the newly formed American Society of Nephrology, however, there was only minor interest in factors controlling the renal circulation. Other issues such as "glomerulotubular balance", volume expansion, and "third factor" seemed to dominate their thoughts. In nephrological circles, renal hemodynamics was championed primarily by those interested in acute renal failure and pathophysiological sodium retaining states. From this perspective, the most fascinating issue was related to the mechanisms responsible for altering blood-flow distribution within the kidney. In spite of this interest, there was great uncertainty about experimental findings based on methods such as inert gas washout or microsphere distribution. Every method used to assess renal blood-flow distribution was recognized as having serious methodological or theoretical flaws which led to substantial controversy about the validity of the results. Thus, early sessions were often heavily focused on methodological concerns related to measurement of renal blood-flow distribution. Nevertheless, there was continued fascination with the possible significance of differences in intrarenal blood-flow distribution in sodium retaining states. Making the jump to normal regulation of sodium excretion seemed a logical next step. From these studies, there emerged an interesting, but as yet to be validated, concept that the deep nephrons were primarily "salt conservers" and superficial nephrons were "sodium wasters" and that changing the distribution of blood flow to the nephron population could serve as a major mechanism regulating sodium excretion. Regardless of its validity, this concept was important in stimulating further work in renal hemodynamics among nephrologists whose primary interests were related to the control of fluid and electrolyte balance.

Several other interesting concepts related to the interaction between the tubular network and circulatory structures were generating enthusiasm as the ASN unfolded. The importance of physical forces within the peritubular environment in the regulation of proximal sodium reabsorption rate was receiving more attention. Also, the availability of means for direct evaluation of glomerular pressure and glomerular filtration rate at the single-nephron level prompted many studies. As several major methodological approaches became available, a burst of activity set the stage for a long and continuous series of studies on control mechanisms regulating the renal circulation. Recognition of multiple humoral, neural, and local intrinsic systems that interacted with each other to control the renal microvasculature stimulated a great deal of research in many areas. These have been divided into five major categories described in the following sections. Ultimately, the quest to understand the cellular basis for renal vascular control mechanisms led to many outgrowths that involved studies with discrete cell populations of mesangial, endothelial, and vascular smooth muscle cells. We are now in an explosive period of investigation using various isolated or cultured cell systems that may yield insights and understandings into vascular control mechanisms at a new dimension.

Intrarenal Distribution of Blood Flow

The concept of an alteration in the intrarenal distribution of blood flow developed from an attempt to explain the augmented renal sodium retention in edema-forming states, notably congestive heart failure. It was known that the dog kidney was composed of outer cortical nephrons with short loops of Henle and juxtamedullary nephrons with long loops of Henle. These morphological differences served as the basis for the notion that the outer cortical short-looped nephrons (sodium wasters) were not as effective in reabsorbing sodium as the juxtamedullary long-looped nephrons (sodium conservers). It was thus proposed that redistribution of renal blood flow and glomerular filtration from the outer cortical sodium-wasting nephrons to the juxtamedullary sodium-conserving nephrons might explain the augmented renal sodium retention of congestive heart failure. It was also postulated that such a redistribution of blood flow and glomerular filtration from outer cortical to juxtamedullary nephrons could account for the discrepancy between the modest reduction in renal blood flow and the marked reduction in urine flow and glomerular filtration rate that characterized acute renal failure.

Investigations regarding this sphere of study were complicated by the wide variety of methods employed to characterize the intrarenal distribution of blood flow. The search for a surrogate marker that faithfully mimicked the rheological characteristics of the red blood cell that would be completely extracted by the kidney in one pass, and that would not itself alter renal blood-flow distribution consumed much time and effort of many investigative groups. Inert gas washout, heated thermocouples, radioisotopically labelled plastic microspheres, frog red blood cells and antiglomerular basement membrane antibodies were some of the methodological approaches. However, with continued assessment of the methods and attempts at reconciliation with existing knowledge of the renal microcirculation, it became apparent that essentially every methodological approach was burdened with one or more fatal flaws. This was particularly apparent during efforts to evaluate intrarenal distribution profiles for both blood flow and glomerular filtration rate (GFR). Under some conditions, the techniques used indicated that the distribution patterns for GFR and blood flow were shifting in opposite directions, yielding extremely high and unrealistic values for outer-cortical filtration fractions. The initial hypothesis concerning the dependency of renal sodium retention in congestive heart failure on the intrarenal redistribution of blood flow and glomerular filtration could not be convincingly substantiated. In fact, an argument against the hypothesis was the finding that the majority of renal vasodilator agents produced a natriuresis in association with a redistribution of blood flow away from the outer cortex to the juxtamedullary nephrons, the opposite of what would be expected if the change in renal blood-flow distribution produced the change in urinary sodium excretion. Thus, in the absence of a reliable method for assessing intrarenal distribution of blood flow, this phase of renal hemodynamic investigation slowly faded, replaced by newer methods that permitted the detailed and more direct study of smaller segments of the intrarenal vasculature. These methods include direct micropuncture of the glomerular microcirculation in the Munich-Wistar rat, endowed with surface glomeruli, isolated perfused renal microvessels and isolated perfused glomeruli (derivatives of the isolated perfused tubule technique), the perfused juxtamedullary nephron preparation, and the hydronephrotic kidney preparation, and the implementation of newer technology such as videometric and laser Doppler methods. These newer methods have been employed with greater frequency to provide new information on various issues. These issues include the effects of increased renal perfusion pressure on the renal papillary circulation (pressure diuresis/natriuresis), effects of vasoactive substances on the glomerular filtration process, and the myogenic and vasoactive responsiveness of isolated renal microvessels. Many reports during recent years have helped to delineate the contribution of preglomerular and postglomerular segments to overall changes in renal vascular resistance during autoregulation or following the administration of vasoactive agents. Studies specifically evaluating vascular characteristics and responsiveness of nephrons from various regions of the kidney are finally helping to resolve differences in function among these units.

"Physical Factors" and the Regulation of Tubular Reabsorption

Interest in peritubular capillary "physical factors" derived as a natural consequence of searches to explain the reductions in proximal tubular reabsorption that occurred following volume or saline expansion and the means by which the medullary circulation could serve as a modifier of renal sodium excretion and urinary concentration. During the early years of ASN, interest was keen on mechanisms of regulation of proximal tubular reabsorption, especially during expansion of the extracellular fluid volume. As it became apparent that known hormonal influences could not consistently explain these phenomena, investigators turned to other possible mechanisms such as alterations in renal plasma flow, filtration fraction, and peritubular and interstitial hydrostatic and colloid osmotic pressures.

At the first HSN meeting in 1967, we find an interesting juxtaposition of symposia and abstracts on natriuretic hormone and glomerulotubular balance while a few abstracts raised questions relating to the role of physical factors in the control of sodium reabsorption. These initial studies utilized both clearance and micropuncture techniques. Studies correlated elevated renal venous wedge hydrostatic pressures with increased NaCl and water excretion during saline expansion and the infusion of renal vasodilators. Although evaluations were indirect, these studies correlated reduced filtration fraction and presumed reductions in peritubular capillary colloid oncotic pressure and elevated capillary hydrostatic pressure with indirect evidence for reductions in proximal tubular reabsorption. Concurrent micropuncture studies utilized elevated renal venous pressure and demonstrated reductions in absolute proximal reabsorption. These findings led to similar conclusions that elevated hydrostatic pressures and reduced colloid osmotic pressures in the peritubular capillary could reduce capillary uptake of reabsorbate and possibly increase passive backleak into the tubular lumen, reducing net proximal tubule fluid reabsorption.

Proponents of the physical-factor hypothesis of the peritubular capillary control of proximal tubular reabsorption were driven by the necessity to provide direct physical evidence for a causal relationship between altered peritubular capillary hydrostatic and oncotic pressures and reductions in proximal tubular reabsorption. This goal served as a strong impetus to develop new techniques for the direct evaluation of pertinent peritubular capillary pressures which therefore resulted in great studies in new micromeasurement technologies. Advances made by investigators interested in the microcirculation were quickly assimilated. During the next five years, increasing numbers of studies employed direct measurements of pertinent hydrostatic and oncotic pressures in peritubular capillaries and the renal interstitium. These studies generally demonstrated correlations between changes in Starling forces for peritubular capillary uptake of reabsorbate and alterations in proximal reabsorption. Peritubular capillary microperfusion techniques demonstrated that perfusion with colloid free solutions were associated with reductions in proximal tubular transport. Other studies demonstrated increased backleak of larger solutes, such as sucrose, into the tubular lumen with elevated renal venous pressures, suggesting that passive mechanisms linked to intrarenal pressures could contribute to the regulation of proximal tubular permeability as well as reabsorption.

More sophisticated approaches were seen explored to further test this interesting physical-factor hypothesis. Measurements of hydrostatic pressures in peritubular capillaries and direct evaluation of interstitial hydrostatic pressures with implanted capsules or newly developed servo-nulling techniques and oncotic pressures with microprotein methods permitted more rigorous evaluation of these forces. When these data were coupled with data on absolute proximal reabsorption, it was possible to derive differential equations that fully described the integrated Starling forces and the peritubular capillary reabsorptive coefficient. These approaches and further in vivo and in vitro microperfusion techniques raised important questions about the importance of an entirely passive system for the control of proximal reabsorption dictated by Starling forces and peritubular capillary uptake rates of reabsorbate. In vitro studies in isolated perfused tubules strongly suggested that if wide variations in peritubular or bath colloid osmotic pressure were to influence proximal reabsorption, it must be the active transport component that was affected rather than simply passive backleak of NaCl and water. The mechanism of this influence remains undefined. Direct measurements demonstrating increased conductances of paracellular shunt pathways with volume expansion stimulated modeling of proximal reabsorption which included the complex lateral interspace. The concept of a rate-limiting step for proximal tubular reabsorption was also seriously considered and evaluated in multicompartment models of tubular lumen, intercellular space, the tubular basement membrane, the complex renal interstitium, and the peritubular capillary.

The pro and con positions that developed regarding the role of physical factors became exceedingly complex as technologies developed for accurate assessment of all of the pertinent pressures, permeabilities, and reabsorptive rates. Microperfusion studies of peritubular capillaries with colloid-containing and protein-free solutions generated major contradictory results. The general opinion evolved that wide variations in basolateral or peritubular capillary colloid osmotic pressure (and presumably hydrostatic pressure) could influence proximal tubular reabsorption rate; but it remained uncertain if smaller changes, observed in vivo, in interstitial or basolateral colloid osmotic and hydrostatic pressures could exert meaningful regulation of proximal tubular reabsorption. Although directional correlations generated from steady-state observations in volume expansion and in pathophysiologic conditions, were usually consistent with the physical-factor hypothesis, causality was difficult to prove in most cases. Primary or nonphysical factor-generated alterations in proximal reabsorption also obligated changes in pressures or permeabilities that dictate uptake of fluid from the renal interstitium into the adjacent peritubular capillary. Since a linkage between pressures, flow, and permeability is determined by the flux equation,

$$J_V = (\Delta\pi_x - \Delta P_x) \cdot LpA_R,$$

it was usually not possible to determine causality from such steady-state micromeasurements, no matter how accurately defined.

How has renal physiology benefited from issues raised pertinent to the physical-factor hypothesis? It seems fair to conclude that the exact role of peritubular physical factors in the normal physiologic regulation of proximal tubular reabsorption still remains poorly defined. That this has been an area of frustration may be reflected by the relative paucity of experimental studies in this area over the past 10 years, even through ASN's first 15 years were characterized by a plethora of innovative studies on this issue. Nevertheless, the benefits of investigation in this area for renal physiology have been abundant. They have provided an enhanced appreciation of the potential that physical events may modify active transport processes independent of external neurohumoral influences. Also, an awareness has developed of the linkage between the process of glomerular ultrafiltration and factors influencing tubular reabsorption. Since variation in filtration fraction is critical to physical-factor control of proximal tubular reabsorption, interest in the process of glomerular ultrafiltration and the role of specific determinants of glomerular ultrafiltration in dictating the filtration fraction increased. The physical-factor hypothesis heightened the awareness of mechanisms of glomerulotubular balance based upon variations in flow of intraluminal fluid and constituents thereof, independent of any mechanisms based on interstitial and peritubular capillary regulation of proximal tubular reabsorption. Potentially of most importance, interest in the peritubular physical factor hypothesis was a major inspiration and driving force for the development of experimental technologies, such as application of accurate methods of measuring hydrostatic pressures in small renal capillaries, development of microprotein methods for assessing protein concentration and colloid osmotic pressure in nanoliter blood samples, application of electrophysiologic methods of assessing low-resistance extracellular shunt pathways, and microperfusion techniques applied to the peritubular capillary circulation. These developments, emanating from a well-developed hypothesis which evolved prior to any directly obtained measurements, contributed to the development of pertinent measurement methods, a trend that stands in contrast to the evolution of glomerular hemodynamics in which technologic developments generated measurements later contributing to hypotheses previously unsuspected or underdeveloped.

Glomerular Hemodynamics

The developments in glomerular hemodynamics were generated not so much by grand hypotheses that required further proof but, rather, because of the fortuitous development of techniques and experimental animal models that permitted accurate evaluation of all the determinants of glomerular ultrafiltration. The developing methodology enabled measurement of glomerular capillary hydrostatic pressure (P_G) and the pressure gradient (ΔP), nephron plasma flow, and systemic and efferent arteriolar oncotic pressures. These measurements permit calculation of the glomerular ultrafiltration coefficient at the single-nephron level. Because of the relative lack of controversies, however, the level of interest in glomerular hemodynamics during the first several ASN meetings was modest at best. This was soon to change! The results Gertz and associates obtained on the basis of stop-flow pressure measurements suggested that glomerular pressure was much higher than was generally held. Various studies utilizing indirect approaches for assessing glomerular pressure suggested that the Gertz valves were excessive; this led to growing controversy regarding even the normal values for glomerular pressure. Initial investigations in this field required the development of servonulling pressure measurement systems which permitted accurate measurements of hydrostatic pressures in small capillaries and the discovery of the "Munich-Wistar rat," a strain with glomeruli on the surface of the kidney.

Methods had been developed to estimate glomerular capillary hydrostatic pressure and ΔP by indirect stop-flow techniques. Although the general process of glomerular ultrafiltration was understood, the rather high indirect estimates of P_G and ΔP implied that glomerular ultrafiltration was an event driven primarily by hydrostatic forces and, thus, regulation of glomerular filtration rate was also assumed to result from changes in P_G and ΔP. Results obtained in the early 1970s using direct measurements of P_G and ΔP in surface glomeruli of the Munich-Wistar rat, in conjunction with accurate measurements of systemic and efferent arteriolar oncotic pressures in the same nephron units, provided interesting conceptual developments. Direct measurements in the Munich-Wistar rat indicated that P_G and ΔP values are much lower than had been previously estimated. Thus, the glomerular ultrafiltration coefficient (LpA or K_f) calculated from these studies was much higher than the previous data would have suggested. Furthermore, lower P_G values in Munich-Wistar rats meant that the glomerular oncotic pressure could increase to values within the glomerular capillary that equal, or nearly equal, the glomerular capillary hydrostatic pressure gradient, ΔP, a phenomenon termed *filtration-pressure equilibrium* when it was proposed originally by Homer Smith. Because of these findings in the Munich-Wistar rat, considerable controversy evolved regarding the presence or absence of filtration pressure equilibrium in other species or under other conditions. The issue has been of particular significance because of implications related to the specific influence of plasma flow on GFR. If the filtration process is characterized by filtration equilibrium, GFR is much more directly dependent on renal plasma flow than when nonequilibrium conditions exist. These controversies stimulated a great deal of additional research which resulted in the recognition that filtration pressure equilibrium is not a universal finding in all species or all strains of rats or in other physiologic conditions such as elevated plasma flow.

Following this early phase characterizing the process of glomerular ultrafiltration, knowledge about the responses of glomerular hemodynamics to various neurohumoral influences and pathophysiologic conditions rapidly expanded. Although the filtration process was defined as being highly plasma-flow-dependent, early studies demonstrated that K_f or LpA could also be reduced in certain pathophysiologic conditions, that is, some forms of acute renal failure, most forms of glomerular immune injury, and during elevated levels of vasoactive agents such as angiotensin II. After infusion of angiotensin II and under conditions of elevated intrarenal angiotensin II generation, the K_f or LpA was found to decrease sufficiently to contribute to reduced-nephron filtration rate. This implied that glomerular cells are capable of responding to angiotensin II and other hormones. Coincident with this new concept, investigators demonstrated the presence of angiotensin II receptors in isolated glomeruli and, specifically, in populations of mesangial cells. Furthermore, it was demonstrated that mesangial cells contract in vitro in response to exposure to physiologic concentrations of angiotensin II. Therefore, various investigative thrusts were developed during the 1970s as a direct consequence of early glomerular hemodynamic observations that pointed to the importance of hormonal interactions. In particular, interest in location, physiologic regulation, and quantification of hormone receptors within the glomerular system increased. In turn, these studies prompted further analysis of signal transduction pathways in glomerular and other renal cells and stimulated interest in the development of in vitro cell culture systems to answer questions complementary to concurrent glomerular hemodynamic studies. As a reflection of activities in this expanding field, symposia of the mesangial cell and glomerular regulation became frequent ASN events beginning in 1974. Into the 1980s, ASN held further subspecialized symposia on the glomerulus. The many complementary studies using hemodynamic and cellular approaches have now clearly established that the glomerulus is remarkable in its responsiveness to a large variety of neural, hormonal, and autocoid systems and can respond rapidly to altered signals via multiple intracellular mechanisms.

Measurements of glomerular hemodynamics were also applied to a variety of pathophysiologic models in the 1970s and 1980s and supplied much needed knowledge regarding these important issues. They also propagated new and exciting areas of research investigation related to mechanisms of acute renal failure, mechanisms of glomerular immune injury, and factors leading to progression of renal disease and glomerulosclerosis after reductions in renal mass. Studies presented at ASN meetings in the 1970s further clarified the respective roles of renal vasoconstriction, glomerular capillary hydrostatic pressure, the ultrafiltration coefficient, tubular backleak of solutes, and tubular obstruction in experimental acute renal failure. Experimental models of glomerular immune injury revealed a remarkable uniformity of glomerular hemodynamic responses, which included increased glomerular hydrostatic pressure gradient and reductions in the glomerular filtration coefficient regardless of the glomerular site of the immune events. These types of studies were prominent at Society meetings in the mid-1970s and early 1980s and affirmed the role of factors such as complement, eicosanoids, and other inflammatory mediators in the complex cascade leading to glomerular immune injury. As a direct spinoff of these glomerular hemodynamic observations, in vitro cell and molecular biologic investigators have flourished and further clarified the important role of these inflammatory mediators as reflected by the increasing importance of these topics at more recent meetings of the ASN.

Some of the more recent studies have combined glomerular hemodynamic observations with other disciplines in models of radical reductions in renal mass and have provided exciting insights into the roles of glomerular capillary hydrostatic pressure, hormonal milieu, renal hypertrophy, and growth factors in the progression of renal disease and evolution of glomerulosclerosis. This important area of research has been strongly highlighted at recent Society meetings and represents a classic example in which the initial observations utilizing physiologic approaches have led to an explosion of expanding interest that has propagated sophisticated investigations in biochemistry, growth factors, regulation of extracellular matrix materials, and the role of lipids and eicosanoids. Indeed, the programs during the last two or three years have been characterized by an ever-increasing number of presentations related to intracellular mechanisms for signal transduction and their interactions with stimuli for growth and increased production of matrix material.

Glomerular hemodynamic observations in vivo have indirectly stimulated the development of newer techniques for the assessment of glomerular macromolecular permeability. Some of the initial experiments helped to validate glomerular sieving approaches and to establish the role of hemodynamics in modifying sieving curves of macromolecules. Further studies focused on the importance of molecular and glomerular membrane charge. Data using these glomerular sieving techniques have provided valuable insights into renal diseases in the human.

The interesting history of glomerular hemodynamics provides an example of how new technologies have opened new fields of knowledge. The glomerulus is no longer viewed as a passive ultrafilter; rather it is recognized as an intricate structure with important cell biologic functions. Issues raised by glomerular hemodynamic studies have rejuvenated interest in protein chemistry of the glomerular capillary membrane and glomerular extracellular matrix materials. Studies on isolated glomeruli and in-vitro cells in culture of glomerular origin have also provided an important area of cell biologic and molecular biologic activity which has furthered our understanding of glomerular immune injury and the mechanisms of progression of renal disease. This multidisciplinary approach has been dramatically in evidence at recent Society meetings and in no investigative area has this multifaceted approach been

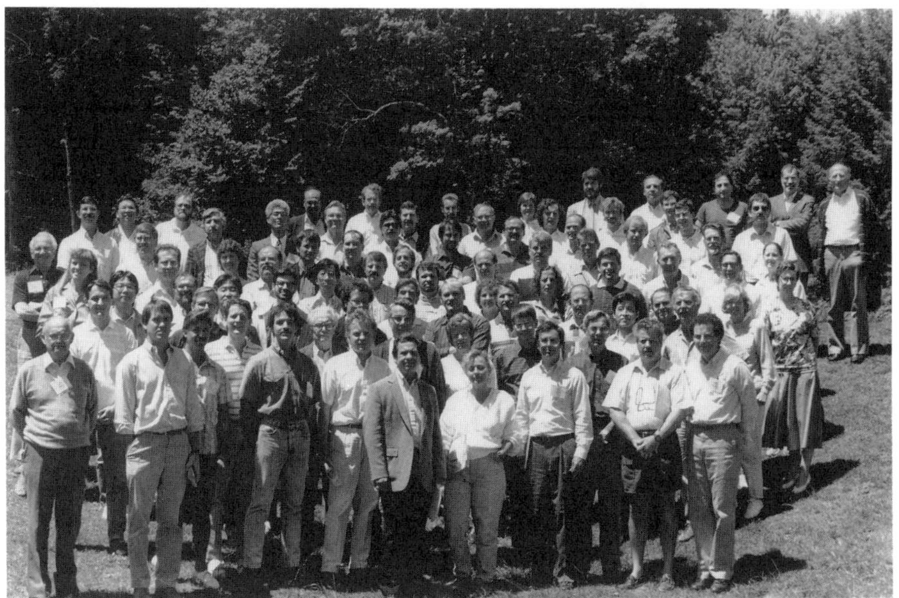

Figure 14.1. Investigators interested in renal hemodynamics had the opportunity to renew friendships and make new friends at the 1989 FASEB Summer Conference on Renal Hemodynamics in Saxtons River, Vermont. Participants at this meeting included senior and younger investigators from several countries.

more in evidence than with the glomerulus. The history of glomerular hemodynamic studies began with physiologic issues which have evolved into complex molecular studies involving cell-to-cell interactions. ASN meetings have the history dramatically chronicled of this evolutionary process.

Tubuloglomerular Feedback

As mentioned briefly in the introduction, investigators interested primarily in renal autoregulation became cognizant of the abundant morphological evidence demonstrating an intimate association between the macula-densa cells of the ascending loop of Henle and the vascular pole of the same nephron. It seemed attractive to postulate that these macula densa cells could act as a sensor of tubular fluid composition and send signals to the smooth muscle cells of the juxtaposed arterioles. The findings from several laboratories that fluid within the early part of the distal tubule was very hypotonic and seemed to be closely regulated regardless of the diuretic state of the animal provided support for this concept. Interestingly, from the perspective of those interested in an explanation for renal autoregulation, it was important to invoke this mechanism as a means of maintaining a constant GFR in response to extrinsic disturbances that might act to alter GFR. From the perspective of renal physiologists interested in the control of sodium excretion, it seemed important to consider the macula-densa feedback system as a mechanism for adjusting GFR in response to alterations in sodium balance because it was becoming increasingly apparent that something in addition to glomerulotubular balance was necessary to link the metabolically determined transport capabilities of the tubules with the hemodynamically determined filtered load.

The notion of the tubuloglomerular feedback mechanism was received with enthusiasm by many European renal physiologists and nephrologists; in particular, developments in this area were heavily influenced by the investigative group from Munich headed by Klaus Thurau. However, this concept developed slowly in the United States; only a few studies related to feedback-induced alterations in glomerular function caused by changes in flow through the loop of Henle were presented at ASN meetings during the formative years. The first paper, presented in 1969 by Fred Wright, Jurgen Schnermann, and their associates, clearly demonstrated that increases in tubular fluid flow through the loop of Henle elicit feedback-mediated reductions in single-nephron GFR. Although this area of research was receiving increased visibility at meetings of the American Physiological Society, the American nephrological community was not particularly enthusiastic about work in this area, and little else on this subject appeared on the ASN program until 1973. As previously mentioned, most of the interest during this early period was focused on peritubular physical factors and intrarenal blood-flow distribution patterns and how these were affected by various vasoactive hormones and drugs. Notably, an interest in the roles of the renin-angiotensin system and prostaglandins in the control of renal hemodynamics emerged. In 1973, additional studies on the tubuloglomerular feedback mechanism were reported by the Duke and Dallas groups. Interestingly, these talks were presented in a session on renal ion transport and not renal hemodynamics. Nevertheless, the demonstration by other laboratory groups of clear-cut feedback-mediated reductions in glomerular pressure and single-nephron GFR in response to changes in distal-nephron perfusion rate provided solid credibility to the tubuloglomerular feedback (TGF) mechanism and prompted increased interest by other groups. As additional investigators became interested in the TGF mechanism, the number of presentations on this subject grew during the rest of the 1970s and into the 1980s. From these studies, it became apparent that the TGF mechanism was a complicated integrative control system that was not going to yield its secrets readily. There emerged a variety of controversies related to just about every aspect of the TGF mechanism. There were heated debates related to the nature of the intraluminal factor that was responsible for the initiation of TGF signals. Some of the data supported the notion that NaCl or, perhaps, just the chloride concentration was the major intraluminal factor that triggered the TGF mechanism. Other studies demonstrated that the magnitude of the TGF response could be altered by changing total solute concentration independent of changes in either sodium or chloride concentrations. Among advocates of the TGF hypothesis, interest increased in the sequence of events responsible for the final effect. Thus, studies focused on specific aspects of the TGF mechanisms, such as the cellular mechanism responsive to the intraluminal factor, the nature of the communicating step between macula-densa cells and the vascular contractile cells, and the mechanism by which signals are transmitted to the vascular contractile cells. Because it is such an intriguing example of a classical negative-feedback control system, the TGF mechanism has provided fertile ground for investigative efforts at all levels ranging from integrative physiology to cell biology. Even today, important issues remain to be resolved. Although the hypothesis emerged as a means of explaining autoregulation of renal blood flow, this issue has remained uncertain to this day. Also, the role of TGF modulation as a means of altering sodium-excretion capability has not been clarified. At the other end of the spectrum, issues related to specific intracellular events involved in the TGF mechanism continue to be the subject of intensive effort.

One of the major spin-offs of studies on the TGF mechanism is that it has prompted investigators to integrate aspects of both tubular transport and vascular control mechanisms. For a complete understanding of the TGF mechanism, the properties of the ascending loop of Henle and the macula-densa cells have to be characterized to the same extent as those of glomerular arterioles and mesangial cells. In addition, the interactions among the determinants of glomerular dynamics as they respond to feedback signals from the macula densa require detailed analysis. Some recent studies have indicated that TGF-mediated reductions in GFR can occur even under conditions where the changes in glomerular pressure are blocked, suggesting at least two effector mechanisms perhaps operating independently. These and related questions have served as an impetus for the development of new techniques and for more sophisticated mathematical analysis. Because the negative feedback nature of the TGF mechanism lends itself to control systems analysis, several highly sophisticated mathematical treatments related to one or more aspects of the TGF mechanism have been presented. In addition, more specific experimental approaches have been utilized to further our knowledge of the steps involved in the TGF mechanism. The isolated perfused tubule methodology has been used to perfuse segments of the ascending loop of Henle with attached macula densa and glomerulus and also to perfuse isolated glomerular arterioles with or without the attached macula-densa segment. Other in vitro preparations such as the isolated perfused juxtamedullary nephron preparation have been developed to enable direct visualization of the vascular structures and macula-densa segments involved in the autoregulatory responses and the tubuloglomerular feedback mechanism. Studies on these preparations, coupled with further studies using traditional microperfusion techniques, continue to provide insights about this fascinating mechanism and how it participates in the control of glomerular function in both normal and pathophysiological conditions.

Neurohumoral Control of Renal Hemodynamics

Interests in neurohumoral control of renal hemodynamics proceeded from initial attempts to characterize the effects of vasoactive agents on renal sodium handling as determined by changes in total renal blood flow and on intrarenal distribution of blood flow. Further studies have characterized the effects of vasoactive agents on glomerular filtration dynamics and the filtration coefficient. In earlier studies, experimental designs consisted of administration of vasoactive drugs which, while eliciting changes in the variables of interest, often represented exercises in pharmacological, rather than physiological, responses. The subsequent availability of more selective and specific pharmacological antagonists allowed an evaluation of the physiological role of the endogenous level of the various neurohumoral systems. For example, competitive angiotensin-II receptor antagonists, which also exerted agonist responses, soon gave way to angiotensin-converting enzyme inhibitors as pharmacological tools for assessing the physiological role of the endogenous renin-angiotensin system. However, this issue has traveled full cycle as more specific receptor antagonists devoid of agonists actions have been developed. Thus, a new wave of reports using more specific angiotensin II receptor antagonists is occurring. The 1990 ASN reported several studies using newly developed nonpeptide receptor antagonists.

Inhibitors of cyclooxygenase (indomethacin and meclofenemate, for example) were initially used to identify the physiological role of the endogenous products of arachidonic acid metabolism. In this regard, an appreciation developed that one had to control for variables that would influence the endogenous activity of various neurohumoral systems, such as dietary sodium intake with its known effect on the activity of the renin-angiotensin system and renal prostaglandin production. In addition, that there were major interactions among the various neurohumoral systems came to be appreciated. For example, renal nerve stimulation would release norepinephrine from renal sympathetic nerve terminals within the kidney. In addition to the adrenergic mediated renal vasoconstriction, there was also an increase in the activity of the renin-angiotensin and prostaglandin systems within the kidney as detected by increases in renal venous renin and prostaglandin release. Their contributions to the renal vasoconstrictor response could be demonstrated when coadministration of agents designed to inhibit the renin-angiotensin and prostaglandin systems substantially modulated the renal vasoconstrictor responses to the same renal nerve stimulation stimulus. In the earlier years, these types of interactive actions seemed to fall within the scope of our experimental designs since were were only considering a few major systems such as renal nerves and adrenergic influences, angiotensin II, a few of the prostanoids, and kinins. Now, the permutations for this type of scenario, which has been replayed many times over the years, seem to be infinite, with the discovery of a seemingly never-ending list of new vasoactive substances. During recent years major advances have been made in the area of vasoactive substances and studies have been reported on the actions of atrial natriuretic peptides, endothelin, endothelial-derived relaxing and constricting factors, platelet-activating factor, a huge assortment of vasoconstrictor and vasodilator prostanoids, and many others. Furthermore, the development of newer agents capable of interfering with the well-known vasoactive systems (renin-angiotensin, kallikrein-kinin, adenosine, prostanoids) has stimulated renewed interest in the role and actions of these systems in the control of renal hemodynamics. Thus, it seems apparent that we are entering a new and very complicated era where it will be necessary to sort through this vast array of endogenous vasoactive substances and render judgments regarding their relative importance in the normal control of the renal circulation as well as their changing influence during altered physiological states or pathophysiological situations. For example, only recently, in the 1989 and 1990, have meetings of the ASN addressed the roles of endothelial-derived relaxing factor and of endothelin in normal control of renal hemodynamics.

Studies at the whole kidney level have now been greatly extended by the development of techniques that enabled specific vascular segments within the renal circulatory bed to be examined. These endeavors led to the appearance of techniques for the direct micropuncture of the glomerular vasculature in the Munich-Wistar rat endowed with surface glomeruli. Other approaches involved evaluation of responses in isolated perfused renal microvessels (a derivative of the isolated perfused tubule technique), isolated perfused glomeruli, and videometric and laser Doppler methods for the study of the renal papillary circulation. Preparations such as the hydronephrotic kidney or the perfused juxtamedullary nephron have enabled direct visualization of the individual arterioles in a flowing system. It is now possible to characterize segments of the renal microvasculature as to their reactivity to pressure and other vasoactive agents. Data from such investigations have furnished new insights into the roles of preglomerular and postglomerular vascular segments in contributing to the overall renal vascular resistance changes that occur during changes in renal perfusion pressure (autoregulation) and in response to administration of vasoactive compounds.

Outgrowth of Interests in Renal Vascular Control Mechanisms

Many of the studies described above have led to the identification of the glomerular mesangial cell as one vasoactive responsive cell resplendent with receptors of many types. It has been postulated that the mesangial cell contributes to many hemodynamic responses, such as changes in the glomerular ultrafiltration coefficient, by determining glomerular filtration surface area and regulating perfusion patterns within the glomerular capillary taft. Because of the potential importance and accessibility of mesangial cells, a marked interest in the biology of the mesangial cell has developed. In turn, this has led to development of techniques for mesangial cell culture and burgeoning studies on mesangial cell biochemistry and cell biology. During recent years, ASN meetings have included many reports on a variety of surface receptors, responses to and production of biologically active materials, and intracellular signaling events. All of these developments have contributed to a more detailed involvement by nephrologists in smooth muscle and mesangial cell control mechanisms and have propagated new fields of investigation in nephrology. These new fields have brought together individuals with diverse interests and backgrounds. The immense complexity of the intracellular signal transduction mechanisms has stimulated the imaginations of many. Endogenous peptides such as angiotensin II may activate multiple intracellular and membrane mechanisms. Some vasoactive agents may directly activate genetic translation and transcription processes and lead to the increased synthesis of various membrane transport proteins or growth factors as well as the more generally appreciated rapid vasoactive responses.

It is now appreciated that those systems that were simplistically recognized as "hemodynamic regulatory mechanisms" may also participate in long-term proliferative responses by way of complex interactions with other intracellular systems. As these more sophisticated concepts develop, so will further need for investigative efforts at all levels of inquiry. It is also being recognized that a variety of peptides and other biologically active molecules initially characterize as being involved in immune inflammatory responses may also have vasoactive properties and may influence renal hemodynamics. As we are able to understand the cellular and molecular mechanisms in more precise terms, we will also have to delineate the relative roles of all these new vasoactive systems in the control of both short-term and long-term renal hemodynamics in physiological and disease conditions. These future challenges will require creative and imaginative approaches blending traditional established integrative techniques with newer cellular and molecular approaches that have generated renewed interest and enthusiasm.

Acknowledgment. The authors thank Agnes C. Buffone for preparation of this manuscript.

15

Advances in Therapeutics

Wadi N. Suki, Manuel Martinez-Maldonado, and William M. Bennett

A Quarter Century

In any medical discipline, such as nephrology, knowledge telescopes with the passage of time so that it becomes difficult to chronicle retrospectively advances that are made. In order to gain a perspective of advances in therapeutics in nephrology during the 25 years of the American Society of Nephrology's existence, it is necessary to take a reference point from which to measure progress. Fortunately, in September 1966, the year preceding the first annual meeting of the ASN, the Third International Congress of Nephrology was held in Washington, D.C. Since large international forums of this type usually serve as the platform for displaying and summarizing the current knowledge in a discipline, the published proceedings of that meeting provide an excellent panoramic view of state-of-the-art renal therapeutics as it was at the time.

As prednisolone had been available since 1955, and the glucocorticoids now in common use had all been in use in 1966, it was not unexpected that an important focus at that time was on the response of the nephrotic syndrome in children and adults to glucocorticoid therapy. Also, since 6-mercaptopurine azathioprine, cyclophosphamide, actinomycin, and other similar drugs were already available and in use at that time, along with corticosteroids, another important emphasis was on the success of renal transplantation. Another area of emphasis was dialysis, both peritoneal and hemodialysis. It must be recalled that in 1966 the teflon/silicon shunt had been in existence for four years and the Cimino AV fistula was first introduced that year.

Of course considerable attention was paid to the conservative management of patients with chronic renal failure, particularly with respect to diet and the proper use of antibiotics in patients with impaired renal function. While diet continues to occupy our attention, the context is certainly quite different. The adjustment of doses of medication in patients with renal insufficiency or failure has become an ever greater challenge with the proliferation of drugs and has necessitated the incorporation of miniaturized guides and manuals into the contents of all physicians' already overweighed pockets.

By the time of the first ASN meeting little had changed in terms of therapeutic emphasis. There was still the emphasis on chronic dialysis and on transplantation. However, a prominent component of the program, both in terms of free communications and symposia, was focused on the problem of reflux and pyelonephritis and the controversy over medical versus surgical therapy for vesicoureteral reflux. The remainder of this chapter profiles specific conditions and abnormalities related to therapeutic trends from 1967 to the present.

Hyponatremia

The ASN has been a critical forum for discussions and presentations relating to the pathophysiology of hyponatremia particularly the syndrome of inappropriate antidiuretic hormone (SIADH) secretion. An early ASN meeting first reported that the volume expansion secondary to the water retention in SIADH leads to increased renal clearance of uric acid and, as a consequence, hypouricemia. The same meeting also emphasized that hyponatremia may be related to resetting of the level of osmolality ("reset osmostat") which triggers the release of ADH from hypothalamic centers. Various treatment strategies for SIADH were also presented at the ASN. Comparison of agents that inhibit the effects of ADH on the distal nephron indicated that lithium, tetracycline, and demeclocycline were able to reduce water reabsorption and thus improve hyponatremia.

The association of SIADH with schizophrenia was first reported at the ASN. In addition, coexistent hypernatremia is a rare but physiologically possible presentation of SIADH, as a result of absence of thirst.

Reports at the ASN indicated that in experimental animals severe hyponatremia for longer than five days could cause a progressive syndrome of limb weakness, paralysis, nystagmus, and a mortality rate greater than 50%. The investigators concluded that in the absence of therapy, hyponatremia could lead to central pontine myelinolysis. Permanent neurological disability was described in women undergoing elective surgery in whom water administration had been excessive. In contrast to the usual setting of hyponatremia associated with serious medical illness, particularly in the elderly, these women were essentially healthy. Appropriate therapy did not prevent permanent neurological disability, or death.

The issue of how quickly should severe hyponatremia be corrected has been discussed extensively at ASN meetings and symposia. Various authors presented data at the meetings suggesting that rapid correction of experimental hyponatremia is associated with central pontine myelinolysis. A similar phenomenon was also reported to occur in patients whose hyponatremia was rapidly corrected. It was relatively safe to correct patients to serum sodium levels of 130 ± 5 mEq/l.

Other investigators reporting on the treatment of hyponatremia indicated that the most appropriate rate of correction of hyponatremia should be less than 0.5 mEq/l/hr. Spinal-cord injury patients were reported to develop a type of hyponatremia that is not the classic SIADH, but rather the result of habitual high fluid intake and mild resetting of the central osmostat. A paper delivered at an ASN meeting was the first presentation that an olfactory neuroblastoma associated with SIADH expressed ADH mRNA.

Severe untreated hyponatremia is associated with a high mortality rate. The prognosis can be improved by rapid correction of serum sodium to mildly hyponatremic levels with hypertonic saline, provided the serum concentration does not rise by more than 25 mEq/l in 24 hours. However, if this rate of correction is exceeded, with resultant normalization of serum concentrations within 24 hours, death will occur. A raging controversy about the rate and degree of correction of hyponatremia was rekindled by a study which revealed that brain damage occurs from relatively rapid correction of mild hyponatremia. During the 1980s the treatment of hyponatremia was the subject of ASN controversy during debates at annual meetings.

Hyponatremia in patients with acquired immunodeficiency syndrome (AIDS) or AIDS-related complex (ARC) was revealed as causing a high mortality rate compared to similarly hyponatremic patients not infected with retrovirus.

The reported increased severity and dangers of its correction in females was questioned at the ASN. This notion was also challenged in experimental animals. Recent authors cannot prove impaired adaptation to hyponatremia in female rabbits.

Hyponatremia occurring posttransurethral resection of the prostate was found to be related to the intravesical administration of glycine with reduced serum sodium concentration similar to that seen with intravesical urea. Mannitol produced less hyponatremia. While glycine has the same volume of distribution as urea (total body water), it does not function effectively as an osmole to prevent water from being reabsorbed from the bladder. As a consequence, hypotonicity and cellular hydration will occur.

Hypernatremia

At the ASN, a retrospective study of 14,133 patients 60 years of age or older revealed that 212 patients (1.5%) possessed serum sodium levels greater than 149 mEq/l. Slow replacement of cumulative water deficits over 48 to 72 hours was associated with the lowest mortality, while replacement within 24 hours appeared to increase mortality. High mortality rates noted in hypernatremic patients was usually evidence of severe underlying disease.

The possibility that prostaglandins may play an important role in nephrogenic diabetes insipidus syndrome was first presented at the ASN. Analysis of the mode of inheritance of congenital nephrogenic diabetes insipidus in surviving ancestors of the ship Hopewell, which sailed to North America in the early 17th century, favored a genetic homogeneity of the disease.

Formation of the ideogenic osmoles that may lead to cerebral edema during correction of hypernatremia revealed accumulation of trimethylamine. Glycerophosphorylcholine and betaine were also found in brain tissue.

Diuretics

Mannitol and bicarbonate were reported to be beneficial in protecting patients who developed myoglobinuria from acute renal failure. Those patients who did not respond suffered a greater degree of muscle damage and volume depletion.

Studies of individuals with idiopathic hypercalciuria divided according to the levels of parathyroid hormone (PTH) revealed that the calciuretic response to an acute calcium load observed in stone formers is not abolished by chronic diuretic therapy.

Beneficial effects of amiloride in the treatment of Bartter's and Liddle's syndrome was first presented at the ASN. In addition, the combined use of metolazone and furosemide to regulate volume expansion (and hypertension) in chronic renal failure was also first reported at the ASN. Furthermore, provocative abstracts delivered at ASN meetings asserted that the hypokalemia of renal tubular acidosis could be reversed by administration of furosemide, presumably by diuretic-induced stimulation of prostaglandin synthesis.

Another important study revealed that amiloride could be natriuretic and antikaliuretic despite marked hyperaldosteronism. Amiloride can thus be used as a tool in the evaluation of hypokalemia. Moreover, it was shown that furosemide may lead to negative body potassium balance when dietary salt is restricted because aldosterone effects persist under these circumstances. Other studies also confirmed that furosemide can be used to evaluate distal acidification and to evaluate cortical collecting duct function in patients with selective aldosterone deficiency. In patients with distal renal tubular acidosis, furosemide has been found to stimulate acidification.

Acetazolamide used in the treatment of glaucoma frequently led to the development of kidney stones. This was dependent on the presence of hyperuricosuria.

The use of diuretics to attempt a conversion from low- to high-output acute renal failure, with improvement, has been debated many times at the ASN.

The diuretics, metolazone and tricrynafen, both made their initial appearances at ASN meetings during the 1970s. Tricrynafen, a uricosuric diuretic was removed from the market because of its hepatotoxic effects.

Metolazone continues to be used and is particularly useful in chronic renal-failure patients since it can potentiate the effect of loop diuretics.

Angiotensin-converting enzyme inhibitors were shown to improve the response of furosemide in congestive heart failure presumably because of their prostaglandin E (PGE) stimulating actions. Furosemide was demonstrated to be more dependent than bumetanide on tubule secretion. Accumulation of endogenously retained weak acids in renal failure may be responsible for the suboptimal response to furosemide in some patients with advanced renal failure.

Thiazides were found to increase microalbumin excretion rates in diabetics and hypertensives alike, suggesting that these agents may be deleterious to the kidney under some circumstances. This provocative finding remains to be corroborated.

Potassium

The role of insulin in the regulation of serum potassium was first discussed at ASN meetings. Poor response to insulin may explain why some diabetics develop hyperkalemia readily, even in the absence of uremia.

A study of sickle-cell disease patients found that a distal type of hyperkalemic hyperchloremic metabolic acidosis may be present. Chronic hyperkalemia was described in other congenital disturbances that exhibited increased renal chloride reabsorption. In addition, the role of alpha and beta adrenergic receptors in modulating extrarenal potassium handling in normal and diabetic subjects was discussed in a series of presentations at the ASN. The possible contribution of calcium channel blockers to potassium homeostasis was elucidated.

Recent ASN meetings recognized the common occurrence of hyperkalemia in AIDS patients, as a result of pentamidine nephrotoxicity, acidosis, or adrenal insufficiency.

In 1989 an evaluation of the clinical causes of hyperkalemia revealed that patients using calcium channel blockers, angiotensin converting enzyme inhibitors, beta-blockers, heparin, and nonsteroidal antiinflammatory agents experienced an increased incidence of hyperkalemia. In addition, patients with advancing age, diabetes, and AIDS now constitute a great percentage of patients referred to nephrologists for hyperkalemia. A study of the use of converting enzyme inhibitors in patients with Bartter's syndrome found that these drugs improved serum potassium, suggesting that hyperaldosteronism is the main cause of hypokalemia in this setting. Insensitivity of the beta-2 receptors to epinephrine contributes to the development of hyperkalemia in fasting control subjects, but not in dialysis patients.

Beta-2 adrenergic receptor inhibitors, as opposed to beta-1 sensitive blockers cause a greater rise in plasma potassium with exercise in chronic renal-failure patients. Dobutamine-induced hyperkalemia was associated with hypomagnesemia, probably through its beta-1 and beta-2 effects.

Lactic Acidosis

Controversy at the ASN over lactic acidosis has revolved around the treatment of this condition. Experimental results revealed that administration of bicarbonate to animals with experimental lactic acidosis did not correct many of the acid-base abnormalities. A dubious therapeutic role for bicarbonate was also reported in patients who developed lactic acidosis as a result of phenformin treatment. Further, hepatectomized animals treated with sodium chloride rather than sodium bicarbonate suffered reduced blood pH, but less mortality. Models of lactic-acid acidosis in dogs also tended to indicate that bicarbonate treatment worsened lactic acidosis. The successful treatment of experimental lactic acidosis with dichloroacetate was first reported at the ASN. In patients with hypoxic heart failure, administration of sodium bicarbonate resulted in systemic hypercapnia, increased production, and decreased extraction of lactate, and increased oxygen desaturation. Infusions of equal volume of isotonic sodium chloride did not cause any adverse changes suggesting that bicarbonate administration had deleterious effects. It should be pointed out that these results vary with the usual response nephrologists observe during the real-life treatment of lactic acidosis.

A study of anion-gap acidosis revealed that neutral organic acids such as lactic acid and ketoacids accounted for approximately 60% of the anion gap; the rest of the gap was caused by organic anions of unknown etiology.

Hypercalcemia

Based on early physiologic data relating calcium excretion to the excretion of sodium and, also, the clinical observation that hypercalcemia patients are often volume-depleted, the administration of saline solutions became a mainstay of the management of these patients in the late 1960s. Sodium sulfate was also administered, based on its known ability to form ionic complexes with calcium in the kidney which enhance calcium excretion. Sodium phosphate was an additional modality which found some utility in patients with well-preserved renal function, because of its properties to inhibit bone resorption and lower serum calcium.

During the ensuing years more was learned and presented at ASN meetings about the renal handling of calcium and the sites in the nephron where calcium is transported. It was learned from micropuncture studies, and subsequently from studies with isolated renal tubules microperfused in vitro, that calcium is reabsorbed passively in the thick ascending limb, secondary to the absorption of sodium and chloride. Consequently, the introduction of diuretics such as furosemide which exert major pharmacologic effects in the thick ascending limb presented an opportunity to enhance renal calcium excretion by pharmacologic means. Thus, furosemide was introduced for the treatment of acute hypercalcemic crisis of malignancy and remains to this day a common approach to the early management of these patients.

Another therapy used in treating hypercalcemia of malignancy was the glucocorticoid group of compounds, although these were not very effective in treating the hypercalcemia of hyperparathyroidism. Following steroids, a number of other agents have been applied to the treatment of hypercalcemia and these include calcitonin, mithramycin or plicamycin, and cisplatin. These compounds, however, especially the latter two, possess a high potential for causing serious side effects. Since the prostaglandins may be involved in bone resorption the prostaglandin synthetase inhibitors enjoyed a brief period of popularity during the 1980s, until they were found to be effective in only a small percentage of patients. More effective and possessing a longer-lasting effect are the diphosphonates which inhibit bone resorption. Etidronate, a member of this group of compounds, is now widely used for the treatment of this disorder. Another promising entry into this arena, and one with much less toxicity, is gallium nitrate, but this remains experimental at the present time.

Stones

As discussed elsewhere in this volume, great strides have been made in the medical therapy of renal calcium stones. Although occurring relatively less frequently, noncalcium-containing kidney stones represent a significant clinical challenge. Oral citrate, which recently has successfully treated calcium stones, does alkalinize the urine if used in sufficient quantities and has been used in treating uric acid stones. When urinary alkalinization and reduction of dietary purine intake have failed to control uric acid stones, allopurinol, a xanthine oxidase inhibitor, has been used successfully.

A challenging medical problem throughout the 25-year history of the ASN has been the management of hyperoxaluria. When mild to moderate, such as that caused by bowel disease, the hyperoxaluria is managed with a low-oxalate diet and a low-fat diet, oral calcium supplements, and cholestyramine. The low-fat diet reduces the concentration in the bowel lumen of undigested medium-chain fatty acids which irritate the colonic mucosa and increase permeability to oxalate. Cholestyramine binds oxalate and also the bile salts, thereby also preventing the irritation of the colonic mucosa. Calcium in the intestinal contents also forms insoluble complexes with oxalate and reduces its absorption. One form of calcium reported useful in treating enteric hyperoxaluria is a marine organic hydrocolloid charged with calcium. Studies presented at the ASN demonstrate that the administration of this natural product reduces urinary oxalate excretion and the calcium-oxalate product in the urine. More severe hyperoxaluria, such as is found in patients with primary hyperoxaluria, is a much more difficult problem and one for which a completely satisfactory treatment has not been developed. Large doses of pyridoxine lower, somewhat, the excretion of oxalate and have been used with some success in the management of these patients. A variety of compounds have been used to inhibit the synthesis of oxalate. One such compound is isocarboxazid, a hydrazine derivative which inhibits the oxidation of 2-amino alcohol to glycolaldehyde, a precursor of glycolic acid. It has been shown in one ASN report to produce significant reductions in oxalate and glycolate excretion, but no further studies of this compound have been reported.

Another type of renal stone disease which presents a challenge to the treating physician is cystine. Hydration is often recommended, but infrequently adhered to by patients because of the large volume of fluids that have to be consumed. Although alkalinization of the urine to a pH of 7.4 has been used and can be successful in preventing or even solubilizing cystine stones, that too is difficult to achieve and may be even hazardous. The consumption of large amounts of sodium bicarbonate to achieve that high of a urine pH results in bloating, which compounds the bloating caused by copious fluid intake. Furthermore, the alkalinization of the urine to this degree causes precipitation of brushite stones. Of interest is the observation that the administration of glutamine, orally, and the restriction of sodium intake result in significant reductions in the excretion of cystine. These measures have been applied to the treatment of cystine stone-formers with some success. However, the most definitive treatment is penicillamine which unfortunately is associated with side effects in some 50% of patients.

Struvite stones also pose a significant challenge. Protracted treatment with antibiotics accompanied by a urease inhibitor acetylhydroxamic acid have been found effective in some patients in controlling and reducing the size of the stones. Acetylhydroxamic acid, however, does have significant complications and complete removal of infected stones followed by prolonged antibiotic therapy seems to be the major definitive approach.

This brings us to the subject of stone removal, where significant advances have been made. Two new approaches, one employing the percutaneous approach using fiber optic instruments and the other using extracorporeal shock wave, have greatly advanced this mode of treatment and greatly reduced morbidity and mortality. An ASN symposium highlighted these new techniques. Extracorporeal shock wave lithotripsy (ESWL) has become widely used alone or in combination with percutaneous nephrolithotomy or lower-urinary-tract endoscopy. Although these techniques have been extremely successful and have changed the manner of treating stones of a size larger than can be passed through the ureter, concerns do exist relative to the effects of these procedures on kidney function and the possible advent of hypertension in the long term.

Parenchymal Renal Disease

Scleroderma. The treatment of patients with progressive systemic sclerosis has been the source of great frustration to physicians for many years, especially those patients presenting with scleroderma renal crisis. This disorder which consists of accelerated hypertension, microangiopathic hemolysis, and gradual deterioration of renal function had frustrated efforts at controlling blood pressure and arresting disease using therapies then available. Early studies revealed that prior to the onset of the renal crisis, and certainly at the height of it, plasma renin levels were markedly elevated. The high renin levels were incriminated in contributing to the vascular disease and the high morbidity and mortality rates for this disorder. In 1973 a report appeared claiming successful treatment of one such patient with bilateral nephrectomy (to remove the source of renin), hemodialysis, and subsequently transplantation. This patient exhibited disappearance of the arthralgias and Raynaud's phenomenon, improvement in the skin changes of scleroderma, and normalization of the blood pressure. This approach was rapidly and widely adopted and was the accepted form of therapy for at least five years thereafter. However, multiple reports began to appear demonstrating successful management of these patients with hemodialysis as well as control of hypertension alone without resorting to nephrectomy. Some of these patients even improved enough and regained sufficient renal function to be able to discontinue hemodialysis. This approach was aided by the introduction of captopril to the therapy of this disorder, beginning in 1979. This drug enabled good control of blood pressure and resulted, in many patients, in arrest of the progression of renal disease and even some improvement in renal function. Using this approach it would now appear that at least 50% of patients with scleroderma renal crisis, a disorder that previously was invariably fatal, can now be conservatively managed and salvaged.

For those patients who do go on to develop renal failure, hemodialysis previously was the main approach and many patients were treated with transplantation as well. Based on a report dating back to 1971, showing that peritoneal clearances of creatinine and of urate were reduced in patients with scleroderma, peritoneal dialysis was thought to be a less adequate approach to the management of these patients. However, multiple reports have appeared since then showing successful therapy of these patients with continuous ambulatory peritoneal dialysis (CAPD) and showing clearances of solutes in these patients not very different from those in patients with other disorders. Consequently, at present, peritoneal dialysis is a valid approach to the treatment of patients with end-stage renal disease secondary to progressive systemic sclerosis.

Multiple Myeloma and Light Chain Disease. The involvement of the kidney in patients with light chain disease and multiple myeloma was very well studied clinically in the early days of nephrology in the mid-1960s. The mechanism of the renal failure secondary to the production and excretion in the urine of light chains has received and continues to receive a great deal of attention. Forced diuresis and alkalinization of the urine were commonly employed by physicians for treating patients with impaired renal function. Steroids and chemotherapeutic agents, such as 1,3bis(2chloroethyl)-1-nitrosourea (BCNU) and melphalan, were widely used and seemed to be effective in stabilizing the disease and renal function when patients were treated before severe renal failure had set in. These approaches were infrequently effective in restoring renal function once the patients had become oliguric and were begun on dialysis. Beginning in 1976, reports began to appear in which, in addition to forced diuresis, chemotherapy, and dialysis, plasmapheresis was employed to remove the circulating light chains. This approach was reported to ASN members in data from at least two randomized prospective clinical trials and has now been demonstrated to be effective in prolonging survival and restoring renal function in the majority of patients. Based on these recent studies from the United States and abroad this should become the accepted approach for the future.

Intractable Ascites, Hepatorenal Syndrome, and Hepatic Failure. Although mostly in the realm of the gastroenterologist, disorders of the liver causing ascites, hepatorenal syndrome, and hepatic coma have preoccupied nephrologists for the entire history of the ASN. Papers on the subject have been delivered at meetings each year. The advent of newer more potent diuretics, and certainly the advent of the potassium-sparing diuretics, did contribute to the management of ascites. However, a group of patients present with ascites resistant to all forms of diuretic therapy. When diuresis is forced, alone, or in combination with paracentesis, renal failure may supervene. A number of approaches were innovated which basically consist of the withdrawal of ascitic fluid, concentrating it and reinfusing it either intravenously or back into the peritoneal cavity. These approaches were associated with reduction of the size of ascites and often with a diuresis and natriuresis. However, this approach is cumbersome and expensive, and when the approach involved direct infusion into the circulation of the ascitic fluid, a febrile reaction often resulted. A breakthrough was made in 1973 with the introduction of a cathether which was used to communicate the peritoneal cavity with the jugular or subclavian vein allowing drainage of the ascitic fluid directly into the venous circulation. This approach was associated with diuresis and remission of the ascites.

Some patients with advanced liver disease developed a form of acute renal failure generally characterized by relatively low systemic arterial pressure, low systemic vascular resistance with a high renal vascular resistance, renal under-perfusion, and avid retention of sodium and water with oliguria. A number of approaches to this problem have been attempted, including the intrarenal arterial infusion of various vasodilators, but with little success. Since low systemic vascular resistance and increased capacitance of the circulation is in large part responsible for this disorder, ornipressin which is an 8-ornithine derivative of vasopressin has been used with remarkable success. This compound increased the systemic vascular resistance and in correspondence, decreased the cardiac index. With these hemodynamic changes the blood levels of atrial natriuretic peptide increased while the levels of catecholamines, renin, and aldosterone decreased. The creatinine clearance increased and sodium and water excretion also increased. Additionally, since these patients have been shown to have markedly reduced prostaglandin excretion, the administration of the prostaglandin analog misoprostil has been shown in preliminary reports to be of some promise. In spite of these encouraging preliminary observations, the management of this disorder remains challenging and often frustrating.

Patients who develop severe hepatic failure and progress into a state of hepatic coma have been managed with remarkable success with the extracorporeal circulation of the blood through charcoal hemoperfusion cartridges. This maneuver diminishes the circulating levels of aromatic amino acids and is associated with improvement of the neurological status in almost 90% of the patients. While this approach does nothing to alter the course of hepatic disease it does allow time for the patient's underlying disease to stabilize for hepatic regeneration to occur, or for hepatic transplantation to be undertaken.

Pregnancy and Renal Disease. It has been noted for many years that in addition to the de novo incidence of preeclampsia and renal disease in pregnant women, pregnancy is often associated with worsening of underlying renal disease. Preeclampsia and pregnancy in the patient with renal disease have come under intensive investigation in the last 25 years with substantial advances. In the first place, it has become recognized from multiple studies that pregnancy per se does not have an adverse effect on renal function; instead it is the hypertension that often accompanies pregnancy that has a deleterious effect on kidney function. A great deal of emphasis has been placed on vigorous and effective control of blood pressure in pregnant women with kidney disease. With such measures, a remarkably large percent of pregnancies can be successful with little or no worsening of the renal function. The choice of antihypertensive medication is unfortunately rather limited because of the many side effects these agents may have in pregnant women. Diuretics, for example, have been shown to reduce placental blood flow and reduce the excretion of dehydroepiandrosterone sulfate, which constitutes evidence of reduced placental function. Other agents such as the converting enzyme inhibitors may be associated with fetal death. At present alpha methyldopa remains the mainstay of antihypertensive therapy in pregnant women. Hydralazine has been used with some success, although chronic administration has been associated with reduced placental blood flow. Beta blockers have also been used but carry the same hazard as hydralazine. ASN symposia over the years have chronicled the pathophysiology, diagnosis, and management of the pregnant women with renal disease and pregnancy-induced hypertension.

With respect to preeclampsia, an important role for thromboxane production has been invoked. In an effort to reduce thromboxane production by platelets without impairing prostacyclin production by endothelial cells, trials using small doses of salicylate have been presented and discussed at the ASN. Both trials have shown that the use of 60 to 100 mg of acetylsalicyclic acid daily prolongs the pregnancy, allows a larger size infant, and is associated with considerably reduced complications.

Tubulointerstitial Renal Diseases

Urinary Tract Infection and Pyelonephritis. Infection of the urinary tract has occupied the attention of investigators for many years, certainly dating back to the inception of the Society and even earlier. Numerous studies have been performed in both men and women and presented since then. In both sexes the major emphasis has been on the efficacy of certain drug regimens in controlling infection and in preventing its recurrence. In women, where urinary-tract infections occur relatively frequently, and most usually without underlying urinary tract disease, therapy has been shown to be relatively simple. Regimens of high doses of cotrimoxazole or of penicillin derivatives given for a period of one to three days have been shown effective in eradicating the infection in the vast majority of patients. In men, however, urinary tract infections are usually superimposed on urinary tract disease, particularly prostatic disease, in the vast majority of patients. In these patients, short-term treatment has been shown to be notoriously ineffective and courses of therapy lasting for as long as six weeks may be necessary. In men with recurrent infections, a large prospective study, carried out with the support of the US Public Health Service, and reported at the ASN, has shown that long-term prophylactic therapy with agents such as nitrofurantoin, cotrimoxazole, and methenamine mandelate does reduce the recurrence rate, reduces the incidence of septic episodes, and may help prevent progression of kidney disease. In addition to these classical antimicrobial agents, the last three to four years have seen the advent of a new class of agents, namely the fluoroquinolines which have proven quite effective in the treatment of urinary tract infections, especially with resistant organisms.

In relation to infection of the urinary tract, vesicoureteral reflux, which predisposes to urinary tract infection and renal scarring, has been a preoccupation of nephrologists for many years, certainly dating back to the inception of the ASN. One of the major points of contention debated at the ASN in the late 1960s has been whether appropriate treatment consists of surgical correction or conservative medical therapy. Evidence on the side of either camp has been presented over the years. However, the preponderance of evidence indicates that recurrent urinary-tract infection, new renal scars, and progressive scarring occur as often in surgically corrected patients as in those treated conservatively. Therefore, in 1990 there seems to be little justification for surgical correction even of severe vesicoureteral reflux.

Miscellaneous Interstitial Disorders. A number of primarily tubulointerstitial disorders have been the subject of investigation over the years. One such disorder is sickle-cell hemoglobinemia which causes interstitial nephritis and papillary necrosis. Even sickle-cell trait can cause a gross hematuria. A number of reports have dealt with the treatment of this disorder and the approaches have varied over the years. These have included vigorous hydration including the intravenous infusion of sterile water. Although the hematuria is self-limited in about 50% of the patients, epsilon aminocaproic acid has been shown to be effective in arresting the hematuria in patients whose hematuria is severe or protracted.

Toxic Nephropathy and Drug-Induced Renal Dysfunction

In 1967, as the ASN was formed, analgesic nephropathy was being defined clinically and experimentally by centers around the world, particularly in Switzerland, Australia, and Scotland. Early meetings of the Society emphasized that the papillary necrosis lesion might relate to the concentration of toxic metabolites in the renal medulla. By 1969 it was obvious that phenacetin could not explain the entire syndrome and that combinations of analgesics were probably involved in the pathogenesis of analgesic nephropathy. Improvement in renal function after drug withdrawal was documented in long-term studies serving as an example of a chronic renal disease that does not progress inevitably to end-stage renal disease. An important paper in 1971 proposed that aspirin inhibited the kidneys' defense against oxidant damage in the renal papilla with phenacetin and its metabolites providing the primary oxidant stress. The frequency and importance of analgesic nephropathy as a cause of end-stage renal disease in the US continued to be debated until 1981 when an epidemiologic study in Pennsylvania lowered previous estimates of analgesic nephropathy causing more than five % of end-stage renal failure requiring dialysis. However, groups from the southeast continued to see new cases of analgesic nephropathy years after phenacetin was withdrawn from compound formulations of analgesics, suggesting that regional, cultural, and, perhaps, climatic conditions were important in the complex etiology of this potentially preventable cause of end-stage renal disease. In 1989 a large epidemiologic study suggested that acetaminophen, a primary metabolite of phenacetin, was associated with an increased relative risk of renal disease. Also in 1989, a study from Europe documented progression of renal disease associated with hidden analgesic use discovered by random urine screening, raising obvious challenges to eradication of this problem simply by physicians' admonitions.

Colistimethate and polymyxin β were the drugs of choice for treatment of serious gram negative infections in the late 1960s. Both were virtually obligate nephrotoxins, and gentamicin, a newly released drug, was being recognized as a much safer alternative. By the mid-1970s the frequency of renal dysfunction due to gentamicin and other newer aminoglycoside antibiotics was being recognized by nephrologists as indicated by multiple papers and symposia at annual ASN meetings. Accumulation of drug by the kidney was documented in man and animals as was the role of the kidney in drug excretion. It also became clear that reliable delivery of aminoglycosides could not be achieved in the urine of end-stage renal disease patients for treatment of urinary-tract infections. Several clinical and experimental studies examined the relative nephrotoxic potential of gentamicin and tobramycin with advocates for each drug sometimes exchanging strongly held convictions based on small studies with widely different experimental designs. Late in the decade the matter was settled clinicallly by the convincing data from the Johns Hopkins group favoring amikacin and tobramycin. Nonetheless, during the 1980s most nephrologists still dealt primarily with gentamicin nephrotoxicity because of the substantial cost differential favoring gentamicin, whose patent had expired. Early diagnostic tests for aminoglycoside and other toxic nephropathies such as enzymuria, cast excretion, immunoassay for tubular epithelial antigens, and electron microscopy of the urinary sediment lacked specificity and were not accepted into clinical practice. Various protective maneuvers for aminoglycoside nephrotoxicity, highly effective in experimental animals, such as sodium chloride, calcium carbonate, and potassium chloride provided insights into cellular mechanisms of injury, but were not practical for patient management.

Other drug-related causes of renal dysfunction were described at ASN meetings. Rifampin, administered intermittently, caused acute renal failure often associated with a severe systemic reaction which included severe myalgia and muscle necrosis. Nitrosoureas used for cancer chemotherapy were implicated in a particularly severe, irreversible form of interstitial fibrosis and glomerular sclerosis. After 30 to 40 years of neglect as an entity worthy of consideration in the US, the renal effects of excess environmental lead exposure were brought to the attention of clinical nephrologists at the ASN meetings in the mid-1970s. Particularly noteworthy were reports of the use of the edetate calcium disodium (EDTA) mobilization test to estimate body lead burden in patients thought to have renal failure on the basis of gout or essential hypertension. Late in the 1980s in vivo fluorescence instruments became available to ascertain body lead burden. This technology could replace the more cumbersome EDTA mobilization test, particularly in end stage renal disease (ESRD) patients.

In 1980 the association of chronic lithium nephrotoxicity manifested by interstitial fibrosis and reduced GFR was brought to the attention of American nephrologists by abstracts submitted to the annual meeting. Confirmatory papers and presentations soon followed. Lithium was also observed to produce vasopressin resistant diabetes insipidus. Indomethacin was useful in controlling polyuria in lithium treated patients. Based on in vitro studies, data were presented documenting the effects of lithium and demeclocycline on water transport in the toad urinary bladder. In addition, data comparing these two drugs in the treatment of eight patients with the syndrome of inappropriate antidiuretic hormone secretion showed superior effectiveness with demeclocycline which caused fewer central-nervous-system side effects in these subjects than lithium.

Anesthetic agents, particularly new fluorinated derivatives such as methoxyflurane and isoflurane, were first recognized in 1970 as causes for a concentrating defect and nonoliguric acute renal failure. Oxalate excretion was increased and was hypothesized by some to be etiologic until it became clear that renal failure was related to the extent of halide metabolism.

A relationship between occupational exposure to hydrocarbons and Goodpasture's syndrome was proposed in 1971. Despite attempts to prove a cause-and-effect relationship over the years this association remains a matter of some controversy in the 1990s. Even the nephrologist's old friend, mannitol, did not escape unscathed from adverse renal reactions. In 1989 seven patients receiving mannitol in large doses for cerebral edema developed reversible acute renal failure presumably secondary to vacuolar change in renal epithelial cells.

In the late 1970s, the physiologic role of prostaglandins in maintenance of renal hemodynamics in disease states such as cirrhosis of the liver, nephrotic syndrome, and congestive heart failure was elucidated. Shortly thereafter, various investigators reported the adverse effects on renal function of the commonly used nonsteroidal antiinflammatory drugs (NSAIDs). Evidence accumulated that nonsteroidal antiinflammatory drugs did not reduce renal function in normal subjects receiving an adequate sodium intake. It gradually became accepted that NSAID-associated renal dysfunction and vasoconstriction was only observed in patients with ineffective circulating plasma volume, high plasma renin and angiotensin II levels, or increased alpha adrenergic neural activity. Presumably, the drug, by cyclo-oxygenase inhibition, reduces renal cortical prostaglandin synthesis and consequent vasodilation in response to vasoconstrictive stimuli. Sulindac sulfoxide, a relatively "renal sparing" NSAID is an active prodrug, reversibly reduced to its active form and then oxidized by the kidney to an inactive sulfone. Several authors, however, reported that sulindac given to high-risk patients could produce renal dysfunction.

Ibuprofen, released for over the counter sales in 1984–1955, created controversy when the FDA did not require the same warning levels as were required of prescription strength ibuprofen. This occurred despite the recommendations of a task force formed by the National Kidney Foundation and the opinions of many experts presented at ASN symposia and presentations. From 1985 to 1990, sporadic reports appeared documenting acute and chronic adverse renal effects of over-the-counter NSAIDs. Suprofen, a nonsteroidal drug similar in structure to the uricosuric thiazide diuretic, ticrynafen, caused many cases of acute renal failure, possibly due to its uricosuric action in previously healthy men. It was withdrawn from the market after pressure was put on the manufacturer by ASN members based on their experience and the expanding number of new cases reported.

Hyperkalemia, due to hyporeninemic hypoaldosteronism, was an additional consequence of NSAID therapy reported first in 1979. Therapeutic advantage was taken of the renal hemodynamic effects of NSAIDs in nephrotic patients who were sodium-depleted to effect major reductions in urinary protein excretion. At the 1979 and 1980 meetings, the first descriptions of minimal change nephropathy and acute interstitial nephritis due to NSAIDs were reported. This fortunately rare adverse event has received widespread notoriety despite its low incidence and presumed idiosyncratic nature. The pathogenesis remains a mystery.

Not long after the introduction of angiotensin-converting enzyme inhibitors in 1979 and 1980, their effects on renal hemodynamics were noted. While renal function generally improved, it was quickly observed that a few patients including those with bilateral renal artery stenosis had marked acute declines in glomerular filtration rate. In 1982, acute renal failure was documented in seven patients with bilateral renal artery stenosis and five patients with a solitary kidney. The role of concomitant diuretic therapy was emphasized. The now-accepted pathogenesis, that angiotensin-converting enzyme inhibition interrupted angiotensin II mediated efferent arteriolar vasoconstriction when perfusion pressure to the entire renal mass was reduced, was proposed in several ASN presentations.

In 1968, renal tubular acidosis was reported in most patients receiving amphotericin B who were stressed with ammonium-chloride loading. A double-blind study ultimately showed the ineffectiveness of mannitol in reducing amphotericin nephrotoxicity, a practice in vogue by extrapolation from ischemic acute renal failure. In the following year, acute interstitial nephritis with acute renal failure was described clinically. Most of the now well-established clinical features, such as delayed onset of fever and renal failure after the drug is discontinued, as well as eosinophilia and a presumed immunologic pathogenesis, were suggested in the original report. Although the initial offenders were most often penicillins and indeed this entity was known as "methicillin nephritis," it soon became clear that a similar type of hypersensitivity reaction could be observed with many drugs. In 1975 a paper was presented which documented the valve of eosinophiluria in diagnosis; this same series still stands today as the only evidence from a controlled study validating steroids as useful in attaining a more rapid improvement in renal function than is observed in patients managed by simple drug withdrawal. This work still frequently cited in the 1990s, stands despite the small number of patients, as the rationale for steroid therapy in acute interstitial nephritis. The diagnostic sensitivity of eosinophiluria was markedly improved by the use of the Hansel's staining technique. In another much cited paper, first presented at the 1980 ASN meeting, it was proposed that Gallium-67 uptake was a useful differential diagnostic tool in separation of acute interstitial nephritis from other causes of acute renal failure. Subsequent reports have somewhat dampened enthusiasm for this technique by pointing out suboptimal specificity. Throughout the 1980s, newly introduced drugs producing acute interstitial nephritis were reported. Nephrologists took the opportunity to share cases, such as those related to the first histamine-2 receptor blocker, cimetidine, at annual ASN meetings.

Early cephalosporin derivatives such as cephaloridine were associated with acute tubular necrosis because of drug accumulation within proximal tubular cells. In an elegant series of experiments, Tune worked out the mechanism of cell uptake and documented uptake inhibition by blockade of organic ion transport. Newer, safer cephalosporins underwent net tubular secretion without intracellular accumulation.

In the late 1960s and early 1970s, imaging of the kidneys in patients with renal insufficiency often depended on large doses of contrast caused by a constant infusion. Several reports given at the ASN meetings in 1975 and 1976 elucidated the risk of contrast studies to the diabetic patient with preexisting renal insufficiency. This fact, combined with the emergence of ultrasound and computed tomography techniques, led to rapid changes in the way nephrologists excluded obstruction and estimated kidney size in their patients. Strong recommendations were made to avoid intravenous pyelography in type-1 diabetics with serum creatinine values greater than 5 mg/dl. Each year papers were presented reiterating the frequency and potential irreversibility of contrast nephropathy in diabetics with preexisting renal dysfunction. Several controlled trials, particularly one reported at the 1981 meetings, documented that mannitol might be of use for prevention in high-risk patients; however, these studies, which generally contained small numbers of patients, were not ideally randomized to treatment and control groups. Calcium antagonists and atrial natriuretic peptide also were proposed to modify nephrotoxicity, although large, properly controlled clinical trials were lacking. Although new nonionic radiographic contrast media were introduced in the late 1980s, large randomized studies could not document a difference in the incidence of contrast nephrotoxicity versus conventional agents, certainly not enough to justify the expense of newer agents based on renal considerations alone.

During the 1980s, various biological agents such as recombinant interleukin-2 and the monoclonal antibody, muromonab-CD3 (OKT3), appeared in clinical practice. Systemic reactions usually included oliguria with low fractional excretion of sodium. This type of "cytokine" nephropathy is presumably due to release of various mediators which cause increased capillary leak, intravascular volume depletion, and, if not modified, acute tubular necrosis.

With the emergence of AIDS as a national health crisis of the mid-to-late 1980s, the antiprotozoal drug pentamidine was rediscovered to treat pneumocystis carinii infections. Twenty-five percent of patients receiving this drug developed serious nephrotoxicity, and hyperkalemic metabolic acidosis was prominent. Although the clinical picture clarified by 1990, the pathogenesis and treatment remain fertile fields for future research.

Cisplatin has produced improved response rates in ovarian and testicular cancer, although higher doses, which would be expected to provide further benefits, are limited by nephrotoxicity. Even adequate hydration and mannitol did not protect from nephrotoxicity at doses of 100 to 200 mg/m^2 of cisplatin. Cisplatinum nephrotoxicity was the subject of many papers throughout the 1980s.

Probably the most investigative effort in therapeutics from a nephrologic standpoint in the 1980s was devoted to the optimal use of cyclosporine. Much of the important work in this field was presented at ASN meetings as oral presentations and posters. Outstanding invited lectures and symposia brought the clinical and basic science aspects of this important drug to the forefront of nephrotoxicity investigation.

With expanded use of cyclosporine in renal, liver, heart, and bone marrow transplantation, dose-related nephrotoxicity emerged as a serious if not inevitable problem. Although glomerular filtration rate usually improved as the dose of cyclosporine was reduced, disturbing chronic tubulointerstitial fibrosis was increasingly reported. This made the long-term outlook for renal function uncertain. Contributions describing the Stanford heart-transplant patients were noteworthy. In addition, hyperkalemic metabolic acidosis due to hypoaldosteronism was common. In renal transplantation, the differential diagnosis of cyclosporine nephrotoxicity from allograft rejection remains difficult and often can only be made retrospectively.

Drugs causing additive or synergistic nephrotoxicity with cyclosporine are ketoconazole, trimethoprim-sulfamethoxazole, aminoglycoside antibiotics, amphotericin B, and acyclovir. The precise pathogenesis of cyclosporine nephrotoxicity is still unknown, although experimental work presented at the ASN strongly suggest a major role for thromboxanes and endothelin. At present, there is no entirely satisfactory model in experimental animals that reproduces the nephrotoxicity observed in humans. The role of monitoring blood levels of cyclosporine in prevention of nephrotoxicity is uncertain and the subject of much debate. Trough cyclosporine levels generally correlate with nephrotoxicity, but there is considerable overlap in blood levels with patients without overt renal dysfunction.

As reported at ASN meetings and symposia in the late 1980s, increases of blood pressure either de novo or from previously hypertensive levels are frequently seen in cyclosporine-treated patients. In cardiac transplantation where renal rejection is not present, the majority of cyclosporine-treated patients are hypertensive when compared with historical azathioprine-treated patients. Although renal function is usually also decreased, this is not uniformly true. In both cardiac and renal allograft recipients plasma renin activity is low and relatively unresponsive to stimulatory maneuvers such as captopril challenge. Conventional approaches to antihypertensive therapy are often ineffective, necessitating multiple-drug regimens. Neurologic symptoms unrelated to hypertension, including focal convulsions and hemiplegia, can be noted with cyclosporine immunosuppression. Calcium channel blockers reversibly increase cyclosporine levels, and careful monitoring of blood levels should be available when these drugs are used in antihypertensive regimens.

Treatment of Overdoses

Treatment of overdoses was often the sole responsibility of the nephrologist in the late 1960s, since extracorporeal removal of toxins and poisons was considered logical and effective. Although conservative means were tried for mild cases, hemodialysis was regularly used for severe intoxications. Barbiturate and salicylate poisonings were the most frequent indications for dialysis treatment of overdoses in the 1960s.

A particularly serious drug overdose during the 1960s to mid-1970s was with the lipid soluble, sleeping medication, glutethimide. Dialysis was often performed using soybean oil as the dialysate because of the belief that clearance would be improved with a lipid dialysate. This process was a nightmare for the nursing staff and aside from theoretical consideration, never validated. Recovery possibly was hastened, although no controlled studies were ever presented and patient survival related to the depth and length of coma on admission. A definitive study of 70 patients in 1970 documented the wisdom of conservative, nondialysis management of overdoses with glutethimide. Fortunately, this agent has been replaced by other drugs which seldom cause lethal problems even when taken in overdose situations.

The profile of overdosage changed with the explosion of psychoactive drugs. The benzodiazepines and tricyclic antidepressants of the 1970s were followed by the drugs of abuse of the 1980s. The clinical presentations of some overdoses changed as well; for example, metabolic acidosis resulted from paint and glue sniffing, and rhabdomyolysis with myoglobinuric acute renal failure was related to intravenous cocaine and narcotic abuse.

The spectrum of renal abnormalities related to i.v.-drug abuse was brought to the attention of ASN members as early as 1971 with further papers defining this entity appearing regularly from large eastern US medical centers. As the drugs of abuse shifted in the late 1980s, so did the nephrologic syndromes. "Crack" cocaine and metamphetamines were reported to produce malignant hypertension, rhabdomyolysis, acute renal and liver failure.

As emergency departments and poison control centers became increasingly sophisticated in resuscitation, information dissemination, and supportive care, the role of hemodialysis and even resin or charcoal hemoperfusion administered by nephrologists became reserved for unusual cases, usually those associated with industrial or accidental poisonings. During the late 1970s, a synthetic resin, amberlite XAD-4, was popular for removal of nonpolar drugs with low intrinsic clearances. Some investigations used resin hemoperfusion for digitalis overdose and toxicity. Even though use of hemoperfusion cartridges shortened the duration of coma or hemodynamic instability in some patients, the achievement of similar patient survival and morbidity with conservative measures has markedly lessened the indications for extracorporeal therapy. Severe ethylene glycol overdoses as well as overdoses with other alcohols such as isopropyl alcohol, methanol, and ethyl alcohol itself were indications for acute hemodialysis because of the ready removal of the toxin.

Pharmacokinetics, Pharmacodynamics, and Renal Disease

The study of drug pharmacokinetics and its application to therapy in patients was severely limited in 1967 because of the relatively crude methods available to quantitate drugs and chemicals in body fluids. One of the first classes of drugs to be studied were the cardiac glycosides. An important paper of that era showed that tritiated digoxin half-life and serum levels were increased in 10 anephric patients. The following year, detailed digoxin dosing recommendations for varying degrees of renal insufficiency were published. The first table of data with recommendations for antibiotic dosage adjustments in renal failure was published in 1967. The "new" drugs at that time were the semisynthetic, penicillinase resistant penicillins, oxacillin and methicillin, which were just coming into common clinical usage. Little or no information existed about the fate of other drugs in renal failure and there was little recognition of the role of the kidney in drug excretion until 1970 when the first comprehensive data was compiled and published in tabular form. About that time dialysis losses of ascorbic acid and water soluble vitamins were documented, forming the basis for vitamin supplements which are now the standard of care in most end-stage renal disease programs.

Over the years, data on specific important drugs used by clinical nephrologists has been presented to the membership each year with subsequent incorporation into widely disseminated references.

In 1980 the first of a series of presentations was given regarding the appearance of antibiotics into cyst fluid from patients with autosomal dominant polycystic kidney disease. Differences in "gradient" and "nongradient" cysts based on sodium concentrations eventually lead to insights regarding cyst growth and transepithelial cyst fluid movement. Lipid soluble antimicrobials such as chloramphenicol, trimethoprim-sulfamethoxazole and ciprofloxacin were shown to kill test bacteria in cyst fluid in vitro after administration to patients.

By the mid-1970s it had become well known and was repeatedly emphasized that blood level monitoring with easily assayable drugs such as the aminoglycosides was necessary to avoid drug accumulation and toxicity. With cardiac glycosides, levels in plasma can overestimate the pharmacologically active drug since endogenous "digoxin-like" substances cross-reacted in the digoxin radioimmunoassay.

Abnormalities of drug-protein binding were described in the presence of uremia. These abnormalities needed to be considered in interpretation of plasma drug levels of anticonvulsants and other agents. A number of investigators reported on the presence of inhibitors of drug-protein binding in the patient with renal insufficiency. Dialysis did not seem to normalize the binding abnormalities in most workers' hands. Changes in drug distribution were reported requiring lowering of initial doses of cardiac glycosides and other agents whose tissue binding and, thus, volume of distribution, were reduced by uremia.

In 1976 an important paper documented the accumulation of the pharmacologically active metabolite of procainamide, N-acetyl procainamide in patients with renal insufficiency. This was the first recognition that metabolites with pharmacologic actions could cause adverse reactions in the renal patient even when the parent compound underwent hepatic metabolism. Another important contribution showed impaired oral absorption of a test drug, D-xylose, in uremic patients. Agents such as iron, commonly prescribed for patients with end-stage renal disease, impaired absorption markedly in the presence of raised gastric pH. It became obvious that each new therapeutic agent released for clinical usage would require sophisticated pharmacokinetic studies in patients with impaired renal function as well as in individuals treated with the various forms of dialysis therapy, if accurate dosing recommendations were to be made for this complex group of patients at great risk of adverse drug reactions.

Essential to proper dosage adjustment in patients with renal insufficiency, particularly the elderly, is an accurate indication of renal function. The effects of varying assay interferences with serum creatinine determinations and competitive inhibition of tubular creatinine secretion were clarified in 1980. Although a variety of nomograms and formulas were proposed for renal function estimation, nothing has supplanted the convenient serum creatinine or a measured endogenous creatinine clearance for purposes of drug dosing adjustment. The formula of Cockcroft and Gault for estimating creatinine clearance without urine collection was validated for a large population of inpatients by using a simultaneously measured creatinine clearance. This formula was readily accepted by many practitioners. Isotopic measures of GFR have not been practical to use in routine practice for drug dosing adjustments.

The importance of proper dosing for renal-failure patients was strongly reinforced in the membership by an extensive study of medication-prescribing practices in dialysis units. The large number of medications prescribed and the potential for drugs to interact and cause adverse side effects was striking. Interactions of angiotensin-converting enzyme inhibitors, beta blockers and salt substitutes to produce hyperkalemia was observed and the role of beta adrenergic control of potassium disposal in uremia emphasized in the late 1980s.

Peritoneal dialysis as a form of maintenance therapy for chronic renal failure was in its infancy in 1970. In an important forerunner of things to come, the utility of the peritoneal route for absorption of insulin in the management of acute renal failure in diabetics was demonstrated in Seattle in 1974 by 75 patients treated with chronic peritoneal dialysis. The report of experience served as a landmark, preceding widespread application of this technique by clinicians. Continuous ambulatory peritoneal dialysis was popularized in 1977. It was soon clear that peritoneal infection limited the success of this procedure. The peritoneal instillation of antibiotics provided surprisingly good systemic absorption and quickly this route was rapidly accepted as standard therapy by patients undergoing self-dialysis and the medical staff caring for them. Each year, papers were presented at ASN meetings regarding detailed pharmacokinetics of individual drugs used in treating peritonitis. Among the first drugs studied were cephalosporins and aminoglycosides. By 1980 it had become common practice to continue peritoneal dialysis during peritonitis while administering loading doses of parenteral antibiotics with simultaneous intraperitoneal maintenance doses in each exchange.

By 1980 resistant staphylococcal infections had become a major problem in nephrology patients, particularly those with access-site infections and peritonitis. The older antibiotic vancomycin was rediscovered for these difficult problems because of superior effectiveness and the negligible losses during routine hemodialysis or CAPD. Proper dosing was ascertained by pharmacokinetic studies presented at ASN meetings.

The importance of accelerated atherosclerosis and its relation to elevated plasma lipids was first addressed therapeutically in the 1970s. Clofibrate used in conventional doses produced muscle necrosis, an adverse reaction subsequently described in patients taking other contemporary hypolipidemic agents. Based on pharmacokinetic studies, a plea for careful dosing in renal failure was first issued at the 1975 meeting. In 1978 one of the first papers documenting the adverse metabolic effects of thiazide diuretics, particularly increases in total cholesterol, was presented. At that time, thiazides were well accepted as standard therapy for most patients with essential hypertension, and clinicians viewed these drugs to be virtually free of adverse effects. The finding of lowered high density lipoprotein (HDL) cholesterol was also noted in patients with renal disease, a full 10 years before the concepts of "good" and "bad" cholesterol became integrated in the common language of the American public. During the late 1980s, the potent lipid lowering agent Lovostatin was used very effectively to treat nephrotic hyperlipidemia. Some posttransplant patients on cyclosporine developed rhabdomyolysis, although many investigators thought that this did not contraindicate the use of this effective drug in reduced dosage.

INDEX